Acute Care Nursing

As populations around the globe continue to grow, healthcare providers face increased demand for acute health services, including management of life-threatening emergencies, management of chronic conditions and routine health issues requiring immediate action. *Acute Care Nursing* provides an accessible and practical overview of the role of the nurse in acute medical and surgical settings in the Australian and New Zealand context.

Linking closely with the Australian *Registered Nurse Standards for Practice* and the New Zealand *Competencies for Registered Nurses*, this text equips students with foundational knowledge of the pathophysiology, treatment and legal and ethical issues associated with common acute conditions. Through the person-centred, collaborative care approach, students will also learn effective communication, decision-making and cultural competency skills that are essential for nurses in any practice context.

Each chapter is enriched with pedagogical features designed to solidify understanding and promote critical thinking, including 'Skills in Practice' case studies, reflections, key terms, review questions, research topics and further readings.

Offering students a relevant and contemporary understanding of the acute care context, *Acute Care Nursing* is an essential companion that can be taken from the classroom into practice.

Julia Gilbert is Lecturer in the School of Nursing at Federation University.

Elisabeth Coyne is Senior Lecturer in the School of Nursing and Midwifery at Griffith University.

Acute Care Nursing

Edited by

Julia Gilbert
Elisabeth Coyne

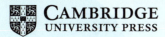

CAMBRIDGE
UNIVERSITY PRESS

CAMBRIDGE
UNIVERSITY PRESS

University Printing House, Cambridge CB2 8BS, United Kingdom

One Liberty Plaza, 20th Floor, New York, NY 10006, USA

477 Williamstown Road, Port Melbourne, VIC 3207, Australia

314–321, 3rd Floor, Plot 3, Splendor Forum, Jasola District Centre, New Delhi – 110025, India

79 Anson Road, #06–04/06, Singapore 079906

Cambridge University Press is part of the University of Cambridge.

It furthers the University's mission by disseminating knowledge in the pursuit of education, learning and research at the highest international levels of excellence.

www.cambridge.org
Information on this title: www.cambridge.org/9781108413039

First published 2018

Cover designed by eggplant communications
Typeset by Integra Software Services Pvt. Ltd
Printed in China by C & C Offset Printing Co. Ltd, June 2018

A catalogue record for this publication is available from the British Library

A catalogue record for this book is available from the National Library of Australia

ISBN 978-1-108-41303-9 Paperback

Additional resources for this publication at www.cambridge.edu.au/academic/acutecare

… …

Contents

Chapter 12 Health emergencies

Elicia Kunst, Jasmine Wadham, Monica Peddle, Susanne Thompson, Elizabeth Elder, Ann-Marie Brown and Amy Johnston

Figures and tables

Figures

Tables

Contributors

Judith Anderson is a highly motivated and committed academic with several national and international publications to her credit. In addition to her national academic profile as an expert in rural nursing, Judith has taught nursing at both undergraduate and postgraduate levels. She has extensive industry experience in management, quality improvement and the clinical area. Judith is also a fellow of the Australian College of Nursing.

Melissa Arnold-Chamney is a Lecturer in the Nursing School at the University of Adelaide. She has worked in the renal care setting for over 20 years, first in the clinical setting and since 2001 in the higher education sector. Melissa is Editor in Chief of the *Renal Society of Australasia Journal*.

Matthew Barton is a Senior Lecturer in the School of Nursing and Midwifery at Griffith University, Australia. He is a member of the Menzies Health Institute Queensland and a research fellow of the Clem Jones Centre for Neurobiology and Stem Cell Research. He is a registered nurse who completed his PhD in Neuroscience in 2014 and has published over 20 peer-reviewed publications. His medical research interests are focused around regenerative therapies for peripheral nerve injury. His teaching interests focus on providing high-quality educational resources in clinical anatomy and the medical biosciences.

Ann-Marie Brown is a Lecturer in the School of Nursing and Midwifery, Faculty of Health, Federation University Australia.

Elisabeth Coyne is a Senior Lecturer and Director of the Master of Acute Care at Griffith University. She has been a registered nurse for more than 30 years and has worked in a range of clinical areas. Her research explores patients' and family members' experience of cancer and works to improve health outcomes for this group. She has developed family nursing videos as a resource to help nurses engage with families in order to provide tailored support during hospitalisation. Ongoing research aims to engage with oncology nurses to provide resources to build the connection with the patients and families in their care.

Rachel Cross is a Lecturer at La Trobe University in Australia. She is a registered nurse with a specialisation in emergency and trauma settings. Rachel has held varying educational leadership positions, including in organisational nursing education. Rachel's primary research area is patient safety in the transition of care, specifically clinical deterioration and clinical handover.

Lyn Croxon is a Lecturer at Charles Sturt University. She has worked in clinical and academic roles for more than 40 years, and has taught across a range of subjects and coordinated the Bachelor of Nursing course across five campuses. Research interests include care of older persons, the impact of delirium, palliative care education and models of clinical placement supervision.

Sally-ann de-Vitry Smith is a Nursing and Midwifery Advisor for the ACT, Chief Nursing and Midwifery Officer and Adjunct Senior Lecturer at Charles Sturt University. Sally has extensive midwifery experience in Australia and internationally. Her special interests include complex pregnancy and hormonal changes related to pregnancy and birth.

Linda Deravin is a Lecturer in Nursing at Charles Sturt University. Throughout her 30-year nursing career, she has worked as a clinical, educator and senior nurse and health manager in a variety of settings. She has a keen interest in Aboriginal and Torres Strait Islander health, chronic care and nursing workforce issues. Linda is a Fellow of the Australasian College of Health Service Managers.

Elizabeth Elder is a Lecturer at Griffith University, Australia and a practising nurse with over ten years of experience in emergency care. She holds a Commonwealth Scholarship to explore factors impacting on emergency clinical staff.

Leeanne Ford currently works in MindBody Healthcare and provides nursing supervision to nurses and nursing students.

Julia Gilbert is a Lecturer and Course Convenor in the School of Nursing and Midwifery, Griffith University, Australia. She has been a registered nurse for over 30 years, working in a variety of clinical and academic settings including acute and chronic care, aged care and midwifery. In addition to her extensive nursing experience, she has completed a Bachelor of Laws and a Graduate Diploma of Legal Practice, and was admitted to the Supreme Court of Queensland as a legal practitioner in 2008.

Amali Hohol is a Lecturer in the School of Nursing, Midwifery and Indigenous Health at Charles Sturt University. She is an experienced clinician with a background in critical care.

Amy Johnston is a Senior Lecturer with over 25 years' experience in teaching the biosciences of acute care. She is currently Conjoint Senior Lecturer in the School of Nursing, Midwifery and Social Work in the Department of Emergency Medicine, Princess Alexandra Hospital Metro South, University of Queensland.

Melissa Johnston is a Clinical Nurse Consultant in Intensive Care in the Western New South Wales Local Health District and a Lecturer in Nursing at Charles Sturt University. Melissa has worked in critical care throughout her career, and has extensive experience and knowledge in both cardiovascular and intensive care nursing.

Janet Kelly is a nurse academic researcher who works collaboratively with Aboriginal and non-Aboriginal colleagues to improve Aboriginal health. Her recent work includes developing patient journey mapping tools with Aboriginal patients and their families, and with providers in urban, rural and remote areas. These tools and case studies enable multiple perspectives to be considered, gaps to be identified and responsive strategies to be developed. Work with renal nurses and doctors has further developed the tools in clinical settings and education toward ensuring high-quality clinical and culturally safe care is provided.

Elicia Kunst is a Lecturer at Southern Cross University, Gold Coast, and a practising nurse with over 15 years' clinical experience in emergency care. She holds a Commonwealth Scholarship to examine best practice in developing acute clinical skills for nursing students.

Sharon Latimer is a Research Fellow (patient safety in nursing) in a conjoint position between Griffith University and the Gold Coast University Hospital. She has more than 30 years of clinical nursing experience in the areas of acute medicine and geriatric rehabilitation. Sharon has spent the past nine years teaching within the Bachelor of Nursing program. Her research interests and experience lie in the areas of medication safety, pressure injury prevention, inter-professional learning and student-centred learning.

Emma Luck is a Nurse Educator in Perioperative Services at the Princess Alexandra Hospital in Brisbane, and has previously been employed as a Sessional Lecturer and Clinical Facilitator for Griffith University. Emma's skills within the main operating theatres translates across all specialties (anaesthetics, instrument/circulating nurse and post-anaesthetic recovery unit). Her background in cardio-thoracic management and surgery has been articulated in her contribution in the cardiac chapter. Emma is deeply passionate about nursing education, and believes that the proliferation of knowledge is paramount to the optimisation of patient-centric outcomes.

Judith Needham is Director of Professional Practice and a Senior Lecturer in the School of Nursing and Midwifery, Griffith University. She has 18 years' clinical experience working in the acute care arena, including medical surgical nursing and special care nursing. Judith has a special interest in promoting clinical education and supporting both students and RNs in the area of clinical placements.

Monica Peddle is the Undergraduate Nursing Courses Coordinator in the School of Nursing and Midwifery at La Trobe University. She has extensive clinical experience at the Alfred Hospital in Melbourne, and widespread academic experience. Monica is currently a PhD candidate. Her thesis focuses on exploring the experience of undergraduate health professionals' interactions with virtual simulated patients to develop non-technical skills. She has completed a Masters of Education and a Graduate Diploma in Nurse Education. Monica has multiple publications related to health professional educational research and has been successful in obtaining numerous grants for funded research projects.

Maryanne Podham is a Lecturer in Nursing at Charles Sturt University, with a passion for student-centred education, continuous improvement in clinical practices and over 20 years' experience in clinical, education and management nursing roles in rural New South Wales.

Sonia Reisenhofer is the Course Coordinator and Academic Program Director of the Bachelor of Nursing degree (Singapore) within the School of Nursing and Midwifery, and Academic Coordinator (Academic Partnerships) in the College of Science, Health and Engineering at La Trobe University. With a background in emergency nursing, Sonia's teaching expertise lies within acute and chronic nursing practice, health assessment, women's health, emergency care and professional nursing practice. Her research interests are primarily within global citizenship/internationalisation of education and the nursing profession, and improving healthcare for women experiencing intimate partner violence.

Ronak Reshamwala finished his medical training at Sardar Patel University at Gujarat, India. His work at the RIKEN Brain Science Institute in Japan during his Masters degree had a particular emphasis on developmental neurogenetics. Currently he is a candidate for a PhD in Neurosurgery from Griffith University, Queensland, Australia. His current work focuses on finding a cure for paralysis caused by spinal cord injuries.

Nang Sein is a Nurse Practitioner practising at a private clinic, in the community and at residential aged care facilities on the Gold Coast, Australia. Nang does sessional teaching in the School of Nursing and Midwifery at Griffith University's Gold Coast campus. She has worked in a clinical leadership role at Wesley Garden (Uniting), Shalom Centre (Baptistcare) and Ozanam Villa (Ozcare) over the past ten years. She worked as a registered nurse at the Children's Hospital Westmead, Allowah Children's Hospital, in the community and in residential aged care facilities. Nang specialises in aged and palliative care, primary care, chronic disease management and mental health.

Lyndal Taylor is a practising nurse in New South Wales.

Susanne Thompson is a highly experienced emergency Nurse Practitioner with over 15 years' experience in critical care and emergency care environments, and extensive academic experience in undergraduate and postgraduate programs. She currently holds the positions of Senior Emergency Nurse Practitioner, Department of Emergency Medicine, Logan Hospital, and Adjunct Lecturer, School of Nursing and Midwifery, Griffith University.

Michael Todorovic is a Lecturer in the School of Nursing and Midwifery at Griffith University, Australia. He is a research member of the Menzies Health Institute and an adjunct research fellow of the Clem Jones Centre for Neurobiology and Stem Cell Research.

Jasmine Wadham practises in the Department of Emergency Medicine at Gold Coast Hospital.

Grant Williams-Pritchard is a Scholarly Teaching Fellow in the School of Nursing and Midwifery at Griffith University. For the past ten years, he has taught human bioscience to nursing students at Griffith University and in a number of other higher education institutes across Southeast Queensland, including Bond University and Southern Cross University. Grant has experience in a wide variety of teaching environments, ranging from large lectures to small problem-based learning (PBL) tutorials, and encourages his students to investigate the links between their bioscience knowledge and clinical practice. He is currently working on his PhD, investigating the role of adenosine and opioid cross-talk in cardio-protection.

Preface

This book presents an overview of the holistic nursing approach to acute care conditions, with twelve chapters providing evidence-based care for acute conditions from emergency to surgical and medical care. This text provides relevant information for both undergraduate nursing students and novice practitioners, in order to guide them through the transition from knowledge to the provision of person-centred nursing care within acute clinical settings.

The use of the Australian and New Zealand Standards of nursing as a structure provides a contemporary overview of the role of the nurse in dealing with acute medical and surgical conditions. Each chapter guides the student through the epidemiology, pathophysiology, simple pharmacology and legislative requirements of the acute care condition. The use of case studies provides clarity around the identified acute condition, and enables the reader to reflect on the challenges, understand the cultural aspects and prepare for the delivery of person-centred care.

The chapters in this book are designed both to be read by individuals and to be used by educators as a basis for course delivery and assessment items. The inclusion of evidence- and outcome-based nursing practice and patient case studies provides all readers – novice or expert – with a reliable, relevant and comprehensive reference to guide their clinical practice.

Acknowledgements

The authors and Cambridge University Press would like to thank the following for permission to reproduce material in this book.

Figure 5.1: © Getty Images/SeanShot; **5.2:** © Getty Images/Blend Images/Erproductions-Ltd; **5.3:** © Getty Images/Janie Airey; **5.4:** © Getty Images/nano; **6.1** and **8.2:** © Getty Images/wetcake; **6.2:** © Getty Images/Encyclopaedia Britannica/UIG; **8.1:** © Getty Images/CSA Images; **8.3:** © Getty Images/Phil Boorman; **9.1:** © Getty Images/Alan Gesek/Stocktrek Images; **9.2** and **11.1:** © Wikimedia Commons/BruceBlaus.

Every effort has been made to trace and acknowledge copyright. The publisher apologises for any accidental infringement and welcomes information that would redress this situation.

The Australian and New Zealand healthcare systems

Linda Deravin, Elisabeth Coyne,
Lyn Croxon and Judith Anderson

LEARNING OBJECTIVES

At the completion of this chapter, you should be able to:

1 describe the Australian and New Zealand healthcare systems
2 explain relevant legislation and policy that influences the acute care health system
3 identify the national health priority areas and strategies for improving health
   outcomes in both Australia and New Zealand
4 describe the healthcare challenges for vulnerable populations including the
   Indigenous populations of Australia and New Zealand, culturally and linguistically
   diverse people and communities that are geographically isolated
5 describe the role of the nurse within the healthcare system.

Introduction

This chapter provides an understanding of registered nurse practice within the Australian and New Zealand healthcare systems. The legislation and registration for nurses is discussed, together with the scope of practice. The national health priorities are presented to enable the student to understand what areas within the health system are targeted. In Australia, the national priorities focus on cancer, cardiac disease, mental health and injury prevention. New Zealand has taken a different approach, with holistic goals around its people and access to healthcare rather than specific disease states. Across the population, there are inequities in health. The determinants of health are described here; these include the economic, social, political and environmental factors that influence the individual's access to healthcare. Particular populations are vulnerable within the healthcare system, including Aboriginal and Torres Strait Islander, Māori, rural, low socioeconomic, and culturally and linguistically diverse – including migrant and refugee – populations. Nurses need to be aware of these vulnerable populations and to understand how to provide appropriate and tailored care for these clients. The nurse's role within the healthcare system accounts for the largest workforce in the system, and it is important for nurses to understand their role in providing care and education to both the patient and their family.

NURSING STANDARDS

The following identifies the national competency standards for the registered nurse from the Nursing and Midwifery Board of Australia (NMBA) and the Nursing Council of New Zealand (NCNZ) that are addressed in this chapter.

Australian Registered Nurse Standards for Practice

Standard 2: Engages in therapeutic and professional relationships

Standard 3: Maintains the capability for practice

Standard 4: Comprehensively conducts assessments

Standard 5: Develops a plan for nursing practice

Standard 6: Provides safe, appropriate and responsive quality nursing practice

(NMBA, 2016b)

New Zealand: Competencies for Registered Nurses

Competency 1.1: Accepts responsibility for ensuring that his/her nursing practice and conduct meet the standards of the professional, ethical and relevant legislated requirements

Competency 1.2: Demonstrates the ability to apply the principles of the Treaty of Waitangi/ Te Tiriti o Waitangi to nursing practice

Competency 1.5: Practises nursing in a manner that the health consumer determines as being culturally safe

Competency 4.1: Collaborates and participates with colleagues and members of the health care team to facilitate and coordinate care

Competency 4.2: Recognises and values the roles and skills of all members of the health care team in the delivery of care

(NCNZ, [2007] 2016)

The Australian and New Zealand healthcare systems

The Australian and New Zealand healthcare systems are complex and continually evolving. These systems have been influenced by both social policy and political decisions, which have shaped the structures we experience today (Duckett & Wilcox, 2015). Acute and community-based services make up the majority of healthcare provision. Although they are interrelated, these services focus on different aspects of healthcare. In this chapter, we are concentrating on the acute care service provision within these healthcare systems. Each of these systems is unique, and a brief description is provided in the following sections.

The Australian healthcare system

In Australia, acute care health services may be provided in large tertiary hospitals that commonly are referred to as teaching or referral hospitals, which provide high-level complex health services. These are usually large hospitals situated in metropolitan areas, where the majority of the population lives. As the population decreases in geographical areas, the level of acute care services decreases to small hospitals such as multi-purpose facilities – a combination of subacute and aged care beds (Anderson & Malone, 2014; Malone & Anderson, 2015) and regional health centres that provide a variety of services, including maternity and surgical care. In more remote areas, smaller health services may be supported by larger referral hospitals through the use of **telehealth**.

Telehealth – A method of enhancing healthcare, public health and health education delivery across a geographical region through using telecommunications technologies.

Funding for acute services is supported by either the government (the public sector) or the private sector. From the acute care perspective, public hospitals are funded by state, territory and federal governments. The federal government provides funding to each state and territory to manage these acute care services. Private hospitals are operated by privately owned companies, which obtain their funding through health insurance companies, accident insurance schemes and directly from patients paying for services (AIHW, 2014).

The public healthcare system also obtains part of its funding through the federally funded system called Medicare. Medicare is a healthcare insurance scheme that was introduced in 1975 to ensure that all Australians had equal access to healthcare across the country. It is not reliant on personal financial circumstances and is designed to ensure that all Australians have access to adequate and affordable healthcare (AIHW, 2014; Hall, 2015). A Medicare levy of 2 per cent is applied to all eligible taxpayers, based on the amount of income they earn. Through the Medicare scheme, Australian residents gain access to a variety of healthcare services and subsidised prescriptions as well as free care within public healthcare services (Australian Government, 2016).

In order to improve the coordination of healthcare services, local health networks have been established to improve access and delivery of healthcare. Local health networks combine small and individual hospitals that share services across a region or within a specialist network across a state or territory (AIHW, 2014). In this way, hospitals can improve their efficiency and provide better care to patients by consolidating their services. To demonstrate that an acute care service is functioning efficiently to improve the safety and quality of care for patients, a system of measurement through key performance indicators may be in place. This will review high-priority areas such as waiting times in an emergency department, infection rates or perhaps surgical waiting times. This is not an exclusive list, and acute care services are subject to a range of other performance measures.

The New Zealand healthcare system

The New Zealand healthcare system is similar to the Australian healthcare system, and obtains its funding from a variety of sources. In New Zealand, funding is sourced through Vote Health, the Accident Compensation Corporation (ACC), other government agencies, local government, and private sources such as insurance and out-of-pocket payments (Ministry of Health NZ, 2016b). The Ministry of Health is responsible for allocating approximately three-quarters of public funds through Vote Health, which is then distributed to District Health Boards (DHBs). These boards administer the day-to-day business of the system. DHBs plan, manage, provide and purchase health services for the people within the boundaries of their district to ensure services are provided effectively and efficiently within New Zealand. With the funding they receive, DHBs provide primary care, hospital services, public health services, aged care services and services provided by other non-government health providers, including Māori and Pacific Island providers (Ministry of Health NZ, 2016a).

Similar to the Australian system, the performance of the healthcare system is measured through key performance indicators such as length of stay in emergency departments and improving access to elective surgery. In this way, the New Zealand system can also demonstrate that it is providing high-quality services to the people within its boundaries.

Legislation and policies

The Australian and New Zealand healthcare systems are guided by legislation with several layers of responsibility at both federal and state government levels for Australia or federal and district levels for New Zealand. The National or Commonwealth Government is responsible for funding and regulation of the national healthcare schemes, such as Medicare, the Pharmaceutical Benefits Scheme (PBS), the national immunisation program, research grants and national registration of health professionals.

In Australia, the *National Health Act* is administered by the Chief Health Officer and sets the standards of care within each state. The states also have specific responsibilities within the healthcare system, which enables the management of the health system at a state level. See Table 1.1 for details of each level.

In 2010, the national registration and accreditation scheme for health professionals commenced. This enabled national registration for nurses in both Australia and New Zealand (AHPRA, 2017). The national registration provided registered nurses with an ability to move between the Australian states and New Zealand using the same registration.

As regulated health professionals, registered nurses (RNs) are responsible and accountable to the Nursing and Midwifery Board of Australia (NMBA). The NMBA has developed a set of **competency standards** for practice under which all RNs work (Figure 1.1). These standards provide information about key areas of practice; critical thinking, therapeutic and professional relationships, capability for practice; assessment; and nursing care planning, provision and evaluation. The standards provide a guideline under which the RN can work to ensure the provision of person-centred and evidenced-based care.

The registered nurse must also follow the Code of Ethics that is relevant to all nurses at any level of practice from clinical care to management, researcher to academic (AHPRA, 2017). This Code is framed by the principles and standards set forth in the United Nations' Universal Declaration of Human Rights, International Covenant on Economic, Social and Cultural Rights and International Covenant on Civil and Political Rights; and the World Health Organization's Constitution (WHO, 2015). There are eight points to the Code of Ethics that nurses must follow in their practice. The Code of Ethics guidelines are to be

Competency standards – Specific activities within nursing may have advanced sets of competency standards above RN standards regarding scope of practice. They include administration of chemotherapy and insertion of intravenous cannulae.

Table 1.1   Legislation responsibilities

The Commonwealth Government has responsibility for:	The states and territories have responsibility for:
<ul><li>Medicare</li><li>the Pharmaceutical Benefits Scheme (PBS)</li><li>the national immunisation program</li><li>aged care services</li><li>medical research grants, the National Health and Medical Research Council</li><li>rebates for private health insurance premiums and regulation of private health insurers</li><li>dental benefits for basic dental services for children and teens</li><li>veterans' healthcare through the Department of Veterans' Affairs</li><li>funding for community-controlled Aboriginal and Torres Strait Islander primary healthcare organisations</li><li>education of health professionals (through Commonwealth-funded university places)</li><li>the Therapeutic Goods Administration (TGA)</li><li>subsidised hearing services</li><li>national coordination and leadership, responding to pandemics and other health emergencies</li></ul>	<ul><li>management and administration of public hospitals</li><li>delivery of preventive services such as breast cancer screening and immunisation programs</li><li>funding and management of community and mental health services</li><li>public dental clinics</li><li>ambulance and emergency services</li><li>patient transport and subsidy schemes</li><li>food safety and handling regulation</li><li>regulation, inspection, licensing and monitoring of health premises</li></ul>

Source: Biggs (2017).

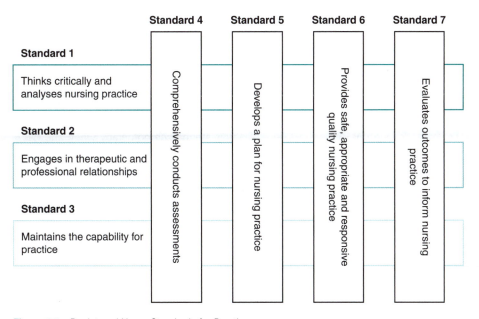

Figure 1.1   Registered Nurse Standards for Practice

Source: NMBA (2016b).

Delegation – Transfer of the activity to a competent person such as an enrolled nurse, a student nurse or a person who is not a nurse. The RN retains the accountability. Delegations are made to meet people's needs and to enable access to healthcare services – to ensure the right person is available at the right time to provide the right service.

Enrolled nurse – A health professional who provides nursing care under the direct or indirect supervision of an RN. ENs are accountable for their own practice and remain responsible to an RN for the delegated care (AHPRA, 2017).

Assistant in nursing – A person who has completed a short healthcare training program to enable them to provide basic cares (activities of daily living) and to support the RN.

Accountability – This means RNs are accountable for their decisions, actions, behaviours and the responsibilities that occur within their nursing role. Activities can be delegated and undertaken by another person who has the appropriate scope of practice to perform the activity; however, the RN who delegates remains accountable. This includes monitoring the performance and evaluating the outcomes of, and completing the documentation for, the activity.

Supervision – Includes managerial supervision, professional supervision and clinically focused supervision.

used in conjunction with the Registered Nurse Standards of Practice to provide a set of fundamental ethical standards AHPRA, 2017).

The *Registered Nurse Standards for Practice* and Code of Ethics should be evident in current practice, and inform the development of scope of practice for RNs. The RN works in a team and provides care to a group of patients for whom the Registered Nurse is accountable. At times, the care of patients will need to be **delegated** to other team members such as **enrolled nurses** or **assistants in nursing** who complete the task; however the **accountability** is retained by the RN.

Code of Ethics for Nurses

1 Nurses value quality nursing care for all people.
2 Nurses value respect and kindness for self and others.
3 Nurses value the diversity of people.
4 Nurses value access to quality nursing and healthcare for all people.
5 Nurses value informed decision-making.
6 Nurses value a culture of safety in nursing and healthcare.
7 Nurses value ethical management of information.
8 Nurses value a socially, economically and ecologically sustainable environment promoting health and wellbeing.

(NMBA, 2016b)

Registered nurses work in a range of different settings. At times various specific policies identify **competency standards** for tasks, which are developed to enable the RN to complete activities within that area, such as PICC line insertion and medication administration. Nursing associations within the specialist areas such as critical care, emergency, oncology and mental health often provide guidelines or information for the advanced practice nurse who is then able to provide a higher level of care to the patient (Ash et al., 2016; Kenison et al., 2015; Moore & Prentice, 2013).

SKILLS IN PRACTICE

Scope of practice

Joanne works as an oncology nurse in a large metropolitan hospital. As a second-year RN on the oncology ward, she is expected to administer chemotherapy to patients under her care. Joanne questions the safety of administering chemotherapy when she has undergone no advanced training in pharmaceuticals. The educator of the oncology ward works with Joanne to help her to complete the module on chemotherapy administration so that Joanne can be deemed competent to deliver chemotherapy under the hospital policy. While working under the **supervision** of the educator, Joanne performs duties that have been delegated to her.

QUESTIONS

- Who retains the responsibility for these activities?
- Is administering chemotherapy within Joanne's **scope of practice** as an RN and what level of training does she need?

- Once Joanne has completed the administering chemotherapy module to the level expected by the health facility, can she administer chemotherapy within her scope of practice and does she retain accountability for the provision of care?
- Can Joanne supervise an EN to administer chemotherapy medications while they are both working in the oncology unit?

Scope of practice – Describes the procedures, actions and processes that a healthcare practitioner is permitted to undertake in keeping with the terms of their professional licence. Specific scope of practice rules may be also set by the health facility policy where the RN works.

REFLECTIVE QUESTION

Why is it necessary to have a code of conduct, code of ethics and competencies or standards of practice to guide nursing practice?

National Health Priority Areas

The national health priority action areas are intended to provide guidance to clinicians and policy-makers in order to strategically target those areas of healthcare where the greatest social and financial benefit can be obtained (Miles, Latham & Biles, 2016). They form goals that are set by governments in order to improve collaborative action within the country in response to the World Health Organization's (WHO) global strategy 'Health for All by the Year 2000' (WHO, 1981). National health priority action areas for Australia and New Zealand, although they tackle the situation very differently, have a strong focus on prevention, maintaining the health of the population and reducing future demands on their health systems (AIHW, 2017a; Ministry of Health NZ, 2016a).

Australia

The Australian government responded to the WHO global strategy initially in 1995, developing the National Health Priority Areas, which aim to build collaboration between state, territory and Commonwealth governments, non-government organisations (NGOs), clinicians and consumers of healthcare. These priority areas were deemed to be of highest priority and cost benefit to Australian society. Further priorities were added as their burden on society was seen to grow (Miles, Latham & Biles, 2016). The National Health Priority Area initiative sought to:

- monitor health outcomes and progress towards set targets
- identify the most appropriate and cost-effective points of intervention
- identify the most appropriate roles for government and non-government organisations in fostering the adoption of **best practice**
- investigate some basic determinants of health, such as education, and socioeconomic status (AIHW, 2017a).

Best practice – Uses the best available evidence to provide clinicians with evidence-informed guidelines to support their clinical practice and guide decision-making in healthcare.

Currently in Australia, there are nine national health priority areas:

- cancer control
- cardiovascular health
- injury prevention and control

- mental health
- diabetes mellitus
- asthma
- arthritis and musculoskeletal conditions
- obesity
- dementia (AIHW, 2017a).

New Zealand

Similarly, in response to the WHO global strategy, the New Zealand government developed health targets with quantifiable outcomes that were cost-effective. These targets are designed to lead to improvements at both the local and national levels, and are aimed at community and hospitals with a strong focus on prevention and the need to address the social determinants of health (King, 2001). The New Zealand government has committed to reviewing its targets each year, so they vary to meet current requirements (Ministry of Health NZ, 2016a).

Recently, the New Zealand action areas were described as:

- people-powered
- closer to home
- value and high performance
- one team
- smart system (Ministry of Health NZ, 2016a).

The New Zealand action areas have a significant focus on the healthcare system, its people, its effectiveness and its accessibility, rather than addressing specific conditions. This aims to be flexible to meet the needs of the population even if they change, and to address determinants of health that may not traditionally be seen as aspects of healthcare (Ministry of Health NZ, 2016a).

Determinants of health

Determinants of health – Any factors that create inequity contributing to the health of an individual, group or community.

Inequalities in health are created by numerous factors that impact individuals, groups and communities. These **determinants of health** are described in a variety of ways, including economic, social, political and environmental. Many of these determinants are linked, and therefore will act together to impact health. Economic determinants include level of income and opportunity for employment, which can impact access to health services, medications and care. Social determinants are less tangible, including gender, culture, ethnicity and life experiences; these can impact the health conditions a person experiences and how much support they receive. Political factors can be extreme, such as those related to civil conflict or those related to government policy regarding provision of social support or taxation, and they impact availability of health services and their quality. Environmental determinants include those that relate to the natural (e.g. air quality) or human-made (e.g. housing or transport) environment, which also directly impact health and access to healthcare services (Guzys & Arnott, 2013). Australia and New Zealand have significant issues related to rurality and Indigenous populations, which impact the health of their populations. These two groups continue to have significant health issues, which have not yet been addressed successfully (Deravin, Francis & Anderson, 2017; Francis et al., 2013; Miles, Latham & Biles, 2016).

Determinants of health impact by creating a gradient that leads to those who are most affected having poorer health than those who are least affected. Overcoming these determinants of health is not easy at any level, but policy-makers and governments often attempt to address those that are most cost-effective (as can be seen in the National Health Priority Action Areas). Nurses may be in the position of having a greater understanding of the impacts of these determinants of health, so they need to advocate for those who are less able to do so (WHO, 2013).

Although determinants of health are usually perceived as being part of primary health-care rather than acute care, it is important for the acute care nurse to understand the impact of determinants of health, as they are often the underlying cause of acute care presentations and readmissions. Addressing the underlying cause will assist in timely discharge and will prevent acute exacerbation of chronic conditions.

REFLECTIVE QUESTION

Focusing on one acute condition, identify at least three determinants of health that could negatively impact a patient experiencing this condition. Explain how this impact may present.

Vulnerable populations

Vulnerable populations include Aboriginal and Torres Strait Islander people in Australia, Māori in New Zealand, those who live in rural areas, culturally and linguistically diverse (CALD) populations.

Aboriginal and Torres Strait Islander people

Based on 2016 Census data, the Australian Bureau of Statistics (ABS, 2017) records the Australian Aboriginal and Torres Strait Islander population as 649 200 people, with one-third of this number living in metropolitan and urban areas. This constitutes 2.8 per cent of the Australian population. The median age for Aboriginal and Torres Strait Islander people is 23 years, compared with a median age of 38 for all Australians. Just over one-third of the number is under 15 years of age and fewer than 5 per cent are over 65 years.

The health of Aboriginal and Torres Strait Islander people is not as good as it is in the general Australian population, with these populations having a higher incidence of hyper-tension, heart disease, stroke, respiratory disease, chronic renal failure, diabetes and cancer. Rates of hospitalisation are 2.4 times greater than for other Australians. Aboriginal and Torres Strait Islander people experience higher mortality at younger ages. In 2015, death rates from intentional self-harm were twice as high for Aboriginal and Torres Strait Islander people than for other Australians (AIHW, 2015).

The Australian government implemented the Close the Gap initiative in 2008 in an attempt to address the health, wellbeing and life expectancy discrepancies that relate to Aboriginal and Torres Strait Islander people compared with the wider Australian community. Based on the WHO strategies and the Ottawa Charter 1986, the aims are to 'reduce Indigenous disadvantage with respect to life expectancy, child mortality, access to early childhood education, educational achievement and employment outcomes' (COAG, 2008; see also Deravin, Francis & Anderson, 2017).

New Zealand Māori population

Māori make up over 15 per cent of the New Zealand population. They have an increased rate of diabetes, cardiovascular diseases and cancers, with an increased mortality rate and shorter life expectancy than the general New Zealand population (Royal Australasian College of Surgeons, 2016; Statistics NZ, 2015). Fewer educational opportunities, more unemployment, less income, poor housing, poor dental care, increased tobacco and alcohol consumption, poor nutrition, more obesity and reduced physical activity are all factors that impact on the health of many Māori people (Ministry of Health NZ, 2015). The cost and availability of health-related appointments and lack of transport to health services are the most common reasons for not accessing health services.

Nurses must play a role to advocate for those in their care to diminish the influence of social inequities experienced by vulnerable populations related to their health outcomes. Having knowledge and an understanding of Australian and New Zealand history and culture, particularly the ramifications of the disempowerment that has resulted from racism, oppression and marginalisation, improves the nurse's practice of cultural competence. Embedding knowledge of a country's First Peoples history, cultural and health issues into nursing education programs and clinical practice experiences can support changes in student attitudes and promote greater cultural sensitivity, leading to improved health outcomes for First Peoples populations (Durey, 2010; Mays, 2013; Webster et al., 2010).

Rural populations

Residents of rural areas are likely to have a decreased lifespan and an increased incidence of illness and disease risk factors than metropolitan populations (AIHW, 2017b). Access to services, waiting times to see medical practitioners and specialists, and the distance that needs to be travelled to access these services are major factors in rural people not accessing health services in a timely manner. A decrease in opportunities around education and employment, and reduced incomes compared with city dwellers further disadvantage the health of rural people.

In Australia and New Zealand, rurality is associated with higher death rates, primarily from cardiovascular disease, chronic obstructive pulmonary disease and motor vehicle deaths, associated with the need to drive on country roads. Increased tobacco and alcohol consumption are evident in rural and remote communities. Issues around mental health, nutrition and physical activity contribute to poor health outcomes for country populations (AIHW, 2017b; Ministry of Health NZ, 2016a).

Those living in remote areas of Australia and New Zealand face increased distance and isolation, and scarcity of health services, which lead to poorer health outcomes. The supply of fresh food, the stress of gaining or maintaining employment, the impact of drought on rural communities, the need for young people to leave the area for education or employment opportunities, limited access to health and dental care and social isolation can all contribute to increased risk to physical health as well as mental and social wellbeing (AIHW, 2017b; Ministry of Health NZ, 2016a).

Culturally and linguistically diverse (CALD) populations

The Australian population is culturally and linguistically diverse. Nearly one-third of the total population was born overseas. As immigration to Australia and New Zealand involves rigorous health checks, migrants generally arrive in Australia in good health (AIHW, 2017; New Zealand Immigration, 2017). However, after 20 years they tend to suffer the same chronic conditions as other Australians (Jatrana, Pasupeti & Richards, 2014). Refugee populations have generally poorer health on arrival in Australia.

There are some mutual problems faced by migrants and refugees. These include loneliness and social isolation, which increase the incidence of mental health issues. Language barriers and poor levels of health literacy result in decreased access to health services and the health resources that are available. This is seen particularly in refugee women, who are fearful or lack understanding about the areas of maternal and child health. For these same reasons, mental health services are also not accessed as needed. Dietary changes in Australia have led to increased obesity in all population groups. Refugee groups may also face developed world problems of vitamin deficiency, tuberculosis, hepatitis B carrier state and Post Traumatic Stress Disorder (PTSD) (Day, 2016). Many CALD communities traditionally have strong links to family groups. The absence of this support can place stress on someone who is new to Australia. Nurses need to be aware of cultural issues that may impact the health of and access to health services by CALD populations.

REFLECTIVE QUESTION

Identify some of the health issues faced by people in marginalised groups such as Aboriginal, Torres Strait Islander or Māori populations, or refugees, on their discharge from an acute care service.

The nurse's role

Nurses make up the largest proportion of the health workforce. This trend continued into 2015 with an 11 per cent increase of RN numbers over this period (AIHW, 2016). The nursing workforce is predominately female. Nurses are an integral part of the health system, providing 24/7 care to vulnerable individuals. The RN acts as a patient advocate, and leads in the detection and escalation of concerns for the deteriorating patient, education of patients and staff, and clinical governance and management.

In Australia, there are two levels of nurse under the Health Practitioner Regulation National Law 2010. These are Division 1, registered nurses and Division 2, enrolled nurses (AHPRA, 2017). Generally, an RN undertakes a university degree at Bachelor level to qualify for registration and enrolled nurses undertake a Diploma level qualification through a vocational and educational training setting. It is necessary for both RNs and ENs to meet standards of practice and abide by a code of conduct and code of ethics as well as demonstrating **continuing professional development (CPD)** and recency of practice hours to maintain registration (NMBA, 2016c).

Australia has a national scheme for the registration and regulation of healthcare professionals. Nurses are one of 14 professions regulated by the Australian Health Practitioners Regulatory Authority (AHPRA). In 2016, 356 417 nurses were registered with AHPRA (AIHW, 2016). Under the national regulatory authority, each profession is registered by a national board – in the case of nurses, the Nursing and Midwifery Board of Australia (NMBA). This board maintains the safety of the public by accrediting and monitoring pre-registration programs and regulating practice through the development of standards, codes and guidelines for practice. Applicants applying for registration must be able to demonstrate that they are of good character. It investigates complaints against the profession and imposes disciplinary or remedial sanctions on nurses if practice falls below the expected standard.

Continuing professional development (CPD) – The means by which nurses maintain, develop and widen their knowledge, expertise and competence, and develop the individual and professional assets necessary to maintain the requirements of their professional lives.

The Standards of Practice for the RN, EN and nurse practitioner (NP) are a guideline for practice for nurses in Australia (NMBA, 2014, 2016b, 2016d). The board also registers nursing students enrolled in entry programs at universities and the vocational education and training sector, such as TAFE. While the educational institutions are responsible for the academic progress and conduct of students, the national board is concerned with students' health impairment or criminal offence issues that may impact on public safety (Chiarella & White, 2013).

In New Zealand, there are two levels of nurses under the *Health Practitioners Competence Assurance Act 2003*. They are registered under the New Zealand Council of Nurses. New Zealand nurses, similarly, are guided by the Competencies for the Registered and Enrolled Nurse, and Nurse Practitioner (NCNZ, [2007] 2016, 2012a, 2012b).

Specialisation in nursing has increased with graduate courses in universities, and colleges, ranging from postgraduate certificates to doctoral-level research as pathways for the RN. Areas of specialisation include acute and critical care, chronic care, education, community health and aged care. The registered nurse can also attain clinical recognition as a clinical nurse specialist (CNS), clinical nurse consultant (CNC), clinical nurse educator (CNE), nurse manager, nurse practitioner (NP), university lecturer, TAFE teacher or nurse researcher. Enrolled nurses similarly can specialise in an area of nursing.

Nurses are relatively evenly distributed geographically across metropolitan, regional and remote areas of Australia, per capita. However, distance travelled to access healthcare is an issue in rural, and particularly remote, areas (Bureau of Health Information, 2016). Due to a shortage of medical practitioners there has been an escalation of skills performed by nurses, as the scope of nurses expand, particularly in the advanced nurse role and nurse practitioner role (Maier & Aiken, 2016). There has also been an increase in the scope of practice of the enrolled nurse (Jacob et al., 2013).

In 2016, there was an average of five RNs to one EN in most Australian states (NMBA, 2016a). There is an increased prevalence of undergraduate nursing students working as assistants in nursing in both acute and aged care settings. Australia has a large number of unregulated care workers, particularly involved in the care of older people, such as in residential aged care, where they work as personal care assistants. Duffield and colleagues (2011) found that health outcomes were better when the proportion of RNs was greater in the hospital staff mix. There is a predicted nursing shortfall from 2014 onwards, with an estimated gap of 110 000 nurses by 2025 (Crettenden et al., 2014; Health Workforce Australia, 2012). This is due partly to the growing ageing population and the retirement of the baby boomer generation of nurses.

The prospects for employment are good for those studying nursing!

SUMMARY

Learning objective 1: Describe the Australian and New Zealand healthcare systems.

Each system is a complex and evolving, multilayered approach to delivering healthcare. Large metropolitan facilities through to small rural hospitals provide a range of services including emergency care and in-patient care. Support to provide these services comes from both the government and the private sector.

Learning objective 2: Explain relevant legislation and policy that influences the acute care health system.

The Australian and New Zealand healthcare systems are guided by legislation with several layers of responsibility across both federal and state government levels for Australia, and federal and district levels for New Zealand. Legislation and policy have a significant influence on the delivery of acute care services.

Learning objective 3: Identify the national health priority areas and strategies for improving health outcomes in both Australia and New Zealand.

Currently in Australia, there are nine National Health Priority Areas:

- cancer control
- cardiovascular health
- injury prevention and control
- mental health
- diabetes mellitus
- asthma
- arthritis and musculoskeletal conditions
- obesity
- dementia (AIHW, 2017).

Recently, the New Zealand action areas were described as:

- people-powered
- closer to home
- value and high performance
- one team
- smart system (Ministry of Health NZ, 2016a).

Learning objective 4: Describe the healthcare challenges for vulnerable populations including the Indigenous populations of Australia and New Zealand, culturally and linguistically diverse people, and communities that are geographically isolated.

Australia's Aboriginal and Torres Strait Islander peoples and New Zealand's Māori population, and communities that are geographically isolated have poorer health outcomes than the wider population. It is imperative that nurses are culturally competent in their care.

Learning objective 5: Describe the role of the nurse within the healthcare system.

Nurses make up the largest proportion of the health workforce. There are two levels of nurse. The registered nurse (RN) acts as patient advocate, and leads in the detection and escalation of concerns for the deteriorating patient, education of patients and staff and clinical governance and management. Australia and New Zealand have national schemes for the registration and regulation of nurses. Practice is guided by competencies or standards of practice.

REVIEW QUESTIONS

1.1 Identify one or two key health targets that are measures within the acute health system which demonstrate quality to people who engage these services.

1.2 For one of the national health priority action areas in your country, identify at least three impacts it will have on your work as an acute care nurse.

1.3 Identify the social and economic factors that are likely to impact the health status of rural populations.

1.4 Describe the benefits of using technology such as telehealth for people in rural and remote areas.

1.5 What are the different levels of nurses and how does their scope of practice differ?

RESEARCH TOPIC

For the Aboriginal and Torres Strait Islander, or the Māori community in your country, identify determinants of health that impact people's ability to access healthcare.

FURTHER READING

Ash, K., Baychek, K., Black, E., Brown, L., Coyne, E., Pascoe, L., … Reid, A. (2016). A scoping exercise by the CNSA Education Committee regarding enrolled nurse (EN) administration of antineoplastic agents. *Australian Journal of Cancer Nursing*, 11(1), 14–18.

Australian Institute of Health and Welfare (AIHW) (2016). *Australia's Health 2016*. Canberra: AIHW.

Cancer Nurses Society of Australia (2018). Publications and resources. Retrieved from https://www.cnsa.org.au/practiceresources/guidelines-position-statements-documents-endorsed-by-cnsa.

Ministry of Health (2016). *New Zealand Health Strategy: Future Direction*. Wellington: Ministry of Health.

Nursing and Midwifery Board of Australia (NMBA) (2018). Regulating Australia's nurses and midwives. Retrieved from http://www.nursingmidwiferyboard.gov.au.

REFERENCES

Anderson, J. & Malone, L. (2014). Suitability of the multi-purpose service model for rural and remote communities of Australia. *Asia Pacific Journal of Health Management*, 9(3), 14–18.

Ash, K., Baychek, K., Black, E., Brown, L., Coyne, E., Pascoe, L., ... Reid, A. (2016). A scoping exercise by the CNSA Education Committee regarding enrolled nurse (EN) administration of antineoplastic agents. *Australian Journal of Cancer Nursing*, 11(1), 14–18.

Australian Bureau of Statistics (2017). *Australian Aboriginal and Torres Strait Islander peoples*. Retrieved from http://www.abs.gov.au/Aboriginal-and-Torres-Strait-Islander-Peoples.

Australian Government (2016). Medicare services. Retrieved from https://www .humanservices.gov.au/customer/subjects/medicare-services.

Australian Health Practitioner Regulation Agency (AHPRA) (2017). Retrieved from http://www.ahpra.gov.au/Registration/Registers-of-Practitioners/Professions-and-Divisions.aspx.

Australian Institute Health and Welfare (AIHW) (2014). *Australia's Health 2014. Cat. no. AUS 178*. Canberra: AIHW.

—— (2015). The health and welfare of Australia's Aboriginal and Torres Strait Islander peoples: 2015. Retrieved from http://www.aihw.gov.au/publication-detail/?id=60129550168.

—— (2016). *Nursing and Midwifery Workforce 2015: Nurses and Midwives, Overview Tables 1–25*. Canberra: AIHW. Retrieved from http://www.aihw.gov.au/workforce/ nursing-and-midwifery/additional.

—— (2017a). National health priority areas. Retrieved from http://www.aihw.gov.au/ national-health-priority-areas.

—— (2017b). Rural health. Retrieved from http://www.aihw.gov.au/rural-health.

Biggs, A. (2017). Health in Australia: a quick guide. Retrieved from http://www.aph.gov .au/About_Parliament/Parliamentary_Departments/Parliamentary_Library/pubs/rp/ rp1314/QG/HealthAust.

Bureau of Health Information (BHI) (2016). *The Insights Series: Healthcare in Rural, Regional and Remote NSW*. Sydney: BHI.

Chiarella, M. & White, J. (2013). Which tail wags which dog? Exploring the interface between professional regulation and professional education. *Nurse Education Today*, 33(11), 1274–8.

Council of Australian Governments (COAG) (2008). *National Partnership Agreement on Closing the Gap in Indigenous Health Outcomes*. Canberra: Australian Government. Retrieved from http://www.federalfinancialrelations.gov.au/content/npa/health_ indigenous/ctg-health-outcomes/national_partnership.pdf.

Crettenden, I.F., McCarty, M.V., Fenech, B.J., Heywood, T., Taitz, M.C. & Tudman, S. (2014). How evidence-based workforce planning in Australia is informing policy development in the retention and distribution of the health workforce. *Human Resources for Health*, 12(1), 1.

Day, G.E. (2016). Migrant and refugee health: Advance Australia fair? *Australian Health Review*, 40(1), 1–2.

Deravin, L., Francis, K. & Anderson, J. (2017). Are closing the gap targets being met? *Australian Nursing & Midwifery Journal*, 24(9), 38.

Duckett, S. & Wilcox, S. (2015). *The Australian Healthcare System* (5th ed.). Melbourne: Oxford University Press.

Duffield, C., Diers, D., O'Brien-Pallas, L., Aisbett, C., Roche, M., King, M. & Aisbett, K. (2011). Nursing staffing, nursing workload, the work environment and patient outcomes. *Applied Nursing Research*, 24(4), 244–55.

Durey, A. (2010). Reducing racism in Aboriginal healthcare in Australia: Where does cultural education fit? *Australian and New Zealand Journal of Public Health*, 34(0), S87–S92.

Francis, K., Anderson, J., Mills, N., Hobbs, T. & Fitzgerald, M. (2013). Advanced roles for nurses working in general practice: a study of barriers and enablers for nurses in rural Australia. *Clinical Nursing Studies*, 1(4), 45.

Guzys, D. & Arnott, N. (2013). The social model of health. In D. Guzys & E. Petrie (eds), *An Introduction to Community and Primary Healthcare in Australia*. Melbourne: Cambridge University Press.

Hall, J. (2015). Australian healthcare: The challenge of reform in a fragmented system. *The New England Journal of Medicine*, 373(6), 493–7.

Health Workforce Australia (2012). *Health Workforce Australia 2012: Health Workforce 2025 – Doctors, Nurses and Midwives – Volume 1*. Adelaide: Health Workforce Australia. Retrieved from https://submissions.education.gov.au/forms/archive/2015_16_sol/documents/Attachments/Australian%20Nursing%20and%20Midwifery%20Accreditation%20Council%20%28ANMAC%29.pdf.

Jacob, E.R., Barnett, A., Sellick, K. & McKenna, L. (2013). Scope of practice for Australian enrolled nurses: Evolution and practice issues. *Contemporary Nurse*, 45(2), 155–63.

Jatrana, S., Pasupeti, S. & Richards, K. (2014). Nativity, duration of residence and chronic health conditions in Australia: Do trends converge towards the native-born population? *Social Science & Medicine*, 119, 53–63.

Kenison, T.C., Silverman, P., Sustin, M. & Thompson, C.L. (2015). Differences between nurse practitioner and physician care providers on rates of secondary cancer screening and discussion of lifestyle changes among breast cancer survivors. *Journal of Cancer Survivorship*, 9(2), 223–9.

King, A. (2001). *The Primary Healthcare Strategy*. Wellington: Ministry of Health.

Maier, C.B. & Aiken, L.H. (2016). Task shifting from physicians to nurses in primary care in 39 countries: A cross-country comparative study. *European Journal of Public Health*, 26(6), 927–34.

Malone, L. & Anderson, J. (2015). Understanding the need for the introduction of the multi-purpose service model in rural Australia. *Asia Pacific Journal of Health Management*, 10(3), GS3–GS6.

Mays, N. (2013). Reorienting the New Zealand healthcare system to meet the challenge of long-term conditions in a fiscally constrained environment. Paper presented at the New Zealand Treasury, Wellington.

Miles, M., Latham, H. & Biles, J. (2016). The Australian and New Zealand healthcare system. In L. Deravin-Malone & J. Anderson (eds), *Chronic Care Nursing: A Framework for Practice*. Melbourne: Cambridge University Press, pp. 64–75.

Ministry of Health NZ (2015). Tatau Kahukura: Māori health statistics. Retrieved from https://www.health.govt.nz/our-work/populations/maori-health/tatau-kahukura-maori-health-statistics.

—— (2016a). *New Zealand Health Strategy: Future Direction*. Wellington: Ministry of Health.

—— (2016b). New Zealand health system. Retrieved from https://www.health.govt.nz/new-zealand-health-system.

Moore, J. & Prentice, D. (2013). Collaboration among nurse practitioners and registered nurses in outpatient oncology settings in Canada. *Journal of Advanced Nursing*, 69(7), 1574–83.

New Zealand Immigration (2017). New Zealand Refugee Quota Programme. Retrieved from https://www.immigration.govt.nz/about-us/what-we-do/our-strategies-and-projects/supporting-refugees-and-asylum-seekers/refugee-and-protection-unit/new-zealand-refugee-quota-programme.

Nursing Council of New Zealand (NCNZ) ([2007] 2016). *Competencies for Registered Nurses*. Retrieved from http://www.nursingcouncil.org.nz/Nurses.

—— (2012a). *Competencies for Enrolled Nurses*. Retrieved from http://www.nursingcouncil .org.nz/Nurses.

—— (2012b). *Competencies for the Nurse Practitioner Scope of Practice*. Retrieved from http://www.nursingcouncil.org.nz/Nurses.

Nursing and Midwifery Board of Australia (NMBA) (2014). *Nurse Practitioner Standards for Practice*. Melbourne: Nursing & Midwifery Board of Australia.

—— (2016a). *Managing Risk to the Public. Regulation at Work in Australia – NMBA 2015/16 Annual Report Summary*. Retrieved from http://www.aphra.gov.au/ annualreport/2016.

—— (2016b). *Registered Nurse Standards for Practice*. Melbourne: Nursing & Midwifery Board of Australia. Retrieved from http://www.nursingmidwiferyboard.gov.au/ Codes-Guidelines-Statements/Professional-standards.aspx.

—— (2016c). *Registration Standard: Recency of Practice*. Retrieved from http://www .nursingmidwiferyboard.gov.au/Registration-Standards.aspx.

—— (2016d). *Standards for Practice: Enrolled Nurses*. Melbourne: Nursing & Midwifery Board of Australia.

Royal Australasian College of Surgeons (2016). *Maori Health Action Plan 2016–18*. Wellington: RACS.

Statistics NZ (2015). Maori population estimates at June 2015 – tables. Retrieved from http://www.stats.govt.nz/browse_for_stats/population/estimates_and_projections/ MaoriPopulationEstimates_HOTPAtJun15.aspx.

Webster, S., Lopez, V., Allnut, J., Clague, L., Jones, D. & Bennett, P. (2010). Undergraduate nursing students' experiences in a rural clinical placement. *Australian Journal of Rural Health*, 18(5), 194–8.

World Health Organization (WHO). (1981). *Global Strategy for Health for All by the Year 2000*. Geneva: WHO.

—— (2013). *The Economics of Social Determinants of Health and Health Inequalities: A Resource Book*. Geneva: WHO.

—— (2015). World Health Organization. Retrieved from http://www.who.int/en.

2

Admitting and assessing medical and surgical clients

Judith Anderson, Monica Peddle,
Sonia Reisenhofer, Judith Needham
and Linda Deravin

LEARNING OBJECTIVES

At the completion of this chapter, you should be able to:

1. define and discuss the process of admission and assessment of the acute client
2. explain the concept of risk management and the importance of patient safety, specifying strategies that exist to increase safety and reduce risk
3. discuss the use of critical thinking to inform clinical decision-making
4. identify and discuss the role of the nurse in providing patient-centred care, including interpretation of diagnostic tests and administration of medication
5. explore and discuss the discharge of an acute client, considering appropriate social, cultural, physical and psychological considerations.

Introduction

This chapter discusses the admission and assessment of medical and surgical patients. It covers the process involved in admission and assessment of these acute clients and explains the concept of risk management, how important it is to patient safety and strategies that can be incorporated to increase patient safety and reduce risks. This is followed by a discussion about critical thinking and how it informs clinical decision-making. The role of the nurse is discussed in relation to patient-centred care, interpretation of diagnostic tests and administration of medication. The chapter concludes with a discussion of the discharge of acute clients, and how this requires consideration of social, cultural, physical and psychological factors.

The following identifies the national competency standards for the registered nurse from the Nursing and Midwifery Board of Australia (NMBA) and the Nursing Council of New Zealand (NCNZ) that are addressed in this chapter.

Australian Registered Nurse Standards for Practice

Standard 1: Thinks critically and analyses nursing practice

Standard 2: Engages in therapeutic and professional relationships

Standard 3: Maintains the capability for practice

Standard 4: Comprehensively conducts assessments

Standard 5: Develops a plan for nursing practice

Standard 6: Provides safe, appropriate and responsive quality nursing practice

(NMBA, 2016)

New Zealand: Competencies for Registered Nurses

Competency 1.4: Promotes an environment that enables health consumer safety, independence, quality of life, and health

Competency 1.5: Practises nursing in a manner that the health consumer determines as being culturally safe

Competency 2.1: Provides planned nursing care to achieve identified outcomes

Competency 2.2: Undertakes a comprehensive and accurate nursing assessment of health consumers in a variety of settings

Competency 2.3: Ensures documentation is accurate and maintains confidentiality of information

Competency 3.1: Establishes, maintains and concludes therapeutic interpersonal relationships with health consumers

Competency 3.2: Practises nursing in a negotiated partnership with the health consumer where and when possible

Competency 4.1: Collaborates and participates with colleagues and members of the health care team to facilitate and coordinate care

Competency 4.2: Recognises and values the roles and skills of all members of the health care team in the delivery of care

(NCNZ, [2007] 2016)

NURSING STANDARDS

Admission and assessment

The **admission** process is pivotal in the establishment of a positive patient experience within the acute healthcare setting. This process should be the beginning or continuation of a therapeutic nurse–patient relationship where patients feel welcome and safe. To this end, part of the admission process includes orientating your patient and their family to the ward staff, environment and routines, explaining relevant procedures and medical equipment, and answering any questions the patient may have.

Assessment is a vital component of nursing care, and is foundational to nursing care plans and interventions. The admission process provides an opportunity for nurses to perform initial assessments of patients to inform clinical decision-making and determine patient goals during the patient's hospitalisation. The admission process is also usually a good time to begin preparing for the patient's discharge from the ward, an element of care discussed later in this chapter.

Admission process and entry points

Patients may be admitted to a ward or unit in a hospital setting as the result of an emergency or planned admission. Emergency admission patients are usually transferred to a ward after presenting to the hospital's emergency department with an acute illness or injury, or an exacerbation of a chronic illness. Planned admission patients may arrive directly at the ward for admission prior to surgery or another health-related procedure. For planned admission patients, ward beds should previously have been reserved for the patient via the treating doctor or surgeon. Both planned or emergency admission patients may be transferred to the ward after surgical or other procedures. In the case of planned surgery, they may have visited the ward or hospital previously as part of their pre-admission process, in which case they may already have some pre-admission assessments completed and may have been orientated to the ward environment.

Health assessment in context

Irrespective of how a patient arrives on your ward, most hospitals will have specific multidisciplinary admission processes and assessments that need to be undertaken. This often commences with a nursing admission interview and preliminary patient assessment, and includes an orientation to the ward. Depending on the patient's condition, learning ability and emotional status, these processes ideally are done immediately upon admission, but must be done within the first twelve to 24 hours of admission, depending on hospital policy (RCHM, 2014; Children's Hospital at Westmead, 2016). During the initial assessment, it is important to consider the patient from a holistic perspective, assessing not only their immediate reason for admission but their mental, physical, emotional, social and spiritual state.

Similarities and differences between medical and surgical clients

Within today's complex healthcare environments, there is often a large overlap between medical and surgical clients. Simplistically, surgical patients will usually have some kind of invasive procedure and their post-operative management often includes a focus on pain management, supporting and managing the patient's ABCs (airway, breathing and circulation) during the immediate post-operative period and then promoting their return to the best level of mobility and independence as they recover. Conversely, medical patients present with an illness not requiring surgical intervention. Medical patients may often have multiple comorbidities and usually present as unplanned emergency admissions. Common examples of medical patients requiring admission include those experiencing acute myocardial infarction, exacerbation of asthma or chronic obstructive pulmonary disease, diabetic foot ulcer or stroke. Care for medical patients often focuses on symptom management, reversal of the underlying disease process where possible, promoting independence and supporting activities of daily living until discharge.

Admission interview and initial patient assessment example activities

When patients first arrive on your ward, you will be required to undertake a number of activities as part of your initial patient assessment and orientation. These may vary slightly depending on your context, the patient's condition, their age and the reason for admission. Many of these activities are related to minimising risk, promoting patient safety, building a therapeutic relationship, proactive health screening, establishing a baseline, detecting abnormalities and promoting patient knowledge, comfort and confidence. Table 2.1 provides examples of activities that the admitting nurse may undertake with the patient and their family.

In conjunction with the assessments a nurse may undertake when admitting a patient outlined in Table 2.1, a number of further orientation activities may be required. These are undertaken to promote patient safety, enhance knowledge, provide comfort and continue to build a therapeutic nurse–patient relationship. To begin, the nurse may provide an introduction to staff, including nursing, allied health, medical and auxiliary supports, who the

Table 2.1 Ward admission assessment activities

Admission assessment activities	Rationale
Identifying the patient and applying identity bands (if not already done) to enable correct patient identification throughout the hospital stay	Promote patient safety. Ensure that the patient is correctly identified to prevent errors in treatment, interventions, medications or other events while admitted.
Confirming the reason for the patient's admission and their understanding of their illness and hospitalisation plan to provide a connection with the patient and family to enable good communication (Bucknall et al., 2016b)	Promote patient safety, detect and prevent communication errors, build a therapeutic relationship and enhance patient/family knowledge related to the patient's illness and planned care during hospitalisation.
Confirming whether the patient has any allergies and applying allergy bands as required	Promote patient safety and prevent medication errors and adverse events.
Confirming the patient's past medical/surgical history and any relevant family history	Baseline data to inform healthcare decisions. Ensure comprehensive health history available and minimise risk of errors/adverse events.
Confirming the patient's current medications, including prescribed medications, over-the-counter treatments and tobacco, alcohol and illicit drug use	Promote patient safety and prevent medication errors and adverse events.
	Often confirming a patient's current medications may provide additional information regarding the patient's health status and past medical history.
Performing a general patient assessment	Establish a baseline for future comparison. Identify abnormalities for more detailed investigation or intervention.

(cont.)

Table 2.1   (cont.)

Admission assessment activities	Rationale
Undertaking vital signs assessment, including pulse, blood pressure, temperature, respirations, peripheral oxygen situation measurements	Establish a baseline for future comparison. Identify abnormalities for more detailed investigation or intervention.
Performing a pain assessment and other symptom assessment – for example, assessing for nausea, vomiting or diarrhoea, shortness of breath or other symptoms experienced by the patient	Establish a baseline for future comparison. Identify abnormalities for more detailed investigation or intervention.
	Provide an opportunity to intervene and promote patient comfort and wellbeing using evidence-based interventions as indicated by assessment findings.
Performing focused assessments related to the patient's presenting complaint and past medical history – for example, a respiratory assessment for a patient admitted with a medical diagnosis of exacerbation of asthma	Establish a baseline for future comparison. Identify abnormalities for more detailed investigation or intervention.
	Provide opportunity to intervene and promote patient comfort and wellbeing using evidence-based interventions as indicated by assessment findings.
Assessing the patient's weight and height	Establish a baseline for future comparison. These parameters may also be used in determining the dose of medications (for example, anaesthetic agents or anti-coagulants).
Performing a urinalysis	Proactive screening. Establish a baseline for future comparison. Identify abnormalities for more detailed investigation or intervention.
Performing a random blood glucose analysis	Proactive screening. Establish a baseline for future comparison. Identify abnormalities for more detailed investigation or intervention.
Performing an electrocardiograph (pre-surgery for patients over 50 years of age, depending on hospital policy)	Proactive screening. Establish a baseline for future comparison. Identify abnormalities for more detailed investigation or intervention.
Performing patient safety assessments including their risk of falling or developing a pressure sore during hospitalisation (discussed below in patient safety)	Establish a baseline for future comparison. Identify abnormalities for more detailed investigation.
	Plan safety interventions or other activities to minimise risk of adverse events while patient is admitted.
Performing a psychosocial and spiritual needs assessment – exploring the patient's normal role(s), support structure, spiritual beliefs and other factors that may impact or be impacted by their hospitalisation	Establish a baseline for future comparison. Identify abnormalities for more detailed investigation.
	Provide an opportunity to intervene and promote patient comfort and wellbeing. Build a therapeutic relationship with patient and family.
Considering referrals to allied health or other services for assessment and management while admitted or upon discharge	Promote patient wellbeing, recovery, and safety during admission and upon discussion. Ensure that the patient will be ready and safe to be discharged in a timely manner.

Admission assessment activities	Rationale
Confirming/suspending any home care services the patient may be using on admission to hospital	Enhanced interprofessional communication, prevent unrequired home visits and allow for workload planning. Patients/families may often overlook notifying home care service providers of patient's admission to hospital – particularly in times of high stress.
Considering home care services or other supports that the patient may need upon discharge	Based on assessment of patient's current and expected discharge health status and supportive needs. Ensure that the patient will be ready and safe to be discharged in a timely manner.
Educating the patient on specific requirements of their admission – for example *nil by mouth* prior to theatre, use the call-bell to ask for assistance prior to mobilising	Promote therapeutic relationship, patient's knowledge, comfort and safety during admission. Assists to prevent adverse events during patient's admission.

patient may encounter during their stay so that the patient is confident about the care being provided. In order to promote patient comfort, an orientation to the physical environment of the ward is also required, which may include an orientation to the bedroom environment, bathroom and toilet location, kitchen and patient lounge area. Additionally, orientation and identification of a safe place for valuables, space for clothing and toiletries, lighting, television and assistance call-bell may assist the patient to feel secure in their new environment.

Each ward tends to have its own routines, so it is often helpful to provide patients with an orientation to activities of daily living and hygiene facilities available, including how to seek assistance if necessary. Providing an overview of the ward schedules, including activities such as when medical reviews occur, mealtimes and visiting hours may assist patients and their families to plan their activities during the patient's hospitalisation.

Finally, being in hospital can be very overwhelming for patients and their families, and the complex medical equipment used may seem frightening to those with limited experience. As such, providing explanations of specific medical/care equipment that the patient is likely to see may be helpful. Such equipment may include intravenous therapy lines and pumps, dressings or drain tubes, monitoring equipment or mobility aids.

The patient admission process is a vital component of patient care. It establishes the therapeutic relationship between the patient and nurse, and provides an opportunity for baseline assessment, proactive health screening and detection of health abnormalities that require further investigation or treatment. It is the first step of the clinical reasoning cycle/nursing process, and is focused on promoting patient comfort and safety, minimising risk and enhancing patient care.

Patient safety and risk management

In the complex clinical environment that exists in today's healthcare facilities, it is imperative that healthcare is provided safely and competently to maximise patient outcomes. **Risk management** and patient safety approaches aim to assist all involved in healthcare to understand the risks involved and to identify and develop effective strategies to manage those risks and maintain patient safety.

Risk management – 'the design and implementation of a program to identify and avoid or minimise risks to patients, employees, volunteers, visitors and the institution' (ACSQHC, 2011, p. 12).

Assessing and managing risk

In clinical practice settings, there are many opportunities and avenues of actual and potential risk. Risk management approaches gather information through feedback, complaints, incidents and adverse event reporting to identify and minimise risks to organisations, patients, visitors and staff (ACSQHC, 2011). Part of the nurse's role in risk management is to identify and address these hazards in order to minimise harm. There are five basic principles of risk management:

1   *Avoid risk.* Identify appropriate strategies that can be used to avoid the risk whenever possible. If a risk cannot be eliminated, then it must be managed.
2   *Identify risk.* Assess the risk by identifying the nature of the risk and who is involved.
3   *Analyse risk.* Do this by examining how a risk can occur, what the likelihood of it occurring is, and the potential consequences of the risk occurring.
4   *Evaluate risk.* Determine how the risk can be reduced or eliminated. Document the process and response/outcomes.
5   *Treat risks.* Manage the risk by determining who is responsible for taking actions, and when and how this will be monitored.

(ACSQHC, 2014b)

When assessing risk, you need to identify:

* who is at risk
* what is involved
* why it can happen
* how likely it is
* the consequences
* what can be done
* whether the solution applied to the situation/risk has been identified (ACSQHC, 2014b).

SKILLS IN PRACTICE

Edith Smith: Admission for fractured neck of femur

Edith Smith is a 68-year-old woman who lives at home by herself after her husband of 40 years, Frank, died last year. Edith has a good overall fitness level but she presented to the doctor last month with low blood pressure. Edith explained to the doctor that she doesn't eat as well as she should now, since Frank isn't around to cook for. Edith is admitted after a fall at home, resulting in a fractured neck of femur. She was found after several hours on the ground in her backyard, by a neighbour who heard her call for help. She seems a bit dehydrated and confused.

QUESTION
Apply the questions listed above to assess Edith's risk of a fall while in your ward for surgical repair of her fractured neck of femur.

Patient-centred care (PCC) – Care provision which acknowledges the patients individual care values and needs.

However, to ensure **patient–centred care (PCC)**, each patient requires an individualised assessment to identify any actual or potential risks that may present a problem for them while they are receiving healthcare. To assist the completion of patient–centred risk assessments, a number of risk-assessment tools have been developed (Table 2.2). These tools gather information from the individual using a checklist or rating scale and summarise it, producing an overall rating on the level of risk. The final rating assists the nurse to determine the appropriate strategies to decrease the risk to the patient.

Table 2.2 Examples of Australian risk-assessment tools

Risk-assessment tools	Example
Falls Risk Assessment Tool (FRAT)	Health.Vic (2018)
Malnutrition screening tools	Queensland Health (2018)
Braden pressure risk assessment tool	SA Health (2018)
Between the flags track and trigger observation charts	Clinical Excellence Commission (2018)

Occasionally things do go wrong, and the response to these errors should not be blame but rather investigation and learning, with the aim of reducing risks for future patients, organisations, staff and visitors (Lord Hunt of Kings Heath, 2002). The occurrence of an **incident** requires an incident report to be completed. Incident reports provide comprehensive data for healthcare facilities to support thorough reviews and root-cause analysis of incidents to identify problems and develop improvement strategies. Incident reports will require responses to questions relating to the who, what, when, where, how and why.

A good report is:

Incident – An 'event or circumstance that resulted, or could have resulted, in unintended and/or unnecessary harm to a person and/or a complaint, loss or damage' (ACSQHC, 2011, p. 10).

- complete
- concise
- specific
- factual and objective
- de-identified where appropriate
- light on abbreviations (DHHS, 2013).

Despite these risk-management approaches, evidence indicates that the complexity of the healthcare system still places patients at significant risk from adverse events and medical error (Kohn, Corrigan & Donaldson, 2000; Makary & Daniel, 2016; Shojania & Dixon-Woods, 2016). Consequences of errors can result in sentinel events, significant morbidity, distress and suffering, and a financial burden for patients and significant others (Ehsani, Jackson & Duckett, 2006; Shojania & Dixon-Woods, 2016).

Sentinel events are a subset of adverse events that result in death or serious harm to a patient. In 2004, the Australian Department of Health developed a core set of sentinel events that were required to be reported by public hospitals to enable reviews of the events and planning for improvements that may be required to prevent the event from occurring again.

Australian national core set of sentinel events

1 Procedures involving the wrong patient or body part
2 Suicide of a patient in an inpatient unit
3 Retained instruments or other material after surgery requiring re-operation or further surgical procedure

4   Intravascular gas embolism resulting in death or neurological damage
5   Haemolytic blood transfusion reaction resulting from ABO incompatibility
6   Medication error leading to the death of patient reasonably believed to be due
    to incorrect administration of drugs
7   Maternal death or serious morbidity associated with labour or delivery
8   Infant discharged to the wrong family

(Department of Health, 2005)

What is patient safety?

Patient safety is a discipline in the healthcare sector that applies safety science methods toward the goal of achieving a trustworthy system of healthcare delivery. Patient
safety is also an attribute of healthcare systems; it minimizes the incidence and impact
of, and maximizes recovery from, adverse events.

(Emanuel et al., 2008)

As part of the healthcare team, it is critical that nurses have background knowledge, skills
and attitudes of the origin of error in healthcare and patient safety approaches to manage
and improve safety challenges in their clinical practice.

Error types and accident causation

Reason (2000) proposes that active failures and latent conditions are associated with
adverse events in healthcare. Active failures are the unsafe acts committed by the healthcare personnel who are in direct contact with the patient and can take the form of slips,
lapses, mistakes and violations (Reason, 2000). These failures have an immediate impact on
the patient. Latent conditions arise from decisions made by healthcare designers, managers and directors that produce inevitable 'resident pathogens' in a system (Reason, 2000).
Latent conditions can lie dormant for some time until combined with active failures and
error-producing factors that result in an accident (Reason, 2000). As depicted in Reason's
(1995) accident causation model (Figure 2.1), adverse events or medical errors occur when
failures appear in a number of layers that momentarily line up to permit the trajectory of
opportunity for an accident.

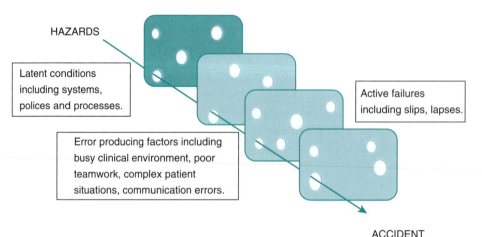

Figure 2.1   Reason's accident causation model
Source: Adapted from Reason (1995).

A key aspect of many adverse events and medical errors is the failure to apply human factors thinking to patient care situations (Walton, 2011). Human factors refer to 'environmental, organisational and job factors, and human and individual characteristics which influence behaviour at work in a way which can affect health and safety' (Flin, Winter & Cakil Sarac, 2009). Four categories and ten topics of human factors have been identified as relevant for patient safety (Flin, Winter & Cakil Sarac, 2009; see Table 2.3).

Table 2.3 Categories and topics of human factors in healthcare

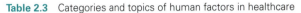

Category	Topic
Organisation/managerial	Safety culture
	Leadership
	Communication
Workgroup/team	Teamwork
	Team supervision
Individual worker	Situation awareness
	Decision-making
	Stress
	Fatigue
Work environment	Work environment and hazards

Source: Flin, Winter and Cakil Sarac (2009).

REFLECTIVE QUESTION

Reflect on the impact that an error could have on an acute patient and their future life. Consider not only immediate pain and suffering but also future earning capacity and the impact on their family and friends.

Australian Commission on Safety and Quality in Health Care

The Australian Commission of Safety and Quality in Health Care (ACSQHC) has identified three safety and quality goals for healthcare in Australia (Table 2.4), along with ten National Safety and Quality Health Service (NSQHS) Standards (Table 2.5) used in the accreditation of healthcare providers to support meeting the stated goals. The standards outline the roles for different groups in healthcare to ensure safe and quality care.

Documentation

Documentation supports vital communication across the healthcare team of the patient's current condition and treatment plan, as well providing information to identify patterns or trends over time that may indicate patient deterioration. While documentation plays an important role in team communication, is also a legal requirement. The Nursing and

Table 2.4 Australian Safety and Quality Health Care Goals

Goal 1: Safety of care – that people receive their healthcare without experiencing preventable harm	
Priority area	**Outcomes**
1.1 Medication safety	Reduce harm to people from medications through safe and effective medication management
1.2 Healthcare associated infection	Reduce harm to people from healthcare associated infections through effective infection control and antimicrobial stewardship
1.3 Recognising and responding to clinical deterioration	Reduce harm to people from failures to recognise and respond to clinical deterioration through the implementation of effective recognition and response systems
Goal 2. Appropriateness of care – that people receive appropriate, evidence-based care	
Priority area	**Outcomes**
2.1 Acute coronary syndrome	Provide appropriate, evidence-based care for people with acute coronary syndrome
2.2 Transient ischemic attack and stroke	Provide appropriate, evidence-based care for people with a transient ischemic attack or stroke
Goal 3. Partnering with consumers – that there are effective partnerships between consumers and healthcare providers and organisations at all levels of healthcare provision, planning and evaluation	

Source: ACSQHC (2012).

Midwifery Board of Australia (2016) Standards for Practice identify that the registered nurse 'maintains accurate, comprehensive and timely documentation of assessments, planning, decision-making, actions and evaluations' and further defines that the nurse is accountable for the documentation completed.

Every clinical facility will have policies and procedure regarding documentation and each nurse must practise by these standards. The essentials of quality nursing documentation have been identified to include seven essential themes (Scruth, 2014). Nursing documentation:

- must be patient-centred
- must contain the actual interventions of the nurse that includes the physical, education and psychosocial support and their effectiveness
- reflects an objective clinical approach of the nurse
- is presented in a logical sequential manner
- is time sensitive
- must reflect the variances in care
- should be clear and concise
- should satisfy legal requirements including
  - handwritten entries must be legible
  - each page must have the patient's name and medical record number
  - each entry must include a time, date and signature with designation
  - each entry must be accurate, including spelling, with correct terminology used

Table 2.5   National Safety and Quality Health Service Standards

Standard	Description
1 Governance for safety and quality in health service organisations	The quality framework required for health service organisations to implement safe systems
2 Partnering with consumers	The systems and strategies to create a consumer-centred health system by including consumers in the development and design of quality healthcare
3 Preventing and controlling healthcare associated infections	The systems and strategies to prevent infection of patients within the healthcare system and to manage infections effectively when they occur, to minimise the consequences
4 Medication safety	The systems and strategies to ensure clinicians safely prescribe, dispense and administer appropriate medicines to informed patients
5 Patient identification and procedure matching	The systems and strategies to identify patients and correctly match their identity with the correct treatment
6 Clinical handover	The systems and strategies for effective clinical communication whenever accountability and responsibility for a patient's care is transferred
7 Blood and blood products	The systems and strategies for the safe, effective and appropriate management of blood and blood products so the patients receiving blood are safe
8 Preventing and managing pressure injuries	The systems and strategies to prevent patients developing pressure injuries and best practice management when pressure injuries occur
9 Recognising and responding to clinical deterioration in Acute healthcare	The systems and processes to be implemented by health service organisations to respond effectively to patients when their clinical condition deteriorates
10 Preventing falls and harm from falls	The systems and strategies to reduce the incidence of patient falls in health service organisations and best practice management when falls do occur

Source: ACSQHC (2011).

- any incorrect entries must be labelled clearly and approved abbreviations must be used
- interventions recorded by the nurse performing the intervention should be documented at the time of the intervention or as close to that time as possible
- the correct ink colour should be used according to facility policy.

(Adapted from Scruth, 2014)

REFLECTIVE QUESTION

Reflect on the positives and negatives of good and bad documentation. What should you document to support yourself when admitting an acute patient?

Clinical decision-making

In the delivery of safe patient care, nurses are required to make decisions. These will be made in a variety of clinical contexts and under a range of circumstances.

What is a decision and why do we need to make them?

A decision is the act of making a judgement or choosing a particular course of action when considering all the available options (Marquis & Houston, 2012; Merriam-Webster. com, 2016). In providing healthcare, patients and clinicians – including nurses – will make clinical care decisions that will affect the outcome of care. It is important that decisions are made about issues that may arise in the delivery of clinical care so that care is not provided in a haphazard way (Swallow, Smith & Smith, 2017).

Critical thinking – The analysis and evaluation of a situation.

Critical thinking, problem-solving and decision-making are key components of any decision-making framework. It is important that clinical practitioners understand why clinical decision-making is significant in the delivery of safe patient care (Swallow, Smith & Smith, 2017). Nurses are accountable for their actions, and these actions are often based on the ability to make a decision, which will be influenced by a nurse's skills, knowledge and experience. Increasingly within the healthcare environment, we are seeing decisions being made in partnership with patients and their carers, together with health professionals working in teams, about the course of clinical care. Nurses are in a pivotal position to influence and make decisions, and for this reason should have an awareness of the decision-making process.

The decision-making process

Clinical judgement – The process by which a decision about care can be made based on the interpretation of available information. In order to make such a judgement, critical thinking and problem-solving are required.

Using **clinical judgement** to effectively make a decision is explained by a number of theories on how a clinical decision may be reached. Some of these theories include traditional knowledge within cultures, trial and error, personal experience, education and research, logical reasoning, intuition and reflective practice (Swallow, Smith & Smith, 2017). As nurses are professionally accountable for their actions and decisions, it is equally important to understand the cognitive steps in the decision-making process:

1 Define the issue.
2 Understand the context within which the decision needs to be made.
3 Identify possible options.
4 Evaluate the consequences of each option.
5 Prioritise the options and make one choice.
6 Review the decision that is made.
7 Enact the decision and deal with any consequences that follow.

(Russell-Jones, 2015)

These steps detail the thought process of making a decision, yet other factors should be considered when making a clinical decision, such as prior and current knowledge. Additional factors include:

• the patient understanding, and possessing the ability to influence, the decision about their own care
• the information that is needed to make a clinical judgement about care

- the impact of the decision on the quality of care
- external influences, which may include the available resources to provide care
- the scope of practice of the person making the decision
- the skills and knowledge of the person making the decision
- whether the decision is being made on the basis of the best evidence available (Swallow, Smith & Smith, 2017).

When decisions go wrong

Even with the best available evidence considered, sometimes a decision is made and the outcome is not what was anticipated. Possible reasons why decisions may go wrong can be attributed to a number of factors, including those listed in Table 2.6.

Table 2.6 Examples of decisions with adverse outcomes

Reasons	Examples
Having the wrong information or data	Incorrect labelling of patient information/incorrect patient
Not receiving the right information or data in a timely manner	Delayed pathology or radiology results influencing clinical diagnosis
Incorrectly interpreting the information or data	Clinician error caused by fatigue or lack of knowledge
Making a decision to avoid conflict rather than addressing the underlying problem	When there is a conflict about treatment regimes and the decision is not based on evidence-based practice
Not using a decision-making framework (process) and making judgements based on best guesses	Not waiting for clinical information to make a judgement – for example, pathology results – and basing judgements on previous experience
Not considering that patients are individuals and that the decision should be based on their unique set of circumstances, the one-size-fits-all rule does not necessarily always apply in practice	Treating with an antibiotic when the patient has been shown not to respond to that antibiotic in the past
Haste – making a decision before all the facts are known	Occurs in emergency or time-pressured situations

Source: Adapted from Swallow, Smith and Smith (2017).

Within your nursing practice, you will be required to make decisions on a daily and sometimes hourly basis. Decisions about clinical care should be made with the best possible information, data and evidence available. Developing skills to interpret this information will improve with more experience (Bucknall et al., 2016a). If there is ever a time when you are unsure about a decision that you need to make, conferring with more experienced practitioners and seeking advice should be considered. Making the best decision based on the information you have, using your critical analytical thinking skills and knowledge, will help to avoid poor decisions, which can have devastating consequences in practice for both patients and clinicians.

Role of the nurse

The role of the nurse is complex in many ways, and is dependent on the reason for admission – for example, a pre-booked surgical admission or surgical admission through the emergency department; or a medical patient admitted acutely for clinical care. Registered nurses are at the frontline of the hospital admission process (Handy, 2016). The nurse's clinical decision-making, particularly how decisions are communicated and documented, enables other healthcare team members to perform their duties while providing accurate care and developing the skills to ensure safe, high-quality care and best practice are achieved.

Assessment is a key component of nursing practice, required for planning and provision of patient- and family-centred care. In 2006, the Nursing and Midwifery Board of Australia (NMBA), in its then current National Competency Standard for Registered Nurses, stated that, 'The registered nurse assesses, plans, implements and evaluates nursing care in collaboration with individuals and the multidisciplinary healthcare team so as to achieve goals and health outcomes.' The current NMBA (2016) standards expand the role of the registered nurse to being person-centred, with the therapeutic interaction including not only the patient but their family and community. The assessment required by the nurse includes: patient history (previous surgery and medical conditions); family history; physical examination (blood pressure, pulse, respiration, temperature, height and weight); electrocardiograph; and current and previous medication history.

What is continuity of care?

Continuity of care – How a patient experiences care over time, including the provision of good interpersonal skills and coordination of care.

Continuity of care involves three types of continuity: informational continuity; management continuity; and relational or interpersonal continuity (CARNA, 2008). All three facets of continuity are paramount to best practice. Informational continuity refers to the transfer of information from one party to another to provide the knowledge that has been accumulated over time, to ensure that the current care is appropriate and ongoing. Management continuity provides a consistent approach to the care of the patient, considering policy and consistent use of care plans, pathways and case management (Haggerty et al., 2003). Relational or interpersonal continuity refers to the ongoing interaction between the nurse, patient and their family, along with other healthcare providers.

Aspinal, Gridley, Bernard and Parker (2012) suggest that continuity of care is the quality care which the registered nurse provides over time. Therefore, the role of the nurse is to ensure that the patient is involved with decision-making in their own care and that services are integrated to provide the best possible care for the patient while also including family members as necessary. Malley and colleagues (2015) point out that the nurse's consideration of the end-users who are discharging the patients back to home is paramount to good care. Both the acute medical and surgical admission process must reflect the care transition of the patient.

The more acutely ill a patient is, the greater the range of needs there will be due to complex requirements; these requirements may include intravenous cannulation for hydration and antibiotics (Hirschman et al., 2015). If a patient has a complicated medical history and extensive information needs to be collected and assessed, this is the role of the registered nurse as the frontline staff member. The registered nurse will perform assessments and report abnormalities to the other health staff for collaboration and clinical decision-making with the team (Paul & Hice, 2014).

Interpretation of diagnostics

Routine testing of patients on admission to the clinical area will require blood work, depending on the diagnosis of the patient for admission. This will include a full blood count (FBC), liver function testing (LFT) and cardiac enzymes, depending on the presentation. Other routine **diagnostics** include blood glucose monitoring, urinalysis and an electrocardiogram (ECG), which are initiated by the nurse on presentation to the healthcare centre (Paul & Hice, 2014). Early intervention and interpretation of diagnostic results improves the quality of care and rapid treatment of patients, providing positive outcomes for the patient.

Diagnostics – Used to help identify a disease, illness or problem.

The opportunity for the nurse to question the patient at the time of admission when undertaking routine observations helps them to clarify and determine any abnormal readings prior to surgery and also during the medical admission. The nurse's role in the admission process is to communicate normal and abnormal diagnostic findings to other healthcare workers, to provide a collaborative approach to patient care and wellbeing.

Administration of medication

The administration of medications to patients is another important role assumed by the nurse, and must be undertaken accurately and competently to promote safe, high-quality care (Handy, 2016). Understanding the patient's diagnosis along with medications prescribed by the medical officers is paramount to achieve best practice in the nursing care of the patient in acute care. Roughead, Semple and Rosenfeld (2013) highlight that medication histories taken at the time of admission remain a point of vulnerability for medication error. The nurse is responsible for ensuring that history and allergy documentation is accurate, including checking the medications with which patients present to hospital. Consequences of ineffective communication and care during the admission process can lead to greater vulnerability for the patient's transition in care (Malley et al., 2015).

REFLECTIVE QUESTION

Reflect on your role as a student registered nurse in the admission process in an acute area, and consider an interaction where you have had difficulty communicating with your patient. What did you do to overcome these difficulties?

Preparation for discharge

Preparation for discharge usually begins when a patient is admitted. The data collected then are useful for discharge preparation, and beginning early allows time to organise services, equipment and education (Hoch & Hamlin, 2015; Palmer & Kresevic, 2014). When a patient is discharged, it is important to ensure that their needs will be met. The more complex the patient's condition is, the more discharge planning will be required – this is particularly the case for elderly patients and those who have comorbid conditions (Sinha et al., 2014). In some instances, another service or agency will assist in the provision of care while the patient is in the community (for this reason, some people refer to discharge as a transfer of care) (Haley, 2014). Good communication with the patient and any carers they may have is essential if this is to be effective (New, McDougall & Scroggie, 2016). Prior to discharge, it is important to assess the patient's needs, possible benefits of involving other health professionals and any education they may need in order to optimise their health outcomes.

Assessment of need

Assessing the patient's needs usually begins with a risk assessment to identify people who will require further assessment and follow-up care before leaving the ward or when they get home. It is important to assess how a patient will cope with the activities of daily living when they return home in order to ensure a positive outcome (Haley, 2014).

Shorter lengths of stay in hospital have several benefits, but this can result in a patient being discharged when they still feel quite unwell and may require family assistance. This means that the ability of the family to provide such assistance may also need to be assessed (some people may not have family or their family members may not be willing to assist) in order to ensure that the person will cope when they return home (Haley, 2014; Hoch & Hamlin, 2015; Pierluissi, Francis & Covinsky, 2014).

People living in Australia and New Zealand may face additional difficulties due to living in rural and remote areas. This extra distance may require assessment when preparing a patient for discharge, as they may not be well enough to travel long distances at the time of discharge and may feel anxious due to the length of time it may take to seek assistance if their condition were to deteriorate. In some instances, road conditions may also be poor or totally impenetrable at some times of the year (e.g. due to flooding) (Anderson & Malone, 2014; Haley, 2014).

Inter-professional involvement

Most health services will have a team of inter-professional staff who can collaborate in preparing patients for discharge. Teams are often varied, and can include case managers, physiotherapists, occupational therapists, dieticians, pharmacists and community nurses. Some of these teams may offer **post-acute care services**, where assistance can be provided to patients after they return to the community. If a wide range of services is available, patients will need to be informed about the relevant services (this varies significantly in different areas), how the services relate to them and what options are available (Sefcik et al., 2016). Patients with complex needs such as comorbidity are more likely to benefit from the involvement of an inter-professional team (Sinha et al., 2014). Even in rural and remote areas of Australia and New Zealand, there are often community nurses who can assist with follow-up care (Anderson & Malone, 2014; Haley, 2014). In order to give the entire team the best opportunity to address patient needs, they should be informed early of the estimated date of discharge. Family and patients themselves should also be informed of this in order to allow them to prepare (New, McDougall & Scroggie, 2016).

Pharmacists can also be helpful when it comes to assisting patients to learn about their medications, how to use them effectively and what side-effects to be aware of. Any change in medication should be addressed so the patient is clear about what has changed (Pierluissi, Francis & Covinsky, 2014). Patients who are being discharged should be provided with written verification of any follow-up appointments with general practitioners, allied health or any other health professionals they will be expected to visit when they have returned to their community, and referrals to such practitioners should be sent (Haley, 2014; Mitchell, 2015).

In some cases, physiotherapy, occupational therapy or nursing assessments can indicate the need for additional equipment (sometimes just in the short term) to assist in caring

Post-acute care services – These healthcare services support patients after they have been discharged from acute care services (e.g. hospitals) to manage at home. Usually access is limited to a number of weeks after discharge.

for someone after they have been discharged. Some health services have equipment available for this purpose, or there may be a leasing company that hires out equipment when required. Organising equipment can take a while, and sometimes patients need to make arrangements to pay for the hire of such equipment – this is one reason why preparing for discharge on admission can help, as nurses will often be aware of the likely outcome of a patient's admission (Haley, 2014).

Social, cultural, physical and psychological considerations

Each patient needs to be considered holistically when discharge is being planned. Social issues can relate to whether a patient has a carer or someone who can take on that role temporarily. Social issues are broad, and also include financial issues, transport, and access to medications and equipment. Culturally sensitive discharge planning is also essential, and can include religious considerations, dietary habits and living arrangements, not only for the patient but for other family members too. It is important to assess a patient's ability to understand the language being used at all times, as we often slip into professional terminology that is difficult for patients to understand. However, when a patient comes from a different cultural background, this is even more important. Asking a patient to explain what you have said in their own words or to demonstrate what you have shown them (teach back) is essential to determine whether they have understood. Interpreter services should be available in all health services (telehealth has made this a much more accessible service) and professionals should be used rather than asking family members to interpret, as cultures often make it difficult for some family members to discuss particular health issues – for example, a child interpreting information about sexual health to a parent (Bowman, Flood & Arbaje, 2014).

Physical considerations for discharge vary depending on the reason for admission. The location of a wound can impact a patient's mobility or their ability to care for themselves. Features of a patient's home that they have never noticed – such as a small step into a shower – may impact them after they have been hospitalised. Assessment of physical considerations therefore needs to be individualised for each patient and their ability on discharge. Similarly, psychological considerations vary. When a patient has a pre-existing psychological condition, support may already be in place, but the hospitalisation may create additional issues that are unexpected. Patients sometimes perceive hospitals as 'safe places' where they can call for help at any time, and are watched and assisted constantly. For some patients, the idea of discharge can cause anxiety as they may feel insecure – particularly if they do not have much social support or are experiencing a great deal of pain (Mitchell, 2015).

Some patients will decide to leave against medical advice. This will probably mean that they are not well prepared, and will make it even more important that some follow-up is undertaken if possible. From a legal perspective, it is important that such a discharge is well documented. Most health services will have a form for these patients to sign, acknowledging that they will not hold the health service liable for any issues that may arise, but some patients will leave without doing so (Alfandre & Schumann, 2013; Haley, 2014).

Education

Health literacy is how well people understand and apply information about their health and healthcare to their lives and make decisions about their health (ACSQHC, 2014a). Part of our role as health professionals is to help patients make effective decisions about their healthcare in an informed way. Such assistance extends to discharge, and often involves education that supports the patient after they have left the health service.

Education may be required for a patient who is returning home and/or for their family members, who will need to provide them with assistance at that time. This may include changing dressings, use of medications, physical care or dietary needs and how to recognise a deterioration in their condition (Haley, 2014). It is also important to ensure that patients are educated about preventing complications of their treatment (Anderson, Deravin-Malone & Anderson, 2016). Any patient who will need to self-manage their care at home, such as those with chronic conditions that are unable to be cured, such as diabetes or chronic obstructive pulmonary disease, will need to be offered education to ensure that they can cope effectively when they return home (Sinha et al., 2014).

As often as possible, verbal education should be supplemented with written education so the patient can return to the material later or if their memory fails (Hoch & Hamlin, 2015). Patient and family education are nursing responsibilities and need to be documented appropriately (Haley, 2014; Hoch & Hamlin, 2015).

Although most patients who are discharged from health services will be independent and not require any follow-up treatment, it is important to assess them thoroughly. In many cases, an admission is a useful window of opportunity to provide education about health generally, how to avoid future admissions and how to recognise a deterioration of their condition, which may require their return to healthcare (Anderson, Deravin-Malone & Anderson, 2016; Haley, 2014).

SUMMARY

Learning objective 1: Define and discuss the process of admission and assessment of the acute client.

The process of admission for a patient to an acute healthcare environment involves providing patients and families with information about the healthcare environment, setting goals for the patient's admission, providing any required patient/family education, initiating referrals and preparing for discharge. It is vital within this process to ensure that the patient feels safe and welcome within your healthcare environment. A fundamental part of the admission process is the initial holistic patient assessment that should provide a benchmark for the patient's hospitalisation.

Learning objective 2: Explain the concept of risk management and the importance of patient safety, specifying strategies that exist to increase safety and reduce risk.

Admission into healthcare presents many risks to patients, and it is imperative that risk management and patient safety approaches are maintained to maximise patient outcomes. Risk-management approaches enable assessment and management of risks to protect patients from accidental injury. Patient safety thinking ensures all members of the healthcare team have common background knowledge, skills and attitudes regarding errors in healthcare, and approaches to manage and improve safety challenges in their clinical practice.

Learning objective 3: Discuss the use of critical thinking to inform clinical decision-making.

Decisions will be made in a variety of clinical contexts and under a range of circumstances. In providing healthcare, patients and clinicians – including nurses – will make clinical care decisions that will affect the outcome of care. Using a decision-making process will support the making of decisions based on the best available information and evidence, and avoid poorly made decisions, which can have devastating consequences for patient care.

Learning objective 4: Identify and discuss the role of the nurse in providing patient-centred care, including interpretation of diagnostic tests and administration of medication.

The nurse's role in the admission process is a complex integration of communication, documentation and education to provide optimal continuity of care. Interpretation of a patient's medical and surgical history, including diagnostics, is paramount to providing optimal care and skills to ensure that safe, high-quality best practice is achieved.

Learning objective 5: Explore and discuss the discharge of an acute client, considering appropriate social, cultural, physical and psychological considerations.

Discharge planning should begin at the time of admission so everyone involved, including the patient and their significant others, can begin preparations. Discharge planning should involve social (e.g. family, transport, financial), cultural (e.g. language, religious habits, dietary habits), physical (e.g. wound care, mobility, pain) and psychosocial (e.g. anxiety, depression, fear) considerations.

REVIEW QUESTIONS

2.1 What are the elements required to orientate a patient and their family to your ward environment?

2.2 What is the nurse's role during an admission assessment?

2.3 Identify some of the possible reasons for clinicians making poor decisions.

2.4 Discuss patient safety and the nurse's role as part of the healthcare team.

2.5 Discuss which type of medications are particularly likely to affect the stay of an acute patient.

2.6 Identify the role of nursing staff in the acute care admission process.

2.7 Identify some issues that may need to be addressed upon discharge after an abdominal surgery.

RESEARCH TOPIC

Investigate which complementary medications are likely to affect an acute patient's stay and how.

FURTHER READING

Australian Commission on Safety and Quality in Healthcare (ACSQHC) (2014). *Risk Management Approach*. Sydney: ACSQHC. Retrieved from https://www.safetyandquality.gov.au/wp-content/uploads/2014/04/Risk-management-approach.pdf.

—— (2017). *Health Literacy: Taking Action to Improve Safety and Quality* (2nd ed.). Sydney: ACSQHC.

Bucknall, T.K., Forbes, H., Phillips, N.M., Hewitt, N.A., Cooper, S., Bogossian, F. & FIRST2ACT Investigators (2016). An analysis of nursing students' decision-making in teams during simulations of acute patient deterioration. *Journal of Advanced Nursing*, 72(10), 2482–94.

Department of Health and Human Services (2013). *A Guide to Completing Incident Reports*. Melbourne: Department of Health and Human Services. Retrieved from https://www2.health.vic.gov.au/about/publications/researchandreports/A-guide-to-completing-incident-reports.

New, P.W., McDougall, K. & Scroggie, C. (2016). Improving discharge planning communication between hospitals and patients. *Internal Medicine Journal*, 46(1), 57–62.

REFERENCES

Alfandre, D. & Schumann, J.H. (2013). What is wrong with discharges against medical advice (and how to fix them). *The Journal of the American Medical Association*, 310(22), 2393–4.

Anderson, J., Deravin-Malone, L. & Anderson, K. (2016). Implementing the micro level of the ICCCF. In J. Anderson & L. Deravin-Malone (eds), *Chronic Care Nursing: A Framework for Practice*. Melbourne: Cambridge University Press, pp. 49–63.

Anderson, J. & Malone, L. (2014). Suitability of the multi-purpose service model for rural and remote communities of Australia. *Asia Pacific Journal of Health Management*, 9(3), 14.

Aspinal, F., Gridley, K., Bernard, S. & Parker, G. (2012). Promoting continuity of care for people with long-term neurological conditions: The role of the neurology nurse specialist. *Journal of Advanced Nursing*, 68(10), 2309–19.

Australian Commission on Safety and Quality in Health Care (2011). *National Safety and Quality Health Service Standards*. Sydney: ACSQHC.

—— (2012). *Australian Safety and Quality Goals for Health Care*. Sydney: ACSQHC.

—— (2014a). *Health Literacy: Taking Action to Improve Safety and Quality*. Sydney: ACSQHC.

—— (2014b). *Risk Management Approach*. Sydney: ACSQHC. Retrieved from https://www.safetyandquality.gov.au/wp-content/uploads/2014/04/Risk-management-approach.pdf.

Bowman, E.H., Flood, K.L. & Arbaje, A.I. (2014). Models of care to transition from hospital to home. In M.L. Malone, E.A. Capezuti & R.M. Palmer (eds), *Acute Care for Elders*. New York: Springer, pp. 175–202.

Bucknall, T.K., Forbes, H., Phillips, N.M., Hewitt, N.A., Cooper, S., Bogossian, F. & FIRST2ACT Investigators (2016a). An analysis of nursing students' decision-making in teams during simulations of acute patient deterioration. *Journal of Advanced Nursing*, 72(10), 2482–94.

Bucknall, T.K., Hutchinson, A.M., Botti, M., McTier, L., Rawson, H., Hewitt, N.A., … Chaboyer, W. (2016b). Engaging patients and families in communication across transitions of care: An integrative review protocol. *Journal of Advanced Nursing*, 72(7), 1689–700.

Children's Hospital at Westmead (2016). Admitting a patient to the ward: Nurses' role in orientating families/carers – procedure. Retrieved from http://www.schn.health.nsw.gov.au/policies/pdf/2006-8008.pdf.

Clinical Excellence Commission (2018). Between the flags track and trigger observation charts. Retrieved from http://www.cec.health.nsw.gov.au/patient-safety-programs/adult-patient-safety/between-the-flags/standard-calling-criteria.

College & Association of Registered Nurses of Alberta (CARNA) (2008). *Annual Report 2007/08*. Alberta: CARNA. Retrieved from http://www.nurses.ab.ca/content/dam/carna/pdfs/Annual%20Reports/annualreport2007-2008.pdf.

Department of Health (2005). National core set of sentinel events. Appendix 8 in *National Safety Priorities in Mental Health: A National Plan for Reducing Harm*. Retrieved from http://www.health.gov.au/internet/publications/publishing.nsf/Content/mental-pubs-n-safety-toc.

Department of Health and Human Services (2013). *A Guide to Completing Incident Reports*. Melbourne: Department of Health and Human Services. Retrieved from https://www2.health.vic.gov.au/about/publications/researchandreports/A-guide-to-completing-incident-reports.

Ehsani, J.P., Jackson, T. & Duckett, S.J. (2006). The incidence and cost of adverse events in Victorian hospitals 2003–04. *Medical Journal of Australia*, 184(11), 551.

Emanuel, L., Berwick, D., Conway, J., Combes, J., Hatlie, M., Leape, L., … Walton, M. (2008). What exactly is patient safety? In K. Henriksen, J. Battles, M. Keyes & M. Grady (eds), *Advances in Patient Safety: New Directions and Alternative Approaches (Vol. 1: Assessment)*. Rockville: Agency for Healthcare Research and Quality.

Flin, R., Winter, J. & Cakil Sarac, M.R. (2009). Human factors in patient safety: Review of topics and tools. *World Health*, 2.

Haggerty, J.L., Reid, R.J., Freeman, G.K., Starfield, B.H., Adair, C.E. & McKendry, R. (2003). Continuity of care: A multidisciplinary review. *British Medical Journal*, 327(7425), 1219–21.

Haley, C. (2014). Community practice and continuity of care. In J. Dempsey, S. Hillege, J. French & V. Wilson (eds), *Fundamentals of Nursing and Midwifery: A Person-centred Approach to Care*. Sydney: Lippincott Williams & Wilkins, pp. 76–93.

Handy, C. (2016). The admission and discharge nurse role: A quality initiative to optimize unit utilization, patient satisfaction, and nurse perceptions of collaboration. Virginia Henderson Global Nursing e-Repository. Retrieved from http://www.nursinglibrary .org/vhl/handle/10755/613233.

Health.Vic (2018). *Falls Risk Assessment Tool (FRAT)*. Retrieved from https://www2.health .vic.gov.au/about/publications/policiesandguidelines/falls-risk-assessment-tool.

Hirschman, K.B., Shaid, E., McCauley, K., Pauly, M.V. & Naylor, M.D. (2015). Continuity of care: The transitional care model. *Online Journal of Issues in Nursing*, 20(3), Article 1. Retrieved from http://www.nursingworld.org/MainMenuCategories/ ANAMarketplace/ANAPeriodicals/OJIN/TableofContents/Vol-20-2015/No3-Sept-2015/Continuity-of-Care-Transitional-Care-Model.html.

Hoch, C. & Hamlin, L. (2015). Nursing management: Postoperative care. In D. Brown, H. Edwards, L. Seaton & T. Buckley (eds), *Lewis's Medical-surgical Nursing: Assessment and Management of Clinical Problems* (4th ed.). Sydney: Elsevier, pp. 330–54.

Kohn, L.T., Corrigan, J.M. & Donaldson, M.S. (2000). *To Err is Human: Building a Safer Health System* (Vol. 627). Washington, DC: National Academy Press.

Lord Hunt of Kings Heath OBE (2002). Patient safety: A major government priority. In S. Emslie, K. Knox & M. Pickstone (eds), *Improving Patient Safety: Insights from American, Australian and British Healthcare*. Brussels: ECRI Europe.

Makary, M.A. & Daniel, M. (2016). Medical error: The third leading cause of death in the US. *British Medical Journal*, 353, i2139.

Malley, A., Kenner, C., Kim, T. & Blakeney, B. (2015). The role of the nurse and the preoperative assessment in patient transitions. *AORN Journal*, 102, 181.e1–181.e9.

Marquis, B.L. & Houston, C.J. (2012). *Leadership Roles and Management Functions in Nursing* (7th ed.). Philadelphia, PA: Lippincott Williams and Wilkins.

Merriam-Webster.com. (2016). Decision. Retrieved from http://www.merriam-webster .com/dictionary/decision.

Mitchell, M. (2015). Home recovery following day surgery: A patient perspective. *Journal of Clinical Nursing*, 24(3–4), 415–27.

New, P.W., McDougall, K. & Scroggie, C. (2016). Improving discharge planning communication between hospitals and patients. *Internal Medicine Journal*, 46(1), 57–62.

Nursing Council of New Zealand (NCNZ) ([2007] 2016). *Competencies for Registered Nurses*. Retrieved from http://www.nursingcouncil.org.nz/Nurses.

Nursing and Midwifery Board of Australia (NMBA) (2016). *Registered Nurse Standards for Practice*. Melbourne: Nursing & Midwifery Board of Australia. Retrieved from http://www.nursingmidwiferyboard.gov.au/Codes-Guidelines-Statements/ Professional-standards.aspx.

Palmer, R.M. & Kresevic, D.M. (2014). The acute care for elders unit. In M.L. Malone, E.A. Capezuti & R.M. Palmer (eds), *Acute Care for Elders*. New York: Springer, pp. 69–97.

Paul, S. & Hice, A. (2014). Role of the acute care nurse in managing patients with heart failure using evidence-based care. *Critical Care Nursing Quarterly*, 37(4), 357–76.

Pierluissi, E., Francis, D.C. & Covinsky, K.E. (2014). Patient and hospital factors that lead to adverse outcomes in hospitalized elders. In M.L. Malone, E.A. Capezuti & R.M. Palmer (eds), *Acute Care for Elders*. New York: Springer, pp. 21–48.

Queensland Health (2018), Malnutrition screening tools. Retrieved from https://www .health.qld.gov.au/__data/assets/pdf_file/0029/148826/hphe_mst_pstr.pdf.

Reason, J. (1995). Understanding adverse events: Human factors. *Quality in Health Care*, 4(2), 80–9.

—— (2000). Human error: Models and management. *British Medical Journal*, 320(7237), 768–70.

Roughead, L., Semple, S. & Rosenfeld, E. (2013). *Literature Review: Medication Safety in Australia*. Sydney: Australian Commission on Safety and Quality in Health Care.

Royal Children's Hospital Melbourne (RCHM) (2014). Nursing Assessment: Clinical Guidelines (Nursing). Retrieved from http://www.rch.org.au/rchcpg/hospital_clinical_ guideline_index/Nursing_assessment.

Russell-Jones, N. (2015). *Decision-Making Pocketbook*. Alresford: Management Pocketbooks.

SA Health (2018). Braden pressure risk assessment tool. Retrieved from https://www .sahealth.sa.gov.au/wps/wcm/connect/b24a8480438d09be9e63dfbc736a4e18/ 2010maybradenrisktool.pdf?MOD=AJPERES&CACHEID=b24a8480438d09be 9e63dfbc736a4e18.

Scruth, E.A. (2014). Quality nursing documentation in the medical record. *Clinical Nurse Specialist*, 28(6), 312–14.

Sefcik, J.S., Nock, R.H., Flores, E.J., Chase, J.A.D., Bradway, C., Potashnik, S. & Bowles, K.H. (2016). Patient preferences for information on post-acute care services. *Research in Gerontological Nursing*, 9(4), 175–82.

Shojania, K.G. & Dixon-Woods, M. (2016). Estimating deaths due to medical error: The ongoing controversy and why it matters. *British Medical Journal of Quality & Safety*, 26, 423–8.

Sinha, S.K., Oakes, S.L., Chaudhry, S. & Suh, T.T. (2014). How to use the ACE unit to improve hospital safety and quality for older patients: from ACE units to elder-friendly hospitals. In M.L. Malone, E.A. Capezuti & R.M. Palmer (eds), *Acute Care for Elders*. New York: Springer, pp. 131–56.

Swallow, V., Smith, J. & Smith, T. (2017). Clinical decision making. In D. Stanley (ed.), *Clinical Leadership in Nursing and Healthcare: Values into Action* (2nd ed.). Chichester: Wiley Blackwell.

Walton, M. (2011). *Patient Safety Curriculum Guide: Multi-professional Edition*. Geneva: World Health Organization.

3

The acute surgical patient

Elisabeth Coyne, Judith Anderson
and Maryanne Podham

LEARNING OBJECTIVES

At the completion of this chapter, you should be able to:

1   define an acute surgical condition and describe the phases of the acute surgical event
2   explore the nursing considerations involved in the management of paediatric, bariatric and elderly patients during the acute surgical event
3   discuss the nurse's role in the delivery of patient-centred and culturally competent care
4   discuss the nurse's role in multidisciplinary collaboration when caring for a surgical patient
5   discuss the nurse's role in the assessment and management of pain, wound care, patient education and discharge planning during the acute surgical event.

Introduction

An acute surgical event is unplanned, can be classified as either major or minor, can require invasive or non-invasive procedures and can involve any part of the body. Also known as an emergency surgery, acute surgery is the focus of this chapter. It can be defined as a procedure that is required to be attended to within 48 hours to:

- remove or repair a body part
- restore or preserve health
- restore function
- prevent further tissue damage
- preserve life.

The degree of urgency is also related to the person's age and general health, including comorbidities, fluid and nutritional state, medications used and mental health status.

The pathway of a patient during an acute surgical event has a similar trajectory to planned or elective surgery; however, the patient experience can be very different (Dillstrom et al., 2017; Schultz et al., 2013). It is therefore imperative that nurses involved in the coordination of the acute surgical patient's journey from the emergency department, through the pre-, intra- and post-operative phases and during rehabilitation act as the **patient advocate** in ensuring that holistic care is provided to the patient and their family as they move through the various phases of peri-operative care (Arzouman, 2016).

> **Patient advocate** – Where the nurse assists the patient to negotiate the health system, particularly by providing plain English explanations to the patient and their family.

The chapter will discuss the nursing considerations for caring for common acute surgical conditions in Australia and New Zealand. The nursing considerations and management of paediatric and bariatric conditions, and care of the elderly patient during the acute surgical event will be presented, together with a discussion of the nurse's role in coordinating multidisciplinary, culturally sensitive and patient-centred care for patients during acute surgical presentations, and in the assessment and management of pain, wound care, patient education and discharge planning during the acute surgical event.

The following identifies the national competency standards for the registered nurse from the Nursing and Midwifery Board of Australia (NMBA) and the Nursing Council of New Zealand (NCNZ) that are addressed in this chapter.

Australian Registered Nurse Standards for Practice

Standard 1: Thinks critically and analyses nursing practice

Standard 2: Engages in therapeutic and professional relationships

Standard 4: Comprehensively conducts assessments

Standard 5: Develops a plan for nursing practice

Standard 6: Provides safe, appropriate and responsive quality nursing practice

Standard 7: Evaluates outcomes to inform nursing practice

(NMBA, 2016)

New Zealand: Competencies for Registered Nurses

Competency 1.1: Accepts responsibility for ensuring that his/her nursing practice and conduct meet the standards of the professional, ethical and relevant legislated requirements

NURSING STANDARDS

Competency 1.2: Demonstrates the ability to apply the principles of the Treaty of Waitangi/ Te Tiriti o Waitangi to nursing practice

Competency 1.5: Practises nursing in a manner that the health consumer determines as being culturally safe

Competency 4.1: Collaborates and participates with colleagues and members of the health care team to facilitate and coordinate care

Competency 4.2: Recognises and values the roles and skills of all members of the health care team in the delivery of care

(NCNZ, [2007] 2016)

The acute surgical event

When the decision has been made that a patient requires an acute surgical intervention (also known as emergency surgery), it is done so to preserve the patient's life, body function or body part. As with elective or urgent surgery, a number of phases occur to ensure that the patient remains safe and everyone involved in the procedure is aware of the patient's needs. The peri-operative acute surgical event consists of the following phases: preoperative preparation; intraoperative considerations; post-anaesthesia care; and post-operative care considerations.

The peri-operative phase

Peri-operative phases – Include pre-operative assessment and documentation, intra-operative procedures, transfer to the post anaesthesia care unit (PACU), and assessment, management and education that occurs during the post-operative phase in the ward to achieve discharge (Zimmerman, 2010).

Table 3.1 provides a summary of patient assessments that may occur during the **peri-operative phase**. These activities are always dependent on the time available, and can be continued in the post-operative care phase.

The patient should be prepared for transfer to theatre; this information is most often collected on a facility pre-operative checklist. This checklist includes information regarding the following aspects:

- *Patient identification, including date of birth and the patient's full name.* These details should be verified as correct with the patient to avoid legal repercussions. The patient should also have an arm band and/or leg band attached with this information (as per facility policy).
- *Fasting.* In adults, it is recommended that solid food be withheld for a minimum of six hours pre-operatively, while clear fluids can be consumed up to two hours before the operative procedure. In the event that the patient requires a life-preserving procedure and the exact time food or drink was consumed is unknown, the anaesthetist will treat the patient as having a full stomach and will put in place interventions to manage this, including the use of a nasogastric tube to decompress the stomach to avoid regurgitation of the stomach contents into the lungs (Hamlin et al., 2016).
- *Consent.* Ask the patient or guardian about their understanding of the procedure and confirm the patient/guardian's signature on the consent form. This maintains legal and ethical aspects of consent. It is the doctor's responsibility to discuss the procedure, including the types of anaesthetic being used.

Table 3.1   Nursing considerations during pre-operative phase

Assessment	Considerations
Medical information	Baseline observations, comorbidities, medications used, nutritional status
Social and emotional wellbeing	Understanding of procedure, possible fears related to the procedure, education about what happens at various phases during the procedure
	Social supports available to the patient, including eligibility for access to assistance resources
Functional capacity	Ability to care for oneself to maintain basic and instrumental activities of daily living
Pre-operative education	Deep breathing and coughing, deep vein thrombosis (DVT) prophylaxis, wound splinting and pain management. Includes rationales to support and encourage the patient to comply with these instructions.
Discharge planning	Consideration of home environment safety, need for rehabilitation and interventions from allied health teams

Source: Adapted from Tollefson and Hillman (2016).

- *Physical assessments.* These include vital signs, weight, height and results of laboratory tests and required investigations, including x-rays, ECG, BGL and U/A.
- *Allergies to drugs, foods, and other substances.* These need to be recorded clearly and accurately. Depending on facility policy, this information may be recorded on arm bands or leg bands.
- *Prosthetics.* All prosthetics, including false teeth, hearing aids, glasses and artificial limbs must be removed, or sent with the patient, depending on facility policy.
- *Specific procedures.* Procedures that may be ordered and recorded on this chart include commencing intravenous therapy (IVT), application of anti-emboli stockings on the patient's legs and, in some instances, administration of medications including pre-operative sedation.
- *Escorting the patient to the receiving area of the theatre.* Here the ward nurse hands over the patient to the anaesthetic nurse, who verifies the patient's identity and consent, and reviews the pre-operative checklist to ensure it is complete. The patient then transitions into the intra-operative phase of the acute surgical event.

(Hoch & Hamlin, 2015; Tollefson & Hillman, 2016)

Intra-operative considerations

During this phase of the acute surgical event, the patient is the shared responsibility of several people, including doctors, nurses and the anaesthetist. The nurse's responsibilities during this time include patient safety during the procedure, accountability for instruments and medications used during the procedure and the transfer of the patient to the post-anaesthesia care unit (PACU) (Farrell, 2017; Hoch & Hamlin, 2015). The care of the patient during this phase is guided by the **surgical safety checklist** (Figure 3.1).

Surgical safety checklist – Used to ensure patient safety during the intra-operative phases throughout the surgical procedure (Hacquard et al., 2013; WHO, 2015).

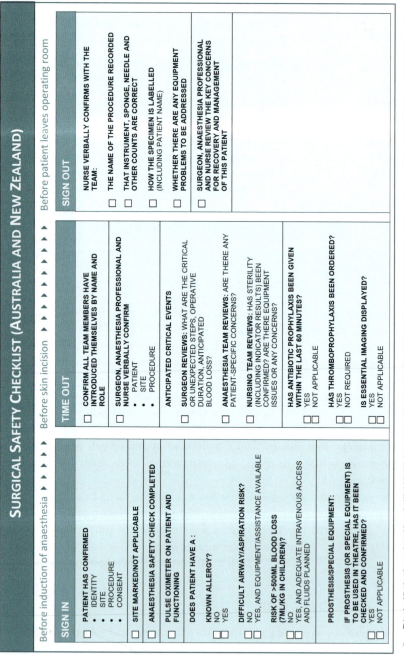

SURGICAL SAFETY CHECKLIST (AUSTRALIA AND NEW ZEALAND)

Before induction of anaesthesia ▶ ▶ ▶ ▶ | Before skin incision ▶ ▶ ▶ ▶ ▶ ▶ ▶ ▶ ▶ | Before patient leaves operating room

SIGN IN

☐ PATIENT HAS CONFIRMED
 • IDENTITY
 • SITE
 • PROCEDURE
 • CONSENT

☐ SITE MARKED/NOT APPLICABLE

☐ ANAESTHESIA SAFETY CHECK COMPLETED

☐ PULSE OXIMETER ON PATIENT AND FUNCTIONING

DOES PATIENT HAVE A :

KNOWN ALLERGY?
☐ NO
☐ YES

DIFFICULT AIRWAY/ASPIRATION RISK?
☐ NO
☐ YES, AND EQUIPMENT/ASSISTANCE AVAILABLE

RISK OF >500ML BLOOD LOSS (7ML/KG IN CHILDREN)?
☐ NO
☐ YES, AND ADEQUATE INTRAVENOUS ACCESS AND FLUIDS PLANNED

PROSTHESIS/SPECIAL EQUIPMENT:

IF PROSTHESIS (OR SPECIAL EQUIPMENT) IS TO BE USED IN THEATRE, HAS IT BEEN CHECKED AND CONFIRMED?
☐ YES
☐ NOT APPLICABLE

TIME OUT

☐ CONFIRM ALL TEAM MEMBERS HAVE INTRODUCED THEMSELVES BY NAME AND ROLE

☐ SURGEON, ANAESTHESIA PROFESSIONAL AND NURSE VERBALLY CONFIRM
 • PATIENT
 • SITE
 • PROCEDURE

☐ ANTICIPATED CRITICAL EVENTS

☐ SURGEON REVIEWS: WHAT ARE THE CRITICAL OR UNEXPECTED STEPS, OPERATIVE DURATION, ANTICIPATED BLOOD LOSS?

☐ ANAESTHESIA TEAM REVIEWS: ARE THERE ANY PATIENT-SPECIFIC CONCERNS?

☐ NURSING TEAM REVIEWS: HAS STERILITY (INCLUDING INDICATOR RESULTS) BEEN CONFIRMED? ARE THERE EQUIPMENT ISSUES OR ANY CONCERNS?

HAS ANTIBIOTIC PROPHYLAXIS BEEN GIVEN WITHIN THE LAST 60 MINUTES?
☐ YES
☐ NOT APPLICABLE

HAS THROMBOPROPHYLAXIS BEEN ORDERED?
☐ YES
☐ NOT REQUIRED

IS ESSENTIAL IMAGING DISPLAYED?
☐ YES
☐ NOT APPLICABLE

SIGN OUT

☐ NURSE VERBALLY CONFIRMS WITH THE TEAM:

☐ THE NAME OF THE PROCEDURE RECORDED

☐ THAT INSTRUMENT, SPONGE, NEEDLE AND OTHER COUNTS ARE CORRECT

☐ HOW THE SPECIMEN IS LABELLED (INCLUDING PATIENT NAME)

☐ WHETHER THERE ARE ANY EQUIPMENT PROBLEMS TO BE ADDRESSED

☐ SURGEON, ANAESTHESIA PROFESSIONAL AND NURSE REVIEW THE KEY CONCERNS FOR RECOVERY AND MANAGEMENT OF THIS PATIENT

This checklist has been adapted from the World Health Organization Surgical Safety Checklist by the Royal Australasian College of Surgeons in consultation with the Australian and New Zealand College of Anaesthetists, the Royal Australian and New Zealand College of Ophthalmologists, the Royal Australian and New Zealand College of Obstetricians and Gynaecologists, the Australian College of Operating Room Nurses and the Perioperative Nurses College of the New Zealand Nurses Organisation; it is not intended to be comprehensive, additions and modifications to fit local practice are encouraged (Oct 09)

Figure 3.1 Surgical safety checklist (Australia and New Zealand)

Source: Tang, Ranmuthugala and Cunningham (2013, p. 149).

Post-anaesthesia care

During this phase, the patient's condition is monitored to ensure optimal patient outcomes. This includes preventing complications, which may prolong the patient's time away from the ward area ('Pre- and post-operative care', 2017). The nurse in this area will receive handover from the anaesthetist involved in the procedure and the peri-operative nurse. This handover includes the procedure, the patient's condition throughout the procedure and the post-operative care orders. The PACU nurse is responsible for ensuring that the patient meets discharge criteria that will allow the patient to be transferred back to the ward. (In some instances, the acute surgical patient may require a continued unconscious state due to the extent of injury or procedure. In this instance, the patient may be transferred to the intensive care unit (ICU), where care will continue until the patient's condition improves).

The discharge criteria from the PACU include:

- a conscious patient who can obey commands, and has a patent airway
- vital observations that fall within pre-operative baseline recordings (or a management plan documented)
- a patient who is pain and nausea free, with appropriate ward-based treatments ordered
- the patient being in a comfortable position in a clean, dry bed
- the documentation of observations and post-operative orders
- drains, IV therapy, indwelling catheters and other attachments appropriately anchored to the patient and patent
- wounds covered with an appropriate dressing and any ooze marked, timed and dated
- all nursing documentation contemporaneous and complete.

When the patient is deemed to be ready for transfer to the ward, the ward nurse is notified and the patient is handed over by the PACU nurse to the ward nurse in the receiving bay of the operating theatre. The patient is then escorted by the nurse back to the ward and the post-operative care phase begins (Farrell, 2017; Hoch & Hamlin, 2015).

Post-operative care phase

On the patient's return to the ward, a thorough assessment is completed, including patient position, **level of consciousness (LOC)** and orientation to the ward, vital observations including blood pressure, respiration rate, pulse, temperature and oxygen saturations and comparison to both pre-operative baseline and the last set collected in the PACU.

Pain and nausea levels are assessed and treated as required; an assessment of the condition of wounds, patency and anchoring or tubes, and neurological and circulatory systems is also completed. Effects of anaesthesia – particularly regional or local – are also assessed.

Post-operative orders including parenteral and non-parenteral medication, dietary requirements, ambulation restrictions and specific instruction related to the procedure are attended to, and the patient is re/educated on deep breathing exercises and DVT prophylaxis.

The frequency of these observations varies between facilities and the nurse is best advised to check the policy of each facility.

Personal hygiene should be attended to, usually four hours after the patient has returned to the ward. The patient should be offered a bed bath, clean gown or comfortable clothes, and have soiled bed linen changed. Mouth care such as teeth brushing or rinsing with mouth wash is also recommended at this time.

Contemporaneous documentation is attended to during this phase, and should include the condition of the patient on return to the ward, any interventions conducted, including

Level of consciousness (LOC) – A measurement of a person's arousability and responsiveness to stimuli from the environment.

pain and nausea management, and evaluation of the effectiveness of these interventions. Post–operative orders should also be discussed (Tollefson & Hillman, 2016; Wagner & Hardin-Pierce, 2015)

REFLECTIVE QUESTION

When receiving a patient into recovery from the operating theatre, what are the key points for consideration?

SKILLS IN PRACTICE

The nurse's role in preparing the acute surgical patient for theatre

Sally is a 32-year-old female who has presented to the emergency department with a 24-hour history of nausea, vomiting, anorexia and severe right lower quadrant abdominal pain with radiation over her periumbilical area. Sally has come in with her husband, John. Sally's mother is minding their three-year-old daughter. Sally states that she has had similar pain over the last two weeks but not as bad as it is now. Following assessment and investigation, Sally has been diagnosed as having acute appendicitis and is scheduled for theatre this afternoon.

The doctor has discussed the operation with Sally and John, and collected her written informed consent. It is the nurse's role to prepare Sally for theatre, which includes the following considerations:

- The patient is aware of the need for nil by mouth (NBM) until otherwise advised by a medical professional.
- Patient hygiene is attended to as condition allows, including removal of jewellery and personal items. The patient is dressed in a surgical gown and instructed to remain on bed rest until transfer to theatre.
- The patient has patent intravenous access and has had medications (including intravenous fluids) as directed.
- All pre-operative baseline assessments have been completed and results recorded in the patient's file. Vital observations have been done, including blood glucose level (BGL), electrocardiography (ECG), height, weight and urinalysis. Pre-operative teaching should also be attended (as appropriate) with regard to what the patient should expect after theatre, including information about deep breathing and coughing exercises, and venous thromboembolism-prevention strategies.

QUESTIONS

- Why is it important to ensure the patient remain nil by mouth and on bed rest until theatre?
- Discuss why it is important to collect baseline assessments from a patient prior to transfer to theatre.

The paediatric, elderly and bariatric patient

Paediatric patients are not merely small adults. Ideally, paediatric patients should be cared for in specialist areas with specialist staff. Such areas would have appropriately designed environments that are child friendly. Consent to attend to the surgery usually comes from parents or next of kin (Carter, 2013). Paediatric patients have a higher potential for fluid loss than adults, so fasting times should be clarified if the acute surgical procedure does not take place immediately and maintenance fluids are provided (Williams et al., 2014). There may be less discomfort for the child if the fluid is warmed (Hausfeld et al., 2015). Often a faces pain scale is used to assess the pain of the paediatric patient. These have been demonstrated to have an acceptable level of validity and reliability for this population, and assessment should be undertaken regularly (some policies recommend this should be hourly for the first 24 hours post-surgery and then every two hours) and be well documented in the patient's notes. Assessment of pain relief should always be undertaken and consistently documented (Twycross, Finley & Latimer, 2013).

Advanced age is associated with poorer surgical outcomes; however, populations are ageing worldwide, so this group is likely to increase in number. One reason for the poorer surgical outcomes is that older people are more likely to have comorbidities, which have negative outcomes for their ability to recover (White, Duncan & Baumle, 2013). Cognitive and functional decline are more common in older people, reducing their ability to recover from acute surgery (Gazala et al., 2013). Nurses need to be aware of these declines, and ensure that they are prevented as much as possible or that negative results are prevented. Nursing considerations for cognitive decline can include measures such as including carers in discharge planning, supporting verbal education with written material and greater involvement of interdisciplinary team members. Nursing considerations for functional decline can include monitoring vital signs, early ambulation, anti-thrombolitic stockings and encouraging coughing and deep breathing (White, Duncan & Baumle, 2013). Older people are more susceptible to delirium, which can be caused by surgery. Delirium is complex and multi-factorial, so is difficult to treat. There are several tools to assist with the assessment of delirium; the confusion assessment method is one that is evidence based and well regarded. While a patient is delirious, it is important to ensure their safety, in particular to watch them closely to ensure that they do not fall or disrupt their recovery in other ways (e.g. removing dressings or IVs) (Phillips, 2013). Older patients are at risk of poor diet and fluid intake, so assessment is important. The nurse should also provide information on a healthy diet and adequate fluid intake to both the patient and carer (Shippee-Rice, Fetzer & Long, 2012). Elderly people are also more prone to vitamin deficiencies. It has been demonstrated that people with low levels of vitamin C, vitamin A or zinc have reduced wound healing, so ensuring a well-balanced diet is essential and the addition of multivitamins can be beneficial for some people (Thomas, 2013).

Obesity is an increasing issue in Australia and New Zealand. Obesity increases the chance of a person having comorbid conditions, which in turn increases the complexity of providing care for them. In acute surgical patients, obesity creates issues around **airway management**, nutritional support, medication doses, procedures and general nursing care. The obese surgical patient requires close assessment with the appropriate-sized equipment. In particular, cardiac and respiratory monitoring is required to due to the increased cardiac and respiratory workload created by obesity and the prevalence of renal issues in bariatric clients (Collins, 2014). Obstructive sleep apnoea is also more common in obese

Airway management – The assessment and maintenance of patency to ensure adequate oxygenation and gaseous exchange between the patient's lungs and the atmosphere.

clients, requiring the nurse to observe the patient (particularly oxygen saturation levels) more closely at night (Cooney, 2016). A nutritional assessment will usually be required by a dietician due to abnormal responses in obese patients, such as higher glucose and cortisol responses to stress and higher normal resting energy expenditure. Mobilisation and positioning create complications, with appropriate furniture not always being available. Skin breakdown and impaired wound healing are also issues about which nurses need to be aware (Collins, 2014).

Australia and New Zealand have significant rural and remote populations. These have vulnerable populations of their own, and distance from definitive care is a big factor in acute surgical conditions. Major trauma in particular has worse outcomes if treatment is delayed (Broman et al., 2016) and there are also issues with the transport of vulnerable populations, such as paediatric patients (who should receive specialist care). Monitoring of patients being transferred is often a specialist responsibility and should include vital signs at a minimum, with the patient being deemed stable before leaving the referral facility (Blakeman & Branson, 2013).

REFLECTIVE QUESTION

Consider your role in assessment of the older patient in the surgical ward. What specific aspects do you need to consider?

The nurse's role in coordinating culturally sensitive and patient-centred care

Cultural sensitivity – To be aware of cultural differences that exist and to not assign a value to them, but rather appreciate the difference.

Patient and family-centred care (PFCC) – 'An approach to the planning, delivery, and evaluation of health care that is grounded in mutually beneficial partnerships among healthcare providers, patients, and families' (IFNA, 2015).

As our society is becoming increasingly culturally diverse, is it important for the nurse to ensure they provide **cultural sensitivity** and patient-centred care. For the nurse to achieve this, they must be aware of their own personal experience and values, as this will influence the way they provide care. The nurse should also acknowledge the importance of family and provide care that is patient focused but also family inclusive. Patient–centred care focuses on the patient in a holistic manner so as to include the family and any cultural considerations. **Patient and family–centred care (PFCC)** is empirically based, and promotes respect and patient autonomy. It is responsive to individual patient preferences, needs and values. PFCC should provide the patient and family with information on which to base decisions and support them with their health adversity from the stages of in-patient to discharge. The provision of PFCC, which is truly supportive of the family, will improve patient outcomes by improving medication compliance and reducing unplanned admissions (van der Meer et al., 2016).

The nurse is the key point of contact for the patient, and is often the first member of the healthcare team to identify patient and family concerns that will influence the patient's condition. The family is defined by the patient, and it is an important consideration to ensure the nurse is talking with the appropriate family member(s) when providing information (Wright & Leahey, 2013). The identification of family members is also strongly related to the cultural composition of the family, as different cultures will define family in very different terms (Shaw, Zou & Butow, 2015).

Understanding and respecting the patient's autonomy is important, as each individual will have different expectations and a different understanding of the information provided.

Even though the patient may be well informed, their preferences may be influenced by personal health beliefs. Remember that you, as the nurse, will also bring your values and beliefs to any patient and family interaction, and how you present information and choices will influence the patient. Nurses subtly influence patients' preferences by framing outcomes in positive (survival) vs. negative (mortality) ways, or by presenting a favoured option first, making it seem like the middle of the road, highlighting its benefits and even using a different tone of voice.

The surgical patient will be cared for by a range of nurses across their surgical trajectory. This highlights the need for nurses to include a patient and family assessment as part of their routine care (Tobiano, Chaboyer & McMurray, 2013). The patient and family assessment provides an opportunity to understand the patient's cultural needs and also an understanding of other needs in relation to this hospital admission. The inclusion of family in this assessment allows for an awareness of the family's functioning and how family members will be able to support the patient at home after discharge (Bail & Grealish, 2016; Wrobleski et al., 2014). The nurse should clarify the patient's and family's understanding of medications and rehabilitation to ensure the patient and family have the ability to care for these aspects at home.

Communication of patient and family assessment and preferences is important with the surgical patient, as failure to communicate clearly when completing transfer information may lead to adverse events for the patient (Tobiano, Chaboyer & McMurray, 2013). Clear communication and transfer of information between nurses and the patient and their family also increases the patient's confidence in the nursing staff. **Clinical handover** at the bedside has been noted as important for the patient and family, as they feel included and this promotes the concept of patient-centred care (McMurray et al., 2011). It is important to gain the consent from the patient prior to handover, and to ensure the patient understands the concept of bedside handover (Anderson et al., 2015). Family members value the chance to participate, and this can ultimately improve the accuracy of handover communication. The type of information shared during bedside handover needs to be considered to ensure no sensitive information is shared in an open environment (Tobiano, Chaboyer & McMurray, 2013).

Clinical handover – The transfer of responsibility and accountability for patient care from one provider or team of providers to another (Chaboyer et al., 2008; Tobiano, Chaboyer & McMurray, 2013).

The nurse has a pivotal role to play in coordinating culturally appropriate and patient-centred care. Ensuring respect, collaboration and information-sharing is integral to providing care. This process has several steps, including assessing and acknowledging the patient and family preferences (Coyne et al., 2017; Mitchell et al., 2009). The Australian Commission on Safety and Quality in Health Care (ACSQHC) identifies the importance of partnering with patients and their families within nine of the ten National Safety and Quality Health Service (NSQHS) standards that drive the implementation of safety and quality systems (ACSQHC, 2011). It is therefore important to care for both the patient and their family, as families are an integral part of the life and wellbeing of patients – particularly during surgical intervention.

REFLECTIVE QUESTIONS

- When providing care to a surgical patient and their family, how can you be sure they have understood the information?
- What are important aspects of surgical care that may need to be repeated at different times during the patient's hospital stay?

The nurse's role in multidisciplinary collaboration when caring for a surgical patient

Interdisciplinary team members' involvement in the peri-operative period begins when it is identified that the patient requires peri-operative intervention. This collaboration involves the collection, analysis, planning and communication of information in order to promote optimal patient care and recovery. These teams support shared decision-making between the patient, their family or caregivers and those involved in the delivery of treatment options that are safe, appropriate, effective and efficient (Deek et al., 2016) (Figure 3.2).

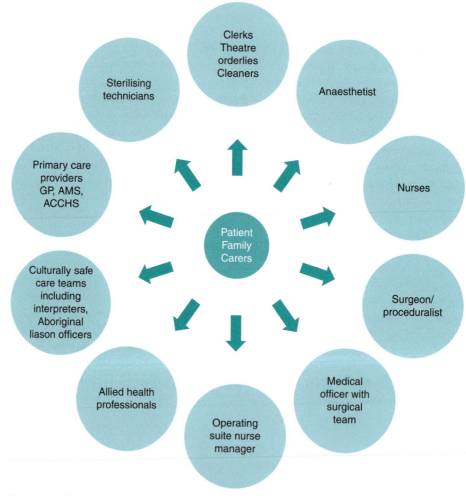

Interdisciplinary team – The integration of knowledge and methods from different disciplines, using a synthesis of approaches to provide the best evidence-based care for the client.

Figure 3.2   The peri-operative multidisciplinary team

Unlike the patient undergoing elective surgery, the acute surgical patient does not always receive an adequate pre-operative workup – hence the liaising between **interdisciplinary team** members often falls to the nurse manager.

The patient and their family/caregivers are usually anxious and extremely vulnerable during the acute surgical event, so it is vital that all team members, regardless of the specialty, work together to ensure that the safety and wellbeing of these people is a priority.

The pre-operative management of the patient involves a number of administrative procedures, which may be done by either a clerk or a nurse; these roles include liaising with the operating theatre staff to ensure the availability of medical and nursing staff to conduct the surgery as well as the equipment available. Post-operative bed availability also needs to be arranged, along with the nursing staff who will care for the patient. Following surgery, a number of other multidisciplinary team members may be required to deliver specialty care to the patient, including but not limited to radiographers, social workers, Aboriginal liaison officers, physiotherapists and speech pathologists.

Patient-centred multidisciplinary ward rounds have been introduced into many Australian hospitals since 2008. These rounds involve a number of **multidisciplinary team** members engaging with the patient and their family at the same time. Overall, the effectiveness of these rounds has improved patient outcomes through improved communication between hospital-based clinicians and available resources in the community. There is also more opportunity for the patient and their family to identify and discuss issues prior to discharge, leading to increased patient satisfaction and positive outcomes.

> **Multidisciplinary team –** Involves a range of health professionals working together to deliver to the patient and their family comprehensive care that improves health outcomes and promotes patient compliance and satisfaction.

Assessment and management of the acute surgical patient

Post-operative assessment is completed frequently in the early post-operative period. To some extent, this will depend on the setting (e.g. how long the patient has spent in the recovery area before returning to the ward) and the patient. The frequency of post-operative assessment – particularly respiratory, neurological and pain assessment – relates directly to the patient's surgery and condition (Estes et al., 2015). Post-operative assessment is usually undertaken every 15 minutes for one hour, then every 30 minutes for one hour, then hourly for four hours, then every fourth hour – as a minimum (Estes et al., 2015). A complete health assessment should be completed on the patient in the first 24 hours, particularly if this has not been completed prior to surgery. This would provide an understanding of the overall patient condition and family assessment (Estes et al., 2015).

Pain assessment

Nurses are the key health professionals who will assess, identify and manage the patient's pain. Pain is an unpleasant sensory and emotional experience that occurs from actual or potential tissue damage (Gosselin et al., 2014). The purpose of pain is to signal tissue damage or potential damage, and protect against further damage. Pain assessment is commonly referred to as the fifth vital sign. Pain assessment involves a holistic view of the patient's pain, including physical, psychological, environmental, cultural and spiritual assessment. Good pain assessment and management lead to better patient outcomes, as the patient mobilises earlier, has fewer psychological symptoms and tends to show increased compliance with treatment (Cooney, 2016).

To assess for pain post-operatively, you need to ask the patient a range of questions, particularly regarding the location, type and duration of pain. Pain is highly subjective, so it is important to always believe what the patient says about their level of pain. Ask the patient to describe their pain, what makes the pain worse and how long they have had the pain.

PQRST – P = Provokes; Q = Quality; R = Radiates; S = Severity; T = Time.

A self-report **PQRST** is considered the gold standard and most accurate measure of pain, enabling nurses to document and evaluate pain assessment. Using this acronym is useful to provide a clear description, assessment and documentation of the patient pain. The numerical pain scale and Wong-Baker scale (Wong-Baker FACES Foundation, 2016) are useful tools for pain assessment (Figure 3.3).

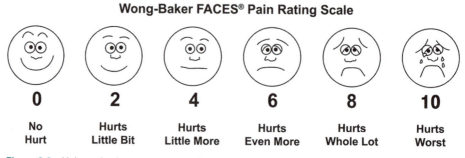

Figure 3.3   Universal pain assessment tool

Source: Wong-Baker FACES Foundation (2016). Retrieved 28 November 2017 with permission from http://www.WongBakerFACES.org. Originally published in Whaley & Wong's Nursing Care of Infants and Children. © Elsevier Inc.

Management of the patient's pain requires a multidisciplinary approach, with the nurse as the key point of assessment. Throughout the assessment phase, communication and reassurance are essential elements. Management should include physical, psychological, environmental, cultural and spiritual elements. The physical management may be pharmacological; however, pain management should include correcting other symptoms such as fatigue, nausea, cough and positioning. Aspects such as lighting, noise, fear and social or cultural aspects should also be considered. Good pain management assists future pain management by establishing a pathway for the patient to express pain and have it controlled. Barriers to effective pain management can be a concern for side-effects, patient attitude, health professional attitude and inappropriate medications.

Wound care

The post-operative wound often has an occlusive dressing, which remains intact for 24 hours to enhance healing and prevention of infection (Downie et al., 2010). Thus assessment of post-operative wounds should be of the surrounding area and dressing to identify changes, swelling, blood loss or bruising. The assessment of the wound site is completed as part of routine post-operative observations with specific assessment of surgical area for swelling, discoloration, blood loss on dressing or around the site, and pain. The extremities should also be assessed regularly to ensure blood flow around and past the site of surgery.

Phases of wound healing

- *The defensive (inflammatory) phase.* Temperature increase occurs immediately after injury, lasting three to four days; haemostasis and inflammation occurs. The patient may experience a raised temperature between 37–38°C. Vasoconstriction platelet aggregation fibrin clot formation occurs at the wound closure to prevent loss of fluids and blood, and prevent entry of micro-organisms. Inflammation is the body's defensive mechanism against tissue injury; this involves vascular and cellular responses. The vascular response includes an increase in blood flow to tissue and increased nutrients and oxygen essential for healing. This removes dead cells, debris and pathogens, and the area becomes red, oedematous and warm. Cellular response neutrophils begin phagocytosis; this is then replaced by macrophages to clean up the area and promote wound healing.

- *The reconstructive (proliferative) phase.* This begins three or four days after injury and lasts two to three weeks. This involves deposition of collagen, angiogenesis, granulation tissue and wound contraction.
- *The maturation phase.* This begins about day 21 and may continue for up to two years or more, depending on the depth and extent of the wound. It consists of scar tissue remodelling. Scar tissue is always weaker than surrounding tissues and it is not as well vascularised.

Patient education

Patient education regarding surgical treatment is intended to ensure that the patient and their family are provided with tailored education to reduce their anxiety and enhance their post-operative outcomes. In particular, pre-operative education should cover:

- what to expect of surgical procedures and routines
- the sensations they may experience
- measures to decrease side-effects of surgery, such as pain and anxiety
- activities to enhance post-operative recovery:
  - deep breathing and coughing, and use of Triflow
  - leg exercises and early mobilisation techniques
  - use of patient-controlled analgesia or pain management.

The amount of teaching depends on client's pre-operative anxiety, their levels of pain and how much they want to know. Too much information given to a client who is already overloaded with information and painful stimuli is not useful, so keep explanations simple and to the point. Including the family is an important aspect of providing nursing care that is patient- and family-centred (Coyne et al., 2017).

Discharge planning

Discharge planning is a process that should begin on admission; however, the nature of acute emergency admissions does not always allow this. Beginning as soon as possible is advisable in order to allow sufficient time to organise the services, equipment and education that may be required (Hoch & Hamlin, 2015; Palmer & Kresevic, 2014). The patient and their family are unlikely to be ready for the situation, and may need additional assistance in preparing the home environment for someone who has had unexpected surgery.

More complex patients, such as the elderly, bariatric patients or people with comorbidities, may have additional requirements with regard to care provision or equipment that is not readily available (Sinha et al., 2014). Wound assessment and pain management may be required in order to plan for care after discharge. Some of these patients may benefit from a transfer of care to community services that may be able to assist them until they are able to care for themselves (Haley, 2014). Communication with the patient and any carers they may have is essential if discharge is to be effective and if education is required to provide them with additional support in the home (New, McDougall & Scroggie, 2016).

SUMMARY

Learning objective 1: Define an acute surgical condition and describe the phases of the acute surgical event.

An acute surgical event (also known as emergency surgery) is conducted to preserve the patient's life, body function or body part. The nurse plays several roles during the peri-operative phases of the acute surgical event. During the peri-operative phase, the patient is prepared for transfer to theatre and the nurse's role is to ensure all information and assessments have been conducted and recorded to ensure the patient remains safe during this journey. Intra-operatively and in the PACU, the nurse is responsible for ensuring that the patient remains safe and regains a similar (or improved) state so as to be able to return to the ward and commence their recovery. On return to the ward, the nurse is responsible for ensuring that the patient is aware of and receives interventions and education to assist them to achieve wellness to facilitate their discharge.

Learning objective 2: Explore the nursing considerations involved in the management of paediatric, bariatric and elderly patients during the acute surgical event.

Nursing considerations should always involve holistic care. Areas where this may involve additional effort for paediatric clients include fluid and pain management; for the elderly, management of cognitive issues and wound healing; and for bariatric patients, management of airways and nutritional support.

Learning objective 3: Discuss the nurse's role in the delivery of patient-centred and culturally competent care.

The nurse has a key role to play in the provision of care that is patient- and family-centred. Care should demonstrate respect, collaboration and shared decision-making. Patient and family assessment provides an opportunity for the nurse to clarify the patient's support persons, cultural issues and learning needs. The nurse's communication with the patient should enable the patient and their family to ask questions and identify their needs.

Learning objective 4: Discuss the nurse's role in multidisciplinary collaboration when caring for a surgical patient.

As the patient moves between areas within their surgical admission, the nurse has a key role to play in ensuring information is passed correctly between health professionals. The nurse needs to be aware of the patient's needs and those of their family to ensure these needs are met from pre-surgical to post-surgical aspects of the admission. This includes the coordination of allied health professionals to enable tailored education and discharge planning.

Learning objective 5: Discuss the nurse's role in the assessment and management of pain, wound care, patient education and discharge planning during the acute surgical event.

The nurse is the crucial link between the patient and the healthcare team. The assessment and management of the patient's pain and wound are designed to ensure good patient outcomes. The provision of good education and discharge planning will ensure the patient and their family are provided with the information to ensure they can manage the patient in the home environment.

REVIEW QUESTIONS

3.1 When the nurse communicates with the doctor about the patient's wishes, what ethical standards are they upholding?

3.2 What is the benefit of using a handover tool when transferring care from one nurse to another nurse?

3.3 What are the five important indicators for a patient's readiness to be transferred from recovery?

3.4 When dealing with obese patients, what factors does the nurse need to consider for their own health and safety?

3.5 When assessing a patient's pain level, what other considerations should be assessed?

RESEARCH TOPIC

Bedside handover has been developed to enable patient- and family-inclusive care. What points does the nurse need to consider when presenting patient handover at the bedside? Read the articles in the Further Reading section to provide a deeper context for bedside handover. There is continuing debate around the benefits and barriers of bedside handover that is patient- and family-inclusive. Research this topic and discuss how you would feel as a patient, a family member and the nurse during bedside handover.

FURTHER READING

Anderson, J., Malone, L., Shanahan, K. & Manning, J. (2015). Nursing bedside clinical handover: An integrated review of issues and tools. *Journal of Clinical Nursing*, 24(5–6), 662–71.

Davoodvand, S., Abbaszadeh, A. & Ahmadi, F. (2016). Patient advocacy from the clinical nurse's viewpoint: A qualitative study. *Journal of Medical Ethics and History of Medicine*, 9, 5. Retrieved from https://www.ncbi.nlm.nih.gov/pmc/articles/PMC4958925.

Tidwell, T., Edwards, J., Snider, E., Lindsey, C., Reed, A., Scroggins, I., Zarski, C. & Brigance, J. (2011). A nursing pilot study on bedside reporting to promote best practice and patient/family-centered care. *Journal of Neuroscience Nursing*, 43(4), E5.

Tobiano, G., Chaboyer, W. & McMurray, A. (2013). Family members' perceptions of the nursing bedside handover. *Journal of Clinical Nursing*, 22(1–2), 192–200.

REFERENCES

Anderson, J., Malone, L., Shanahan, K. & Manning, J. (2015). Nursing bedside clinical handover: An integrated review of issues and tools. *Journal of Clinical Nursing*, 24(5–6), 662–71.

Arzouman, J. (2016). A culture of safety and the role of the medical-surgical nurse. *MEDSURG Nursing*, 25(2), 75–6.

Australian Commission on Safety and Quality in Health Care (ACSQHC) (2011). *Patient-centred Care: Improving Quality and Safety through Partnerships with Patients and Consumers*. Sydney: ACSQHC.

Bail, K. & Grealish, L. (2016). 'Failure to maintain': A theoretical proposition for a new quality indicator of nurse care rationing for complex older people in hospital. *International Journal of Nursing Studies*, 63, 146–61.

Blakeman, T.C. & Branson, R.D. (2013). Inter- and intra-hospital transport of the critically ill. *Respiratory Care*, 58(6), 1008–23.

Broman, K.K., Hayes, R.M., Kripalani, S., Vasilevskis, E.E., Phillips, S.E., Ehrenfeld, J.M. … Nealon, W.H. (2016). Interhospital transfer for acute surgical care: Does delay matter? *The American Journal of Surgery*, 212(5), 823–30.

Carter, H. (2013). *Paediatric Surgery Manual of Peri-operative Care: An Essential Guide*. Chichester: John Wiley & Sons, pp. 263–70.

Chaboyer, W., McMurray, A., Wallis, M. & Chang, H.Y. (2008). *Standard Operating Protocol for Implementing Bedside Handover in Nursing*. Brisbane: Griffith University.

Collins, J. (2014). Nutrition and care considerations in the overweight and obese population within the critical care setting. *Critical Care Nursing Clinics of North America*, 26(2), 243–53.

Cooney, M.F. (2016). Optimizing acute pain management in the obese patient: Treatment and monitoring considerations. *Journal of PeriAnesthesia Nursing*, 31(3), 269–76.

Coyne, E., Grafton, E., Reid, A. & Marshall, A. (2017). Understanding family assessment in the Australian context: What are adult oncology nursing practices? *Collegian*, 24(2), 175–82.

Deek, H., Hamilton, S., Brown, N., Inglis, S.C., Digiacomo, M., Newton, P. J. … FAMILY Project Investigators (2016). Family-centred approaches to healthcare interventions in chronic diseases in adults: A quantitative systematic review. *Journal of Advanced Nursing*, 72(5), 968–79.

Dillstrom, M., Bjersa, K. & Engstrom, M. (2017). Patients' experience of acute unplanned surgical reoperation. *Journal of Surgical Research*, 209, 199–205.

Downie, F., Egdell, S., Bielby, A. & Searle, R. (2010). Barrier dressings in surgical site infection prevention strategies. *British Journal of Nursing*, 19(20), S42–S46.

Estes, M.E.Z., Calleja, P., Theobald, K. & Harvey, T. (2015). *Health Assessment and Physical Examination* (2nd ed.). Melbourne: Cengage.

Farrell, M. (ed.) (2017). *Smeltzer & Bare's Textbook of Medical-Surgical Nursing* (4th ed.). Sydney: Wolters Kluwer.

Gazala, S., Tul, Y., Wagg, A., Widder, S.L. & Khadaroo, R.G. (2013). Quality of life and long-term outcomes of octo- and nonagenarians following acute care surgery: A cross-sectional study. *World Journal of Emergency Surgery*, 8(1), 23.

Gosselin, E., Bourgault, P., Lavoie, S., Coleman, R.M. & Méziat-Burdin, A. (2014). Development and validation of an observation tool for the assessment of nursing pain management practices in an intensive care unit in a standardized clinical simulation setting. *Pain Management Nursing: Official Journal of the American Society of Pain Management Nurses*, 15(4), 720–30.

Hacquard, P., Cunat, C., Toussaint, C., Auclair, A., Malecot, M.A., Ginet, M.F., … Piriou, V. (2013). Assessment of the checklist in the operating room: Perceptions of caregivers and physicians (level II assessment). *Annales Françaises d'Anesthésie et de Réanimation*, 32(4), 235–40.

Haley, C. (2014). Community practice and continuity of care. In J. Dempsey, S. Hillege, J. French & V. Wilson (eds), *Fundamentals of Nursing and Midwifery: A Person-centred Approach to Care*. Sydney: Lippincott Williams & Wilkins, pp. 76–93.

Hamlin, L., Davies, M., Richardson-Tench, M. & Sutherland-Fraser, S. (2016). *Peri-operative Nursing: An Introduction* (2nd ed.). Sydney: Elsevier.

Hausfeld, K., Baker, R. B., Boettcher-Prior, P., Hancock, D., Helms, C., Jablonski, T., … Morris, M. (2015). *Journal of Pediatric Nursing*, 30(6), e3–e9.

Hoch, C. & Hamlin, L. (2015). Nursing management: Postoperative care. In D. Brown, H. Edwards, L. Seaton & T. Buckley (eds), *Lewis's Medical-Surgical Nursing: Assessment and Management of Clinical Problems* (4th ed.). Sydney: Elsevier, pp. 330–54.

International Family Nursing Association (IFNA) (2015). IFNA Position Statement on Generalist Competencies for Family Nursing Practice. Retrieved from https://internationalfamilynursing.org/2015/07/25/ifna-position-statement-on-generalist-competencies-for-family-nursing-practice-2.

McMurray, A., Chaboyer, W., Wallis, M., Johnson, J. & Gehrke, T. (2011). Patients' perspectives of bedside nursing handover. *Collegian (Royal College of Nursing, Australia)*, 18(1), 19–26.

Mitchell, M., Chaboyer, W., Burmeister, E. & Foster, M. (2009). Positive effects of a nursing intervention on family-centered care in adult critical care. *American Journal of Critical Care*, 18(6), 543–52.

New, P.W., McDougall, K. & Scroggie, C. (2016). Improving discharge planning communication between hospitals and patients. *Internal Medicine Journal*, 46(1), 57–62.

Nursing Council of New Zealand (NCNZ) ([2007] 2016). *Competencies for Registered Nurses*. Retrieved from http://www.nursingcouncil.org.nz/Nurses.

Nursing and Midwifery Board of Australia (NMBA) (2016). *Registered Nurse Standards for Practice*. Melbourne: Nursing & Midwifery Board of Australia. Retrieved from http://www.nursingmidwiferyboard.gov.au/Codes-Guidelines-Statements/Professional-standards.aspx.

Palmer, R.M. & Kresevic, D.M. (2014). The acute care for elders unit. In M.L. Malone, E.A. Capezuti & R.M. Palmer (eds), *Acute Care for Elders* (pp. 69–97). New York: Springer.

Phillips, L.A. (2013). Delirium in geriatric patients: Identification and prevention. *MEDSURG Nursing*, 22(1), 9.

Pre- and post-operative care (2017). *Australian Nursing and Midwifery Journal*, 25(2), 22–3.

Schultz, H., Qvist, N., Mogensen, C.B. & Pedersen, B.D. (2013). Experiences of patients with acute abdominal pain in the ED or acute surgical ward: A qualitative comparative study. *International Emergency Nursing*, 21(4), 228–35.

Shaw, J., Zou, X. & Butow, P. (2015). Treatment decision making experiences of migrant cancer patients and their families in Australia. *Patient Education and Counseling*, 98(6), 742–7.

Shippee-Rice, R.V., Fetzer, S.J. & Long, J.V. (2012). *Gerioperative Nursing Care: Principles and Practices of Surgical Care for the Older Adult*. New York: Springer.

Sinha, S.K., Oakes, S.L., Chaudhry, S. & Suh, T.T. (2014). How to use the ACE unit to improve hospital safety and quality for older patients: From ACE units to elder-friendly hospitals. In M.L. Malone, E.A. Capezuti & R.M. Palmer (eds), *Acute Care for Elders*. New York: Springer, pp. 131–56.

Tang, R., Ranmuthugala, G. & Cunningham, F. (2013). Surgical safety checklist: A review. *ANZ Journal of Surgery*, 84(3), 148–54.

Thomas, D.R. (2013). The role of nutrition in the management and prevention of pressure ulcers. In D.R. Thomas & G. Compton (eds), *Pressure Ulcers in the Aging Population: A Guide for Clinicians*. Totowa, NJ: Humana Press, pp. 127–42.

Tobiano, G., Chaboyer, W. & McMurray, A. (2013). Family members' perceptions of the nursing bedside handover. *Journal of Clinical Nursing*, 22(1–2), 192–200.

Tollefson, J. & Hillman, E. (2016). *Clinical Psychomotor Skills* (6th ed.). Melbourne: Cengage.

Twycross, A., Finley, G.A. & Latimer, M. (2013). Pediatric nurses' postoperative pain management practices: An observational study. *Journal for Specialists in Pediatric Nursing*, 18(3), 189–201.

van der Meer, D.M., Weiland, T.J., Philip, J., Jelinek, G.A., Boughey, M., Knott, J. … Kelly, A.M. (2016). Presentation patterns and outcomes of patients with cancer accessing care in emergency departments in Victoria, Australia. *Supportive Care in Cancer*, 24(3), 1251–60.

Wagner, K.D. & Hardin-Pierce, M.G. (2015). *High-Acuity Nursing* (6th ed.). Sydney: Pearson.

White, L., Duncan, G. & Baumle, W. (2013). *Medical Surgical Nursing: An Integrated Approach*. New York: Cengage.

Williams, C., Johnson, P.A., Guzzetta, C.E., Guzzetta, P.C., Cohen, I.T., Sill, A.M., … Murray, J. (2014). Pediatric fasting times before surgical and radiologic procedures: Benchmarking institutional practices against national standards. *Journal of Pediatric Nursing*, 29(3), 258–67.

Wong-Baker FACES Foundation (2016). *Wong-Baker FACES® Pain Rating Scale*. Retrieved from http://www.WongBakerFACES.org.

World Health Organization (WHO) (2015). World Health Organization. Retrieved from http://www.who.int/en.

Wright, L.M. & Leahey, M. (2013). *Nurses and Families: A Guide to Family Assessment and Intervention* (6th ed.). Philadelphia, PA: F.A. Davis Company.

Wrobleski, D.M., Joswiak, M.E., Dunn, D.F., Maxson, P.M. & Holland, D.E. (2014). Discharge planning rounds to the bedside: a patient- and family-centered approach. *MEDSURG Nursing*, 23(2), 111–16.

Zimmerman, P.G. (2010). Peri-operative nursing: An introductory text. *AORN Journal*, 92(3), 370–1.

The acute medical client

4

Rachel Cross, Ann-Marie Brown
and Nang Sein

LEARNING OBJECTIVES

At the completion of this chapter, you should be able to:

1   define the concept of acute medical illness and explore demographics, risk factors
    and social determinants associated with the typical acute medical client
2   discuss sociocultural influences on client perceptions of health and illness and the
    development of cultural competency among healthcare professionals
3   explore the nursing assessment, interventions and management of the acute
    medical client with reference to the paediatric, elderly and bariatric client
4   understand the impact of comorbidities on the care of the acute medical client
5   understand the importance of chronic illness management for achieving good
    outcomes for the acute medical client.

Introduction

Management of the acute medical client is complex. Clients suffering from medical conditions often require acute care, so nurses need to provide holistic, patient-centred care to both the client and their family. Clients with medical conditions often have differing levels of wellness. Collaboration with other members of the healthcare team is crucial for the acute medical client, and understanding the role of the nurse within this team is important. Medical clients are not defined by age, socioeconomic status or culture, and nurses must integrate these considerations when providing client care. The complexity of the acute medical client also extends to sociocultural influences about client perceptions of health, as these can influence client care for acute medical conditions.

This chapter provides an overview of the surrounding ailments relevant to the provision of nursing care for clients with acute medical conditions. The nurse's role in coordinating multidisciplinary, culturally appropriate and patient-centred care will be presented, as well as the role of the nurse in assessment, management, education and discharge planning during the acute medical event.

NURSING STANDARDS

The following identifies the national competency standards for the registered nurse from the Nursing and Midwifery Board of Australia (NMBA) and the Nursing Council of New Zealand (NCNZ) that are addressed in this chapter.

Australian Registered Nurse Standards for Practice

Standard 1: Thinks critically and analyses nursing practice

Standard 2: Engages in therapeutic and professional relationships

Standard 3: Maintains the capability for practice

Standard 4: Comprehensively conducts assessments

Standard 5: Develops a plan for nursing practice

Standard 6: Provides safe, appropriate and responsive quality nursing practice

Standard 7: Evaluates outcomes to inform nursing practice

(NMBA, 2016)

New Zealand: Competencies for Registered Nurses

Competency 1.1: Accepts responsibility for ensuring that his/her nursing practice and conduct meet the standards of the professional, ethical and relevant legislated requirements

Competency 1.2: Demonstrates the ability to apply the principles of the Treaty of Waitangi/ Te Tiriti o Waitangi to nursing practice

Competency 1.5: Practises nursing in a manner that the health consumer determines as being culturally safe

Competency 4.1: Collaborates and participates with colleagues and members of the health care team to facilitate and coordinate care

Competency 4.2: Recognises and values the roles and skills of all members of the health care team in the delivery of care

(NCNZ, [2007] 2016)

Acute medical conditions

An acute medical condition can best be described as a sudden onset of an illness that is unpredicted, and that is of short duration, often requiring **hospitalisation**. Some of these acute hospitalisations may lead to a long-term chronic illness in some medical clients. Clients across all age groups who have a medical condition will at some stage during their disease suffer from an acute exacerbation, requiring specialist care. Conditions such as asthma and COPD may require clients to seek urgent hospitalisation and management. Every client will have a different journey, requiring differing lengths of stay. Older clients aged over 65 years are more likely to require an acute hospitalisation for treatment of their disease (AIHW, 2016b), but some acute exacerbations can also be managed in primary healthcare settings. However, those requiring acute hospitalisation can predispose the medical client to further health decline. The incidence of delirium and functional decline for the older client increases with each acute care presentation requiring hospitalisation (Department of Health Victoria, 2012).

Hospitalisation following an acute presentation can have a significant impact on the medical client, including increasing incidence of falls, pressure injuries and altered nutrition. Clients can also experience depression and a loss of independence (Department of Health Victoria, 2012). Early identification and recognition of signs and symptoms for these conditions is therefore essential for nursing assessment and individualised client care planning. Hospitalisation for acute illness presentations also contributes to the economic burden for healthcare systems. Implementation of chronic illness frameworks at both the macro and micro levels is therefore required to address the complexities of chronic diseases (Deravin-Malone & Anderson, 2016; NHC, 2007).

Clients with medical conditions have these conditions all the time – they live, breathe and sleep with them. This makes the care quite complex, and requires early assessment and management to prevent complications. Older clients with medical conditions often have multiple medical illnesses that require specialist care for each individual issue. Side-effects of medications and treatments can often exacerbate other illnesses, leading to further complications.

Many medical clients have secondary conditions associated with their primary condition that may require acute intervention, such as cellulitis as a result of long-term diabetes, urinary sepsis from a urinary tract infection or acute pulmonary oedema resulting from heart failure.

It is imperative that the nurse is involved with the care of the client throughout their journey from the emergency department through to the ward, whether this is in ICU or general ward, and finally onto discharge to either rehabilitation settings or home and long-term management.

Exacerbation management

Ongoing care for the medical client with a chronic disease often includes exacerbation management. While the medical client may require acute hospitalisation for exacerbation of a chronic disease, ongoing client management is largely undertaken in the community by multiple providers within the primary healthcare team. This multidisciplinary approach seeks to ensure that each client with a chronic illness has a **multidisciplinary team** who can provide an individualised holistic plan of care based on their disease and illness pattern. Depending on the level of involvement with the client, members of the multidisciplinary team can include:

Hospitalisation – An episode of hospital care that starts with the formal admission process and ends with the formal separation process (being discharged home or into another type of care).

Multidisciplinary team – Involves a range of health professionals working together to deliver to the patient and their family comprehensive care that improves health outcomes as well as patient compliance and satisfaction.

- nursing staff
- medical staff
- dietitian
- occupational therapist
- physiotherapist
- speech pathologist
- social worker (Chang & Johnson, 2015).

Nurses are pivotal to this team and the management of the exacerbation event. Nurses can provide education on disease management for both the client and their family and/or carer, promote both physical and psychological wellbeing, liaise with members of the multidisciplinary team to enable coordination of care and contribute to health-promotion activities (Deravin-Malone & Anderson, 2016). Nurse practitioner models of care are also becoming more crucial for the medical client with a chronic illness.

Social determinants of health

Social determinants of health are becoming increasingly relevant and a growing priority in healthcare. Like the continued push toward patient-centred care, the need to explore client health outside of the hospitals is growing far more prevalent (Department of Health, 2017). Social determinants of health can include socioeconomic status, transport, race/culture, education, early life, disability, food and nutrition, social support, genetics and responses by the health system to the person with disease (ACSQHC, 2018a; WHO, 2018). As a nurse, it is essential to consider these determinants when planning interventions for a client's care.

Socioeconomic factors are important determinants of health and wellbeing in Australia. The Australian Bureau of Statistics (ABS, 2011) reports that people in lower socioeconomic groups are among those with the highest rates of illness. Socioeconomic status has three variables: education, income and occupation (ABS, 2011). To best influence a positive health journey and outcome for patients, the nurse needs to consider the possible impact of these when planning, implementing and evaluating care. The World Health Organization (WHO, 2018) identifies that higher income and social status are linked to better health. The greater the gap between the richest and poorest people, the greater the differences in health. The higher a person's income, education or occupation level, the healthier they tend to be – a phenomenon often termed the 'social gradient of health' (AIHW, 2016c).

People who are in the lower socioeconomic group have been identified as smoking at a higher rate than those in the more affluent group. In 2013, 20 per cent of those aged fourteen and over in the lowest socioeconomic group smoked daily, a rate three times that of people in the highest socioeconomic group (6.7 per cent) (AIHW, 2016c). This can lead to COPD, chronic lung conditions, cardiovascular disease and cancer. People in lower socioeconomic groups access medical services at a greater rate than higher socioeconomic groups. There are fewer GPs, with a greater number of patients in lower socioeconomic areas. This leads patients to present frequently to the local hospital for assistance and treatment. There is a relationship between lower socioeconomic households and poorer health outcomes for the people with chronic medical conditions living in lower socioeconomic areas (ABS, 2008).

A person's employment situation can be a determining factor in their ability to be admitted or remain in hospital for an optimal duration. A person in a highly competitive work environment may perceive time away from work as detrimental to their career, and therefore wish to discharge early. Some people are in employment situations where they are unable to financially afford to take time off, or work in a casual position receiving no sick leave benefits. There is also the situation where the work environment is not conducive to good health. A patient who has experienced a myocardial infarction through detrimental lifestyle factors would have decreased health outcomes if they returned to work in a stressful environment; however, for some people with financial commitments, simply leaving a work environment is not an option and it is essential that the registered nurse respects and honours the patient's situation and perspective on what is of value to them.

Income can determine a client's ability to afford treatment options offered, and can impact on compliance with any treatment plans and future health outcomes. It is essential for nurses to remember that not all clients are able to afford prescribed treatments, or access transport to pharmacies to adhere to medication prescriptions; nor can all people afford nutritious food and time off work to recover fully. With these factors in mind, a collaborative approach to care, which includes all members of the healthcare team, needs to be applied in many situations.

The healthcare system can be very challenging to navigate and to understand, and the lowest level of **health literacy** is most prevalent in clients from lower socioeconomic populations (NHHRC, 2009). The health literacy of a person needs to be determined, as these people may not have the ability to understand what is asked of them or the ability to comprehend the consequences of not adhering to prescribed treatment plans. It is essential for the nurse to assume the role of patient advocate and ensure that the patient genuinely is informed at a level suitable to their individual capacity to understand. A person's health literacy can be a determinant in their experience and in their health outcomes.

Health equity can be achieved by addressing the social determinates of health. Health equity is identified as all people having the opportunity to attain their full health potential and no one being 'disadvantaged from achieving this potential because of their social position or other socially determined circumstance' (Department of Health, 2017).

> **Health literacy** – The cognitive and social skills that determine the motivation and ability of individuals to gain access to, understand and use information in ways that promote and maintain good health.

Communication

Therapeutic rapport requires the nurse to be non-judgemental and empathetic in all aspects of communication to clients, despite their gender, race, culture or socioeconomic status. Effective nursing care requires open communication from a client, and when a client feels safe and not judged, they are more likely to disclose their actual situation and any issues (Gilbert, 2010). Clients and their families need to inform the nurse of any challenges to adherence to the prescribed care. This ensures clients and their families can be provided with options and education about the best treatment plan for them. It also allows the nurse to work with the client and the family to develop the best and most effective outcome. The client and family need to be actively involved with the care and management of the client to achieve a positive, collaborative outcome.

Communication also needs to be extended to all members of the healthcare team. This may also include case conferences with family members, allowing all aspects of care to be considered. Effective communication also involves follow-up procedures and education, management of acute exacerbations and times where respite care may be needed.

Excellent communication develops the relationship between the nurse and the patient, so the patient can freely communicate what is meaningful and valuable to them in terms of treatments and outcomes. Effective communication also provides an opportunity for the patient to increase their knowledge of their own health conditions and options and facilitates their involvement in their own care, which enhances adherence to prescribed treatments and therefore leads to better outcomes and a more positive patient experience (Kitson et al., 2013).

Inherent inequalities exist in the nurse–patient relationship, and they can create an unequal power differential (Corless, Buckley & Mee, 2016) – for example, the client may not get to choose the nurse they are dependent on for care and information. The nurse must be aware of this differential and have the goal of partnership and collaboration in order to empower the patient to make choices that meet their own unique needs regarding their health moving forward. This approach means that patients are more likely to adhere to treatment plans into which they have had input, and therefore have better health outcomes, better control over their symptoms and a greater degree of management.

Assessment of the acute medical client

The assessment of the medical client can often be lengthy and complex. Health assessment is an ongoing process, and forms the foundation of all nursing care. This evaluates the person as a whole – their physical, mental, psychosocial and functional wellbeing (Estes et al., 2016). A number of specific physical assessments need to be completed by the attending nurse undertaking assessment of the medical client. There are also many other areas of assessment that are required to be undertaken in determining overall care of the client.

A general survey of the client regarding the client's general condition can be observed by the nurse watching the client. This would include the stated age versus the apparent age of the client, the general appearance, the body fat, stature and motor activities; these are all important assessments that can be observed by the nurse prior to undertaking any hands-on assessment.

The stated age versus the apparent age may lead the nurse to question whether the client may have a disorder of the endocrine system – is the client small for their age or large? Do they appear older or younger? Often clients with a long-term chronic illness may look older due to facial changes, but in fact may still be quite young. This is often difficult when assessing children and adolescents, where the size and weight of the patient does not reflect the age.

The appearance of the client is important, as this gives a nurse an idea of the level of wellness (Estes et al., 2016). Does the client have gross motor issues, or walk with a frame or stick? How is the client positioned – do they sit over a table to assist with breathing; do they have a paralysis or facial droop? The nurse needs a keen eye to observe the client in a normal setting and to compare one side of the body with the other, looking for symmetry. If there are any changes, further investigations may be warranted.

The body fat should be distributed evenly. Observing the client to be obese or underweight is an important factor when planning nursing care. Some disease processes, such as hypothyroidism or long-term steroid therapy, cause a client to be obese. Other clients could be quite emaciated or have decreased fat stores, which can be a result of long-term chronic illness, changes in metabolic states of the body and certain diseases such as anorexia nervosa. This is important for nurses to recognise, as often these clients require multidisciplinary team input for acute hospitalisation. The nurse can therefore make appropriate referrals for the acute medical client.

Other areas of assessment may also include body or breath odour. These may be the result of a disease process or poor hygiene practices. A dishevelled and unkempt client may be due to a mental health condition, poor self-esteem or a homeless lifestyle. This also may be an indication of neglect by the caregiver. All these areas should be addressed by the nurse and included in the care of the client.

Facial expressions and client alertness should be appropriate to the surroundings of the client. Changes in expressions may be lacking in clients with feelings of lethargy or sadness, or the client may have dementia with an inappropriate expression. Observe for a client with Bell's palsy, showing a paralysis of the facial muscles or mouth droop.

As part of a physical assessment, vital signs provide data surrounding the client's general health. These include temperature, heart rate, blood pressure, respirations, oxygen saturations and oxygen flow. Pain is also considered a vital sign, as this may affect the physical, emotional and mental health of each client (Estes et al., 2016).

A number of specific areas of assessment need to be focused on for acute medical clients. These include:

- neurological
- cardiovascular
- respiratory
- gastrointestinal
- renal
- musculoskeletal
- skin.

Using the techniques of inspection, palpation, auscultation and percussion will allow the nurse to make a thorough and accurate assessment of the client.

Often the admission of a medical client is quite long and complex. An accurate complete client history, which includes other illnesses, medications and previous hospitalisations, also needs to be assessed. From the information gathered, a plan of care will need to be developed.

Other assessments should include:

- family health history
- social history
- previous medical/surgical conditions
- lifestyle
- mental status
- cultural and spiritual assessment.

Comorbidities

The Australian Institute of Health and Welfare (AIHW, 2017) defines **comorbidity** as 'any two or more diseases that occur in one person at the same time'. Healthcare professionals are required to be aware of multiple coexisting disease in management of a person's health. Comorbidity has an influence on an individual's life and a potential impact on their complex healthcare.

Comorbidity – Any two or more diseases that occur in one person at the same time.

What is a comorbidity?

People with a comorbidity require frequent medical professional attendance, often recurrent hospital admissions and longer lengths of hospital stay. The cost to the healthcare system and the time spent with clinicians are increasing, due to multiple medications and complex treatment requirement by people with comorbidities.

The Australian Department of Health (2017) reports that one in three Australians aged 65 years and over has three or more chronic diseases. Several chronic diseases are listed as common and significant health problems presenting with comorbidity:

- cardiovascular disease (CVD)
- cancer
- arthritis
- back problems
- diabetes
- chronic obstructive pulmonary disease (COPD)
- asthma
- mental health conditions.

Multiple comorbidities impact on the person's physical functioning, social life and work. Furthermore, they increase a person's living expenses and healthcare costs, creating a burden for Australia's healthcare system (ACAM, 2011).

The term 'multimorbidity' (Wallace et al., 2015), which is a client presenting with two or more chronic diseases or conditions, is relatively new worldwide. Increasing numbers of diseases increases the number of medications, and therefore the side-effects, and the potential for adverse drug interactions also increases.

Length of stay in hospital

Multimorbidity – The new term for comorbidity (Wallace et al., 2015), a client presenting with two or more chronic diseases or conditions; this is relatively new worldwide.

Multiple comorbidities have very complex clinical management and require extensive use of health services. Comorbidities increase the length of stay of clients in hospital. Gruneir and colleagues (2016) suggest that hospitalisations also become more complicated with increasing **multimorbidity**. This is demonstrated by longer stays, increased frequency of non-medical discharge delays and a greater likelihood of multiple hospital admissions, including re-presentations within 30 days of discharge. For example, people presenting with coronary heart disease and COPD require complex management due to the impact on coronary heart disease of the treatment of COPD by using beta-blockers. The length of average stay for people with both CVD and chronic kidney disease (CKD) recorded 10.8 days compared with 5.4 days for CVD patients and 4.9 days for CKD patients (AIWH, 2017).

These findings reinforce the need for better integration of patient-centred care practices both within and across healthcare sectors and the sharing of information to support care for those with multimorbidity (Gruneir et al., 2016).

Patient- and family-centred care

The Institute of Medicine (IOM, 2011) defines patient-centred care as, 'Providing care that is respectful of, and responsive to, individual patient preferences, needs and values, and ensuring that patient values guide all clinical decisions'. When the patient's family is also included, the term becomes patient- and family-centred care (PFCC), defined as 'an approach to the planning, delivery, and evaluation of health care that is grounded in mutually beneficial partnerships among healthcare providers, patients, and families' (IFNA, 2015).

To meet Nursing Council Standards and Competencies in Australia and New Zealand, it is essential that the registered nurse provides care centred on the client's own individual preferences, and that the client and their family are empowered to make their own choices. The nurse can only truly ascertain a person's preferences by developing the skill of excellent, non-judgemental empathic communication, as described earlier in this chapter (Rossiter, Scott & Walton, 2014).

Patient-centred care is an evidence-based approach that results in increased quality of life for clients and their families, reduced morbidity, improved patient experience and outcome (Levett-Jones et al., 2014).

Manley, Hills and Marriot (2011) found that keeping the client central to the planning, implementation and evaluation of care is also beneficial for increasing the meaning and purpose that the nurse derives from their job, creating greater job satisfaction.

Discharge planning

Following an acute presentation requiring hospitalisation, comprehensive discharge planning for the medical client is required. The preparation for a successful discharge needs to commence on a client's admission. Nurses should ensure that the discharge planning includes all members of the multidisciplinary team caring for the client, education relating to discharge instructions for both the client and their family/carer, and documentation and communication with primary healthcare providers to enable the continuation of care outside the acute healthcare setting.

For effective discharge planning, the registered nurse needs to consider social factors such as the client's ability to transport themselves to scheduled outpatient appointments, and to the pharmacy to collect prescribed medications. The nurse also needs to determine and consider the client's level of social support at home and to make referrals accordingly. It is helpful to involve family and close friends in the ongoing care of the client after discharge. A client with diabetes will have better outcomes if their family supports them in developing and maintaining healthy eating and exercise habits. A client who has disabilities can require extensive support. Caregivers need to be identified and supported in the process by external agencies so they can provide the care required on an ongoing basis. Referrals to community agencies are vital and can prevent increased hospitalisations.

Discussion with the discharge planner and multidisciplinary team may be required to assess and coordinate all aspects of care and support required. This may include home visits and alterations to access to the home, as well as extra care that may be needed.

Chronic illness management

Chronic diseases are the leading cause of mortality in the world (WHO, 2014). However, in the majority of cases these deaths are preventable. In New Zealand, chronic conditions are the leading cause of illness and are responsible for more than 80 per cent of deaths in the population (NHC, 2007). In Australia, over half of the population suffers from one chronic disease, with 20 per cent affected by multiple chronic conditions (AIHW, 2015). Chronic disease and illness also constitute a significant economic burden (NHC, 2007). Between 2008 and 2009, 36 per cent of the allocated healthcare expenditure in Australia was for chronic disease (AIHW, 2014), yet the impact on the quality of life for clients and their families is difficult to quantify.

Chronic disease can have many definitions; however, as stated by the Australian Institute for Health and Welfare (AIHW, 2012a, 2012b), diseases often include aspects of the following:

Chronic illness/disease – A group of diseases that tend to be long lasting and have persistent effects.

- complex illness trajectory with multiple factors leading to their onset
- prolonged course of illness that may progress to other complications
- a long development period, during which there may be no symptoms
- associated functional impairment or disability.

Illness patterns for chronic diseases can follow acute (onset is sudden) and/or chronic (slower onset) trajectories. These patterns directly affect primary healthcare treatment and management and hospitalisation for acute care treatment, as well as representing a financial and psychosocial burden for both the client and their family. The impact of chronic disease and illness patterns for the client and their family, however, is difficult to measure and can be influenced by many factors, including:

- disease progression
- frequency of acute care hospitalisation
- impact upon quality of life
- acute and chronic nature of individual disease and illness
- the presence of psychological support.

To provide holistic patient–centred care, nurses must have an understanding of the individual impact that chronic disease and illness has on the client and their family. Understanding this can enable a more individualised nursing care plan to be prepared and implemented.

Age-related considerations

While the prevalence of chronic disease does increase with age, younger people are also affected. In 2012 more than 40 per cent of all chronic illness deaths in the world were for people aged under 70 years (WHO, 2014). Therefore, an ageist view that only older people suffer from disease is no longer true. It is not solely the older population that is affected by chronic illness: clients of all ages can suffer from one or more chronic diseases. In Australia, nearly 40 per cent of people aged 45 years and over suffer from two or more chronic diseases (AIHW, 2015). The burden of chronic disease for both the healthcare system and the individual client also changes across the lifespan. Clients aged from birth to fourteen years are more likely to experience illness burden due to pre-term/low-birthweight complications, asthma and birth trauma/asphyxia compared with coronary heart disease, COPD, dementia and cancer for clients aged 65 years and over (AIHW, 2016a).

Age-related considerations are essential for nurses to understand, as these can have a direct impact on nursing assessment and management, and treatment and participation in care. Often, clients will require management and treatment for childhood chronic illnesses that progress into adulthood – for example, cystic fibrosis, diabetes, epilepsy, asthma and cerebral palsy. It is therefore important for nurses to collaborate with clients and their families to understand the individual nature of the client's chronic illness pattern. Understanding these patterns can assist with client education, and with ongoing care and management in both the acute and primary healthcare settings.

Overweight and obesity

AIHW (2017) states that overweight and obesity are risk factors for poor health and increase the risk of one or more chronic diseases, such as cardiovascular disease, high blood pressure, type 2 diabetes, sleep apnoea and osteoarthritis. Over a million Australians over the age of two have been diagnosed with diabetes (AIHW, 2014).

In 2014–15, 63 per cent of Australians were considered obese (AIHW 2017). Obesity can be determined by body mass index (BMI) calculation. A BMI of over 25 indicates that a person is overweight and a BMI of over 30 indicates that someone is obese. Measuring overweight and obesity, BMI is calculated by dividing a person's weight (in kilograms) by their height (in metres) squared, which uses the BMI classifications for adults defined by the World Health Organization (WHO).

Obesity is split into three classes, according to severity, with more severe obesity associated with a higher risk of comorbidities (WHO, 2018). Waist circumference is another commonly used measure of overweight and obesity. A wider waist is associated with a higher risk of metabolic complications. Different waist circumference cut-off points might need to be considered for certain population groups other than white Caucasian people, such as South Asian, Chinese and Japanese populations (NHMRC, 2013). The nurse will assess the client on admission and assist with referrals to a dietitian if that is requested by the client.

Coexisting diseases: Tobacco smoking, alcohol and illicit drugs

The WHO (2014) suggests that tobacco smoking, alcohol and illicit drugs are preventable causes of poor health and increase the risk of acute and chronic diseases – for example, chronic respiratory conditions, cardiovascular disease, liver disease and mental health. Excessive use of alcohol is a major risk for liver, heart conditions and mental health, contributing to motor vehicle accidents and physical violence. In adolescence and young adulthood, certain lifestyle decisions such as cigarette smoking, excessive alcohol, use of illicit drugs, lack of exercise and dietary choices can establish multiple comorbidities of health. The WHO (2014) estimates that 'tobacco use will account for approximately 10 million deaths each year, of which 70% will occur in developing countries by 2030'.

Client participation in shared decision-making

Client participation in decision-making is integral for the treatment of chronic disease. Having an informed and activated patient – that is, where a patient is actively engaged with their healthcare team in shared decision-making – is advocated by the chronic care model (Wagner et al., 1999). Clients have also stated that they prefer to be involved in decisions made about their own care (Chewning et al., 2012). The nature of chronic illness demands a multidisciplinary approach for care and management (Chang & Johnson, 2015). All relevant members of the multidisciplinary team should be included alongside the client and their family for shared decision-making.

Age considerations must also be taken into account for client participation. The inclusion of family and/or carers may be required. Nurses need to be aware of individual client considerations to ensure that, even in the presence of others, the client has participated in their care and contributed to shared decision-making. Clients with a chronic disease are of divergent ages, have different illness patterns and may also have cultural and linguistic diversity. These factors are important to recognise, as they affect the ability of the client to participate in decision-making about their care.

Medication management

The aim of pharmacology treatment is to treat symptoms or to prevent deterioration of a person's illnesses. The medication management process in a clinical setting includes receiving medication orders, ordering medication from the pharmacy, liaising with a medical doctor and patient, administering medication, monitoring the outcome of administration, recording the outcomes, appropriate storage and discarding of unwanted medications.

Health professionals must follow the National Medication Policy and the Quality Use of Medicines (QUM), such as judicious, appropriate, safe and efficacious care (ACSQHC, 2018a). Nursing staff who are responsible for medication management must ensure that they act within their legal framework for medicines to ensure patient safety. Knowledge of medications through the rights for medication administration – dose, drug, patient, time, route, clinical scenario – is very important for the registered nurse, as this can help with detection of adverse events and potential harm to patients.

Prior to discharge, medication management and education are very important. The client and their caregiver need to meet with the pharmacist to understand the medications and their possible side-effects. The pharmacist can also offer advice about dosing and managing medications, possibly with pre-packed medications from the client's local pharmacy.

Polypharmacy

Polypharmacy is the use of five or more medicines. These can also include over-the-counter medications, those prescribed by a general practitioner and traditional/complementary medicines. Patients with a chronic illness often use an array of medicines to assist their disease process and manage their symptoms. However, with each medicine the risk of adverse drug reactions increases. Nurses must be aware of potential medication interactions when multiple drugs have been prescribed to prevent medication incidents. The older client may also be more vulnerable to adverse effects of certain medications, such as aspirin, clopidogrel, warfarin, insulin or oral hypoglycaemic (Budnitz et al., 2011). Nursing staff who are responsible for administering medications need to maintain their knowledge of safe use of medication and adverse effects, as an incident could potentially be harmful, particularly for older people and young children (Steinman, Handler & Gurwitz, 2011). Engagement with a pharmacist is helpful for the medical client, as they can review the patient's medication and ensure that both the patient and their family receive the appropriate education for safe medication management upon discharge.

Advance care planning

Clients are not always in a state whereby they can communicate effectively. In the field of palliative care, an advance care plan is a document that contains the client's preferences should certain eventualities arise. An advance care plan can help ensure that the client's own personal values and preferences are taken into account when planning, implementing and evaluating the care offered. The advance care plan can differ between states, but it has a primary role in the promotion of the autonomy and dignity of an individual in providing high-quality, patient-centred care (Department of Health, 2017). Many clients in aged care facilities have an advance care plan or directive in place when admitted to hospital. These are used in conjunction with other factors after discussion with the client and family to determine the best and optimal care for the client.

Advance care planning is completed not to control medical decisions, but in the hope of allowing a person to live well and die with dignity, and with their own personal decisions respected. Many are completed in stages – they are begun when the person is well, but may alter as the person becomes unwell and enters the palliative care stage. An advance care directive differs from the advance care plan in the sense that the advance care directive is *part* of the advance care plan. A client may decide, as part of their advance care plan, not to be resuscitated or not to have CPR if they become very unwell and their heart stops. The advance care directive will state this information, which forms part of the overall advance care plan.

Culture and self-awareness

The culture with which we identify is deeply embedded in us and forms our values, beliefs, perceptions, attitudes and behaviours. Without self-reflection, our cultural beliefs bias us, so it is vital that the determinants of **cultural safety** are discussed with each individual client and their family in the context of care. Rossiter, Scott and Walton (2015) state that therapeutic communication needs to be an empathetic, genuine exchange in order for the patient's needs to be heard as they were intended. Lack of awareness of our own cultural determinants can lead to the nurse assuming that their own beliefs, values and preferences are also those of the patient (Martinez, 2014).

Cultural safety – Culturally safe care is inclusive of ethnic groups, age, gender, occupation, socioeconomic status, ethnic origin, religious or spiritual beliefs and disability.

Culturally safe care in New Zealand has its roots in honouring the Treaty of Waitangi to ensure better health status of Māori. The New Zealand Nursing Council also considers culturally safe care to be much broader than just racial identity. It includes a much wider range of cultural determinants to meet cultural competence (Richardson & Williams, 2007).

The Australian community has a rich mixture of cultural and linguistic diversity, and the *Registered Nurse Standards for Practice* identify the registered nurse's ability to recognise the importance of the history and culture to health and wellbeing. This practice reflects a specific understanding of the impact of colonisation on the cultural, social and spiritual lives of Aboriginal and Torres Strait Islander peoples, which has contributed to health inequity in Australia (NMBA, 2016). Registered nurses are responsible and accountable to the Nursing and Midwifery Board of Australia (NMBA, 2016), as they are considered health professionals. These are the national *Registered Nurse Standards for Practice* for all registered nurses.

Clients must feel safe and respected in their environment, without facing any risk of assault. With this in mind, the nurse should ensure a welcoming environment and open and honest communication, and allow clients to access language interpreters. Clients should also be assured that their staff/carers have been offered ongoing training regarding culture and diversity.

REFLECTIVE QUESTIONS

Take some time to think about these clients below and attempt the questions that follow:

- a two-year-old male child with asthma
- a 65-year-old female with breast cancer who is non-English speaking
- a 16-year-old female with cystic fibrosis
- a 78-year-old male with dementia.
- Can these clients participate in shared decision-making about their care? If not, who can or who should act on behalf of the client?
- Which members of the multidisciplinary team should be involved in shared decision-making for each of these clients?

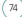

Preparations and administration: Blood transfusion

Blood is a precious resource that can be used to save the lives of thousands of patients every year. Preparation and administration of blood and blood products require both theoretical knowledge and technical skill from nurses. Nurses must be aware of blood components and the differing equipment needed for blood product administration. Blood and blood product transfusion are associated with patient risk, so careful consideration for preparation and administration is imperative. In Australia, national safety and quality health service standards exist to provide health service organisations with a framework for accreditation and quality assurance and improvement mechanisms. One national standard is Blood and Blood Products (ACSQHC, 2018b). This standard provides guidance for the safe preparation and administration of blood and blood products.

Blood and blood products require a documented legal order from a qualified endorsed practitioner. Prior to administration, however, nurses are responsible for ensuring that the right blood product is administered to the right patient at the right time via the right route and at the right dose. Nurses must also be aware of and possess knowledge of local health service guidelines and policies relevant to their practice. Close monitoring of the patient during the transfusion procedure is a key responsibility of nurses, as early recognition of blood transfusion reactions is critical for patient safety. There are numerous resources available to assist nurses in the preparation and administration of blood products. *Flippin' Blood: A BloodSafe Flip Chart* is published by the Australian Red Cross Blood Service to help make transfusion straightforward (BloodSafe, 2012).

SKILLS IN PRACTICE

Noel Goolagong

Noel Goolagong is a 57-year-old Aboriginal man living in a rural town. He has been a heavy smoker for over 40 years, and currently smokes 35 cigarettes per day. He was recently diagnosed with small cell lung cancer on a recent check-up and chest x-ray. He also has a history of type 2 diabetes mellitus and has had foot and leg ulcers for a number of weeks. Noel lives with his wife, Cindy, who is 55 years old and also smokes. She has been diagnosed with COPD and has limited mobility due to breathlessness.

Noel presents to the local hospital stating that he is more tired than usual and having more difficulty with his breathing. He also states that he has been passing some blood from the 'back passage' and has a terrible cough. He has a sore on his leg that won't heal and he has been putting a bandage on it. The triage nurse assesses Noel's vital signs:

- temperature – 36.8°C
- pulse – 112 and regular
- blood pressure – 105/53
- respirations – 22 and showing increased WOB
- oxygen saturation – 88% on room air.

A full blood count was taken and it was found that Noel had a haemoglobin level of 75 g/L.

QUESTIONS

- Looking at the haemoglobin level, identify the issues and the management of this level.
- Identify the pathophysiology and management of a client with lung cancer, especially small cell cancer.
- What are the outcomes?
- What is the short- and long-term care required?
- Does this client require an advance management plan and how would you, as the nurse, be able to assist in the implementation?
- What supports will Noel and Cindy need when Noel is discharged?
- Noel asks you, 'Am I going to die?' and you need to respond. What might you say?
- Thinking of his Aboriginal culture, identify any issues that will impact Noel's care.

SUMMARY

Learning objective 1: Define the concept of acute medical illness and explore demographics, risk factors and social determinants associated with the typical acute medical client.

Acute medical conditions are described as the sudden onset of an illness that is unpredicted, of short duration and often requiring hospitalisation. Clients across all age groups who have a medical condition will at some stage suffer from an acute exacerbation. This may result from the primary condition or may be associated with a secondary condition. Clients over the age of 65 are more likely to require hospitalisation. This can have significant impacts on clients, and it is vital for nurses to be involved with the care of the client from the emergency department through to the ward, and onto discharge to either a rehabilitation setting or home and long-term management.

Learning objective 2: Discuss sociocultural influences on client perceptions of health and illness and the development of cultural competency among healthcare professionals.

Social determinants of health and their effect upon patient care and the health society are multifaceted. Social determinants of health can include socioeconomic status, transport, race/culture, education, early life, disability, food and nutrition, social support, genetics and responses by the health system to the person with disease (AIHW, 2016c; Mitrou et al., 2014; WHO, 2018). As a nurse, it is essential to consider these determinants when planning interventions for a client's care. The provision of patient-centred communication and effective discharge planning is therefore integral to the medical client.

Learning objective 3: Explore the nursing assessment, interventions and management of the acute medical client with reference to the paediatric, elderly and bariatric client.

Nurses are a crucial part of the multidisciplinary team caring for clients with medical conditions, and the focus of a team approach is to provide holistic patient-centred care. Shared decision-making is integral to treatment of chronic disease, and it is important for nurses to advocate for the inclusion of the client and their family/carers in this process. Following hospitalisation, the significance of effective discharge planning is again highlighted in this chapter as an important role of the nurse.

Learning objective 4: Understand the impact of comorbidities on the care of the acute medical client.

Comorbidities for the medical client increase the chance of acute hospitalisations and prolong hospital stays. The economic burden caused by this is significant for policy-makers; however, the impact upon the client and their family cannot be quantified.

Learning objective 5: Understand the importance of chronic illness management for achieving good outcomes for the acute medical client.

Chronic illness and acute exacerbation were presented in this chapter to highlight that chronicity cannot be typified by older age. Nurses must consider the impact of the age span trajectory for care of chronic conditions and the medical client. Acute hospitalisations for chronic illness treatment and management are common; however, exacerbation management for acute presentations of medical conditions can be complex.

REVIEW QUESTIONS

4.1 Why are considerations of age in relation to the acute medical client important for nurses to understand?

4.2 Why do nurses need to understand the efficacious and safe use of medicines?

4.3 What knowledge and skills should nurses learn to provide care for a client with comorbidity?

4.4 Which members of the multidisciplinary team should be included in the care of the acute medical client?

4.5 As nurses, how can we begin to gain an awareness of our own cultural beliefs to ensure they are not assumed to be all people's beliefs?

4.6 What strategies can a nurse practise in order to stay present with a client during uncomfortable communications?

RESEARCH TOPIC

You are a nurse in a hospital on a medical ward caring for William Jones, a 79-year-old man who has been diagnosed with an exacerbation of his COPD. William has a past medical history of hypertension, angina, osteoarthritis and type 2 diabetes. William is to be discharged home and he lives alone. What is the current evidence supporting best practice for effective discharge from hospital? Use the following resources to jumpstart your research:

Braet, A., Weltens, C. & Sermeus, W. (2016). Effectiveness of discharge interventions from hospital to home on hospital readmissions: A systematic review. *JBI Database of Systematic Reviews & Implementation Reports*, 14(2), 106–73.

Kamermayer, A.K., Leasure, A.R. & Anderson, L. (2017). The effectiveness of transitions-of-care interventions in reducing hospital readmissions and mortality: A systematic review. *Dimensions of Critical Care Nursing*, 36(6), 311–16.

FURTHER READING

Advance Care Planning (2018). Website. Retrieved from http://www.advancecareplanning .org.au/for-health-and-care-workers/starting-the-conversation.

AMH (2018). *Australian Medicines Handbook*. Adelaide: Australian Medicines Handbook.

Australian Commission on Safety and Quality in Health Care (ACSQHC) (2018). *National Safety and Quality Health Service (NSQHS) Standards*. Retrieved from https://www .safetyandquality.gov.au/publications/national-safety-and-quality-health-service-standards.

National Blood Authority (NBA) (2018). Website. Retrieved from https://www.blood.gov.au.

NPS MedicineWise (2018). Website. Retrieved from https://www.nps.org.au.

Nursing Council of New Zealand (2002/2011). *Guidelines for Cultural Safety, the Treaty of Waitangi and Māori Health in Nursing Education and Practice. Te whakarite i ngaā mahi tapuhi kia tiakina ai te haumaru aā-iwi*. Wellington: Nursing Council of New Zealand.

World Health Organization (2014). *Global Status Report on Noncommunicable Diseases*. Retrieved from http://www.who.int/nmh/publications/ncd-status-report-2014/en.

REFERENCES

Australian Bureau of Statistics (2008). *Australian Social Trends: Health and Socioeconomic Disadvantage*. Cat. no. 4102.0. Retrieved from http://www.abs.gov.au/AUSSTATS/abs@.nsf/Lookup/4102.0Main+Features30Mar+2010.

—— (2011). *Measures of Socioeconomic Status*. Cat. no. 1244. 0.55.001. Retrieved from http://www.ausstats.abs.gov.au/Ausstats/subscriber.nsf/0/367D3800605DB064CA2578B60013445C/$File/1244055001_2011.pdf.

Australian Centre for Asthma Monitoring (ACAM) (2011). *Asthma in Australia 2011*. Retrieved from http://www.aihw.gov.au/publication-detail/?id=10737420159.

Australian Commission on Safety and Quality in Health Care (ACSQHC). (2018a). *Safety and Quality Improvement Guide Standard 7: Blood and Blood Products*. Retrieved from https://www.safetyandquality.gov.au/publications/safety-and-quality-improvement-guide-standard-7-blood-and-blood-products-october-2012.

—— (2018b). *National Safety and Quality Health Service Standards*. Retrieved from https://www.safetyandquality.gov.au/our-work/clinical-communications.

Australian Institute of Health and Welfare (AIHW). (2012a). *Indicators for Chronic Diseases and their Determinants*. Canberra: AIHW.

—— (2012b). *Risk Factors Contributing to Chronic Disease*. Cat. no. PHE 157. Canberra: AIHW. Retrieved from http://www.aihw.gov.au/publication-detail/?id=10737421466.

—— (2014). *Australia's Health 2014*. Cat. no. AUS 178. Canberra: AIHW.

—— (2015). 1 in 5 Australians affected by multiple chronic diseases. Retrieved from http://www.aihw.gov.au/media-release-detail/?id=60129552034.

—— (2016a). *Australian Burden of Disease Study: Impact and Causes of Illness and Death in Australia 2011*. Canberra: AIHW. Retrieved from http://www.aihw.gov.au/publication-detail/?id=60129555173.

—— (2016b). *Admitted Patient Care 2014–15: Australian Hospital Statistics*. Cat. no. HSE 172. Canberra: AIHW.

—— (2016c). *Australia's Health 2016*. Cat. no. AUS 178. Canberra: AIHW. Retrieved from https://www.aihw.gov.au/reports/australias-health/australias-health-2016/contents/determinants.

—— (2017). *Chronic Diseases*. Canberra: AIHW. Retrieved from http://www.aihw.gov.au/chronic-diseases.

BloodSafe (2012). *Flippin' Blood: A BloodSafe Flip Chart to Help Make Transfusion Straightforward*. Sydney: BloodSafe and the Australian Red Cross. Retrieved from http://resources.transfusion.com.au/cdm/ref/collection/p16691coll1/id/20.

Budnitz, D.S., Lovegrove, M.C., Shehab, N. & Richards, C.L. (2011). Emergency hospitalizations for adverse drug events in older Americans. *New England Journal of Medicine*, 365(21), 2002–12.

Chang, E. & Johnson, A. (2015). *Chronic Illness and Disability* (2nd ed.). Sydney: Elsevier.

Chewning, B., Bylund, C.L., Shah, B., Arora, N.K., Gueguen, J.A. & Makoul, G. (2012). Patient preferences for shared decisions: A systematic review. *Patient Education and Counseling*, 86(1), 9–18.

Corless, L., Buckley A. & Mee, S. (2016). Power inequality between patients and nurses. *Nursing Times*, 112(12–13), 20–1.

Department of Health (2017). Chronic conditions are the leading cause of illness, disability and death in Australia. Retrieved from http://www.health.gov.au/internet/main/publishing.nsf/content/chronic-disease.

Department of Health Victoria (2012). *Best Care for Older People Everywhere: The Toolkit.* Melbourne: Victorian Government. Retrieved from www.health.vic.gov.au/older.

Deravin-Malone, L. & Anderson, J. (2016). *Chronic Care Nursing.* Melbourne: Cambridge University Press.

Estes, M.E., Calleja, P., Theobald, K. & Harvey, T. (2016). *Health Assessment and Physical Examination* (2nd ed.). Melbourne: Cengage.

Gilbert, P. (2010). *The Compassionate Mind: A New Approach to Life's Challenges.* Oakland, CA: New Harbinger.

Gruneir, A., Bronskill, S.E., Maxwell, C.J., … Wodchis, W.P. (2016). The association between multimorbidity and hospitalization is modified by individual demographics and physician continuity of care: A retrospective cohort study. *BMC Health Services Research*, 16, 154.

Health Quality and Safety Commission New Zealand (HQSCNZ) (2017). *National Medication Chart.* Retrieved from: http://www.hqsc.govt.nz/our-programmes/ medication-safety/projects/national-medication-chart.

Institute of Medicine (US) Committee on Quality of Health Care in America (2011). *Crossing the Quality Chasm: A New Health System for the 21st Century.* Washington, DC: National Academies Press.

International Family Nursing Association (IFNA) (2015). IFNA Position Statement on Generalist Competencies for Family Nursing Practice. Retrieved from https://internationalfamilynursing.org/2015/07/25/ifna-position-statement-on- generalist-competencies-for-family-nursing-practice-2.

Kitson, A., Marshall, A., Basset, K. & Zeitz, K. (2013). What are the core elements of patient-centred care? A narrative review and synthesis of the literature from health policy, medicine and nursing. *Journal of Advanced Nursing*, 69(1), 4–15.

Levett-Jones, T., Gilligan, C., Outram, S. & Horton, G. (2014). Key attributes of patient safe communication. In T. Levett-Jones (ed.), *Critical Conversations for Patient Safety: An Essential Guide for Health Professionals.* Sydney: Pearson.

Manley, K., Hills, V. & Marriot, S. (2011). Person-centred care: Principle of Nursing Practice B. *Nursing Standards*, 25(31), 35–7.

Martinez, M. (2016). *The Mindbody Code.* Boulder, CO: Sounds True.

Mitrou, F., Cooke, M., Lawrence, D., Povah, D., Mobilia, E., Guimond, E. & Zubrick, S.R. (2014). Gaps in Indigenous disadvantage not closing: A census cohort study of social determinants of health in Australia, Canada, and New Zealand from 1981– 2006. *BMC Public Health*, 14(1), 201.

National Advisory Committee on Health and Disability (NHC) (2007). *Meeting the Needs of People with Chronic Conditions. Häpai te whänau mo ake ake tonu.* Wellington: NHC. Retrieved from https://www.health.govt.nz/publication/meeting-needs- people-chronic-conditions-0.

National Health and Hospitals Reform Commission (NHHRC) (2009). *A Healthier Future for All Australians: Final Report of the National Health and Hospitals Reform Commission.* Canberra: Commonwealth of Australia.

National Health and Medical Research Council (NHMRC) (2013). *Clinical Guidelines for the Management of Overweight and Obesity in Adults, Adolescents and Children in Australia.* Retrieved from https://www.nhmrc.gov.au/guidelines-publications/n57.

Nursing Council of New Zealand (NCNZ) ([2007] 2016). *Competencies for Registered Nurses.* Retrieved from http://www.nursingcouncil.org.nz/Nurses.

Nursing and Midwifery Board of Australia (NMBA) (2016). *Registered Nurse Standards for Practice*. Melbourne: Nursing & Midwifery Board of Australia. Retrieved from http://www.nursingmidwiferyboard.gov.au/Codes-Guidelines-Statements/ Professional-standards.aspx.

Richardson, S. & Williams, T. (2007). Why is cultural safety essential in health care? *Medical Law*, 26(4), 699–707.

Rossiter, R., Scott, R. & Walton, C. (2014). Key attributes of therapeutic communication. In T. Levett-Jones (ed.), *Critical Conversations for Patient Safety: An Essential Guide for Health Professionals*. Sydney: Pearson.

Steinman, M.A., Handler, S.M. & Gurwitz, J.H. (2011). Beyond the prescription: Medication monitoring and adverse drug events in older adults. *Journal of the American Geriatrics Society*, 59(8), 1513–20.

Wagner, E.H., Davis, C., Schaefer, J., Von Korff, M. & Austin, B. (1999). A survey of leading chronic disease management programs: Are they consistent with the literature? *Managing Care Quality*, 7(3), 56–66.

Wallace, E., Salisbury, C., Guthrie, B., Lewis, C., Fahey, T. & Smith, S. (2015). Managing patients with multimorbidity in primary care. *British Medical Journal*, 350, h176. doi:10.1136/bmj.h176.

World Health Organization (WHO) (2014). Global status report on noncommunicable diseases. Retrieved from http://www.who.int/nmh/publications/ncd-status-report-2014/en

—— (2018). About the WHO. Retrieved from http://www.who.int/en.

Acute respiratory conditions

5

Melissa Johnston, Amali Hohol
and Grant Williams-Pritchard

LEARNING OBJECTIVES

At the completion of this chapter, you should be able to:

1 demonstrate understanding of the underlying pathophysiology, risk factors and incidence of common acute respiratory conditions
2 describe a comprehensive nursing assessment for the patient with common acute respiratory conditions
3 utilise comprehensive assessment findings to plan and develop evidence-based management strategies
4 describe patient education and discharge planning interventions required to assist a person with acute respiratory conditions
5 understand the concepts of multidisciplinary collaboration, cultural awareness and patient-centred care in caring for patients with acute respiratory conditions.

Introduction

Acute respiratory conditions are a common occurrence within the acute care setting, and alterations of the respiratory system not only increase the number of hospitalisations in Australia and New Zealand, but also greatly contribute to mortality rates (McDonald & Penola, 2015). More broadly, the global burden of respiratory disease is significant. For nurses to provide quality patient care, a thorough understanding of the common acute respiratory conditions is vital, as the role of the respiratory nurse has expanded to include a range of advanced practice skills (Ferkol & Schraufnagel, 2013). Nurses and other health professionals must appreciate that a vast range of acute respiratory conditions exist, and that it is through understanding disease processes and carefully and systematically examining the clinical presentation of the patient that best-practice treatment strategies are identified and implemented (Schraufnagel & Turino, 2010).

This chapter discusses several key elements of the care of the acute respiratory patient. This includes the underlying pathophysiology of a range of acute respiratory conditions, as knowledge of the physiological changes that occur to the respiratory system in the presence of respiratory illness is important in order to better manage presenting symptoms. Furthermore, the role of the acute care nurse in the assessment, planning and treatment of acute respiratory conditions will be explored to encourage the application of holistic nursing care in the acute setting, promote the integration of preventative measures into treatment plans and minimise the impact of respiratory illness on the patient.

NURSING STANDARDS

The following identifies the national competency standards for the registered nurse from the Nursing and Midwifery Board of Australia (NMBA) and the Nursing Council of New Zealand (NCNZ) that are addressed in this chapter.

Australian Registered Nurse Standards for Practice

Standard 1: Thinks critically and analyses nursing practice

Standard 2: Engages in therapeutic and professional relationships

Standard 3: Maintains the capability for practice

Standard 4: Comprehensively conducts assessments

Standard 5: Develops a plan for nursing practice

Standard 6: Provides safe, appropriate and responsive quality nursing practice

Standard 7: Evaluates outcomes to inform nursing practice

(NMBA, 2016)

An evidence-based practice framework is an essential component of the criteria in this standard; the utilisation of the best available evidence presented on the care and management of acute respiratory conditions will assist registered nurses to make decisions and provide safe quality nursing care for acute respiratory patients. In addition, a person-centred approach to the care of the acute respiratory patient is required to facilitate multidisciplinary collaboration and improve patient outcomes. Reflection is an essential skill for nurses to develop their practice, assist in consolidating their knowledge and provide culturally competent care for acute respiratory conditions.

New Zealand: Competencies for Registered Nurses

Competency 1.1: Accepts responsibility for ensuring that his/her nursing practice and conduct meet the standards of the professional, ethical and relevant legislated requirements

Competency 1.2: Demonstrates the ability to apply the principles of the Treaty of Waitangi/ Te Tiriti o Waitangi to nursing practice

Competency 1.5: Practises nursing in a manner that the health consumer determines as being culturally safe

Competency 4.1: Collaborates and participates with colleagues and members of the health care team to facilitate and coordinate care

Competency 4.2: Recognises and values the roles and skills of all members of the health care team in the delivery of care

(NCNZ, [2007] 2016)

Pathophysiology

Acute respiratory conditions constitute a variety of diseases that involve rapid pathophysiological changes to both the airways and lung parenchyma (alveoli). These conditions ultimately tend to affect gas exchange, often resulting in decreased plasma oxygen (hypoxaemia) and increased plasma carbon dioxide (hypercapnia). In some instances, the patient will be experiencing an acute crisis – for example, a tension pneumothorax. In other cases, the patient will be suffering from an acute exacerbation of a chronic condition, such as asthma or chronic obstructive pulmonary disease (COPD) (Criner, 2013). Acute respiratory conditions will generally develop over minutes to hours, and often the individual will present with extreme symptoms as intrinsic compensatory mechanisms have not had sufficient time to adapt to the altered respiratory system (Criner, 2013). Therefore, well-developed clinical skills are required to ensure positive patient outcomes.

Acute respiratory conditions – A range of conditions that affect either the upper or lower respiratory tract and generally develop over minutes to hours.

Asthma

It is estimated that over 2.5 million, or one in ten, Australians have asthma (National Asthma Council Australia, 2016a). Asthma is generally considered a chronic respiratory disease with acute exacerbations, known as asthma flare-ups or 'asthma attacks' (National Asthma Council Australia, 2016a). Asthma flare-ups are hypersensitivity reactions triggered by external (e.g. moulds or animal dander) or internal (e.g. exercise or cold air) stimuli (Grossman & Porth, 2014). With external or allergic asthma, the allergen stimulates activation of mast cell degranulation, resulting in the release of a suite of inflammatory mediators, including histamine and prostaglandins (Copstead & Banasik, 2013). Ultimately, asthmatic reactions cause three main changes in the large airways: parasympathetic stimulated constriction of smooth muscle; increased vascular permeability leading to mucosal oedema; and increased mucus production (Grossman & Porth, 2014). This combination of changes can result in severe airway obstruction. The airway obstruction – whether partial or total – results in a number of common clinical manifestations. For instance, there is a subjective awareness that breathing requires an increased amount of effort, commonly known as dyspnoea (Bullock & Hales, 2013). The dyspnoea, along with a non-productive cough, may be the result of irritation of the airway receptors by the increased presence of mucus. Upon auscultation, a high-pitched wheeze is often evident as expired air rushes through the narrowed bronchioles. Partial obstruction may result in hyperinflation as air becomes trapped in the lower airways, while with total obstruction the trapped air eventually diffuses out, leading to collapse of the affected lung region (VanMeter, Hubert & Gould, 2014). In both cases, the subsequent hypoxaemia reduces oxygen delivery to tissues, which is further exacerbated by the increased oxygen demand of over-worked respiratory accessory muscles. The reduced oxygen content of the blood also results in central cyanosis, characterised by a blue or purple discolouration of the tongue, lips and mucus membranes. Finally, the reduced diffusion of carbon dioxide out of the blood may cause respiratory acidosis (VanMeter, Hubert & Gould, 2014).

Respiratory infections

Infections of the respiratory system are initially categorised as affecting the upper or lower respiratory tract. More specifically, they can be described on the basis of the exact structures they affect – for example, rhinitis (nose), bronchitis (bronchi) and pneumonia (lung parenchyma = alveoli and bronchioles). These infections may be caused by a virus, bacterium or fungus (VanMeter, Hubert & Gould, 2014).

Pneumonia, a common respiratory infection, is categorised by inflammation of the lung parenchyma, usually caused by pathogens but occasionally due to aspiration of irritating substances such as gastric contents (Bullock & Hales, 2013). In 2012, pneumonia accounted for over 77 500 hospitalisations and 1.7 per cent of deaths in Australia (ABS, 2012; Lung Foundation Australia, 2017). For those aged 65 years and older, hospital stays averaged thirteen days (Lung Foundation Australia, 2017). Regardless of the cause (infection or aspirated irritant), epithelial damage triggers inflammation and subsequent alveolar oedema. With excessive parenchymal inflammation, consolidation may develop due to the accumulation of exudate and cellular debris (Bullock & Hales, 2013). The build-up of fluid in the alveoli leads to decreased diffusion of oxygen into the pulmonary capillaries and several clinical manifestations often seen with pneumonia: hypoxaemia, tachypnoea, dyspnoea and tachycardia (Bullock & Hales, 2013). The pulmonary oedema of the airways often produces a productive cough (especially if caused by bacterial infection) and crackles (rales) upon inspiration as blocked airways are forced open.

Acute respiratory distress syndrome

The incidence of acute respiratory distress syndrome (ARDS) is relatively low at about 34 cases per 100 000 persons; however, the hospital mortality rate can be as high as 40 per cent (Walkey et al., 2012). ARDS is an acute interstitial lung disease caused by either pulmonary (e.g. pneumonia or aspiration of gastric contents) or extrapulmonary (e.g. severe sepsis or pancreatitis) causes (Bullock & Hales, 2013). During the initial inflammatory stage of ARDS, fluid rich in plasma proteins, neutrophils and inflammatory cytokines accumulates in the interstitium and alveoli (Grossman & Porth, 2014). There is decreased production of surfactant and increased deposition of collagen fibres, both leading to increased stiffness of the lung (Walkey et al., 2012). The combination of alveolar oedema and diminished lung compliance results in hypoxaemia, dyspnoea and cyanosis.

Acute respiratory failure

Acute respiratory failure (ARF) is defined as an inadequate exchange of gases required to meet the metabolic demands of the body at rest, and is the end result of many pulmonary disorders rather than a specific disease. The two types of ARF are described in Table 5.1.

Table 5.1   Types of acute respiratory failure

Type	Causes
Type I Hypoxaemic (PaO_2 <60 mmHg)	Decreased partial pressure of oxygen in inspired air • Breathing at altitude Decreased ventilation • Bronchoconstriction • Atelectasis (alveolar collapse) Decreased perfusion • Reduced blood flow to pulmonary capillaries – pulmonary embolism Decreased rate of oxygen diffusion • Pulmonary oedema – pneumonia and ARDS

Type II
Hypercapnic/hypoxaemic
($PaCO_2$>50 mmHg,
PaO_2 <60 mmHg)
	Decreased ventilation
	Reduced central ventilatory drive
	• Brain stem compression, overdose of depressant
	  drugs (e.g. anaesthetics)
	Decreased neuromuscular transmission
	• Spinal cord injury, multiple sclerosis and myasthenia
	  gravis
	Musculoskeletal conditions
	• Altered spine curvature – kyphoscoliosis
	• Reduced function of respiratory muscles – fatigue
	Inability to expand lungs
	• Pneumothorax and morbid obesity

Sources: Bullock and Hales (2013); Matthay and Slutsky (2016).

The clinical manifestations of ARF are consistent with hypoxaemia and include cyanosis, fatigue, dyspnoea, restlessness, confusion and cardiovascular effects such as tachycardia and increased blood pressure (Grossman & Porth, 2014).

Comprehensive respiratory assessment of the acute care patient

Acute respiratory illness can potentially be life threatening. It is imperative that nurses and allied health professionals can identify clinical signs that indicate a serious respiratory condition (Talley & O'Connor, 2014), such as those outlined in Table 5.2. Purposeful and skilled clinical assessment is what guides clinical management, determines treatments and prevents adverse events from occurring. Using only clinical data gathered from traditional

Respiratory assessment
– The evaluation of the function and condition of a patient's respiratory system, which includes a number of physical examination skills such as inspection, palpation, percussion and auscultation.

vital signs is inadequate, so comprehensive **respiratory assessment** is required to prevent the patient deteriorating from a potentially preventable cause (Elliot & Coventry, 2012). Nurses should recognise that the primary survey should lead the assessment process to ensure that essential information about the patient is identified, and that treatment strategies can be determined in order of clinical priority. Once the patient is stable, the clinician should then progress into a more focused secondary assessment (Schoenwald & Douglas, 2017).

Table 5.2 Common symptoms of respiratory distress

Cyanosis
Reduced SpO$_2$
Inability to speak in sentences
Tachycardia
Increased drowsiness
Reduced air entry/silent lung fields
Use of accessory muscles
Significantly increased or decreased respiratory rate
Chest trauma
Stridor

Source: Adapted from Elliot and Coventry (2012).

Patient history

A comprehensive respiratory assessment looks beyond the act of respiration. Respiratory assessment should commence with a thorough patient history, including presenting respiratory problems, symptoms, and personal and family history (Ringdal & Gullick, 2016). Careful questioning on the topic of dysponea is fundamental, and exploring the characteristics of breathlessness can assist in diagnosis (Talley & O'Connor, 2014). The duration, type and associated factors relating to a cough should be identified, while the colour, consistency and amount of sputum produced must be determined (Elliot & Coventry, 2012). Identification of whether the patient has suffered any chest pain associated with respiration, or haemoptysis, is important as both symptoms can indicate a serious respiratory problem (Ringdal & Gullick, 2016; Talley & O'Connor, 2014). In addition to the patient's health history, patient data involving the hands, face, trachea, cardiovascular system and further lung function must be gathered to ensure that all relevant information is identified (Talley & O'Connor, 2014). A structured approach should be employed when performing a physical examination using the techniques of inspection, palpation, auscultation and percussion.

Inspection, palpation, auscultation and percussion

When inspecting, rate, rhythm, symmetry and depth of respiration should be observed. Clinicians should be aware that even a slight alteration in rate can denote impending respiratory distress (Elliot & Coventry, 2012). Chest expansion should be symmetrical, and cyanosis (either peripheral or central) can be indicated via the patient's colour. Cyanosis of the lips and mouth are late but reliable signs of hypoxia, while pursed lips, nostril flaring and use of accessory muscles all evidence respiratory difficulty (Ringdal & Gullick, 2016;

Smith & Rushton, 2014). Examining the hands for signs of clubbing or staining can also provide relevant information on respiratory health (Talley & O'Connor, 2014).

The chest should first be palpated methodically for symmetry. Following this, palpate to detect tenderness, injury, subcutaneous emphysema and tactile fremitus, as these are all symptoms associated with respiratory illness. Skin temperature should be noted, as clammy, hot or cold skin is abnormal. Gentle palpation of the trachea is necessary to identify whether any deviation has occurred, thus indicating a life-threatening issue such as a tension pneumothorax (Ringdal & Gullick, 2016). Chest expansion should be assessed to identify reduced chest movement or respiratory fatigue, remembering that it is common for a patient with restrictive lung disease to have little to no chest expansion (Chellel, 2010).

When listening to lung sounds, a systematic approach should be used by auscultating from the lung apices to the bases, and comparing opposite sides of the chest (Eisel & Kent, 2017) (Figure 5.1). Often respiratory decline will be accompanied by abnormal breath sounds during either inspiration or expiration. Common abnormal respiratory sounds include wheezing, stridor, crackling or gurgling. While dissimilar, these auditory symptoms signify different types of airway obstruction. For example, bronchospasm, a narrowing of the airways, is a common symptom of asthma and is indicated by the presence of inspiratory and/or expiratory wheezing. Stridor, an abnormal high-pitched sound, can be associated with a partial airway obstruction of the larynx or trachea, and is more commonly heard on inspiration (Eisel & Kent, 2017).

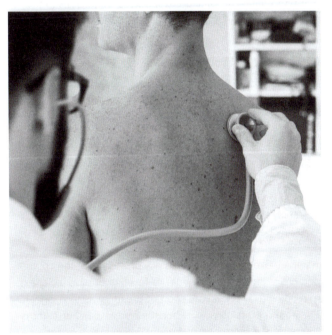

Figure 5.1 Auscultation

Percussion is performed to determine the density and aeration of the lungs. This assessment technique can assist in the identification of air, fluid or sputum consolidation in the lung spaces (Eisel & Kent, 2017). Commonly, percussion is performed indirectly: the middle finger of the non-dominant hand is placed against the patient's chest and the tip of the middle finger of the dominant hand strikes against the distal phalanx to elicit sound (Elliott, Aitken & Chaboyer, 2011). Resonance, a low-pitched sound, is heard over normal lungs, whereas a flat, high-pitched percussive sound may indicate a pleural effusion, or a dull, medium-pitched percussive sound may point to atelectasis or pulmonary oedema (Ringdal & Gullick, 2016).

Additional assessment

Spirometry – A method of determining lung function by measuring the amount of air inhaled in one breath.

Pulse oximetry – The measurement of oxygen saturation of arterial blood, which gives an indication of oxygenation status.

As Harle and Dudgeon (2012) explain, identification of the underlying pathophysiological cause of respiratory dysfunction can be achieved through in-depth clinical investigation. Lung function assessments and **spirometry** complement the physical assessment. Spirometry is particularly useful when differentiating between obstructive and restrictive lung disease (Harle & Dudgeon, 2012). **Pulse oximetry** is considered a reasonably accurate non-invasive method of measuring levels of arterial blood oxygenation; however, clinicians must remember that oxygen saturations can be within normal parameters, yet inadequate oxygenation may continue to be an unidentified problem (Harle & Dudgeon, 2012). Several factors can interfere with the reliability of pulse oximetry, including issues with signal transmission (e.g. motion artefact, reduced peripheral perfusion) or the presence of substances (e.g. acrylic nails) (WHO, 2011).

Arterial blood gas (ABG) sampling is considered a superior measurement of respiratory function to pulse oximetry, as it is more accurate and provides data on parameters of metabolic function. Information obtained via ABG sampling is often used to inform clinical decision-making, and for this reason nursing staff must be able to interpret ABG results accurately (Chellel, 2010). Chest x-ray, ultrasound, computed tomography, magnetic resonance imaging and ventilation/perfusion scanning are medical imaging techniques that, in conjunction with arterial blood gas (ABG) sampling and pathology, can be used to support the assessment and diagnosis of acute respiratory conditions (Talley & O'Connor, 2014).

SKILLS IN PRACTICE

Community acquired pneumonia

Samantha is a 41-year-old female who is admitted to the respiratory ward with community acquired pneumonia (*Streptococcus pneumoniae*). Samantha has adult onset asthma with no other medical history. She uses a regular preventer for her asthma and is also prescribed a reliever and reports she does not have to use her reliever often. She has an allergy to cats, but no medication allergies. Samantha is a childcare worker in a local childcare centre. She states she has been fatigued lately as she has been doing a lot of overtime for work.

This morning, when Samantha woke up, she felt generally unwell. Over the course of a few hours, she developed chills and an abrupt onset of fever, with pleuritic chest pain that was worse on deep breathing. She felt very short of breath, was tachypnoeic and developed a wheeze. She took several doses of her reliever as per her asthma action plan, which did not improve her shortness of breath. Following this, she presented to the emergency department. Samantha also reports having a productive cough, with mucopurulent sputum that is rusty in colour.

QUESTION

Samantha's presentation could initially be considered an exacerbation of her asthma. Explain how a comprehensive nursing assessment will assist in establishing a definite diagnosis, and which immediate and long-term nursing interventions should be implemented.

Care planning and nursing management of the acute respiratory patient

Care planning for the acutely ill respiratory patient cannot occur until after a comprehensive assessment has been completed (Shelledy & Peters, 2014). Treatment interventions are continuously reassessed and improvement in ventilation and oxygenation, pulmonary function, arterial blood gases or work of breathing may indicate that patient care needs to be altered accordingly. As Shelledy and Peters (2014) explain, treatment interventions are based on assessment findings and will generally include:

- therapy goals
- diagnostic testing
- medications to be administered
- special procedures
- method of oxygen delivery
- oxygen concentration
- secretion management
- lung expansion therapy.

Oxygen administration

Oxygen therapy is considered a drug, and as such should be prescribed by a medical physician at a dose expected to achieve a desired outcome (a specific oxygen saturation range). It is important that this be determined, as both insufficient and excessive administration of oxygen therapy can result in adverse patient outcomes (Pilcher & Beasley, 2015). For example, research evidence informs clinicians that oxygen has the potential to cause vasoconstriction of the coronary vessels, and in patients suffering from acute coronary syndrome this may worsen cardiac ischemia. Therefore, clinicians should not apply oxygen therapy until oxygenation has been confirmed via pulse oximetry (Asha, Kenneally & Hodge, 2015).

Oxygen administration is indicated when a patient is unable to maintain oxygen saturation at a specified target range on room air (Pilcher & Beasley, 2015). Low-flow and high-flow oxygen-delivery devices are available (Figures 5.2, 5.3 and 5.4), and the choice of device is dependent upon the individual patient's condition (Cone, 2016). Low-flow devices, such as nasal prongs, provide 1–3 L/min of flow, while high-flow devices, such as a Venturi mask, can provide oxygen at a rate of up to 15 L/min (Asha, Kenneally & Hodge, 2015). Nursing staff are responsible for ensuring that equipment is correctly fitted, as well as for management of the flow rate and monitoring of the patient's response to treatment (Williams & Hopper, 2015).

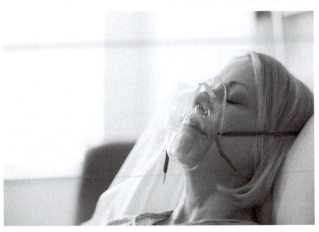

Figure 5.2   Hudson mask

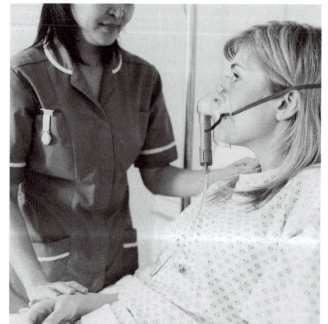

Figure 5.3   Venturi mask

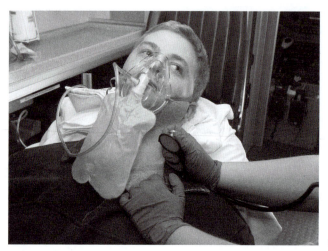

Figure 5.4   Non-rebreather mask

Enhancing airway patency and lung expansion

Suctioning – Use of negative pressure and a device to remove respiratory secretions obstructing the nasal and oral passages.

As Brinton and Fenton (2015) explain, the acutely unwell respiratory patient can lack the ability to clear respiratory secretions, including blood, saliva, vomitus and/or sputum. Under such circumstances, **suctioning** can be performed to minimise the incidence of infection, atelectasis and consolidation. Respiratory secretions can be present in the oropharyngeal space extending down into the trachea (Cone, 2016). It is necessary to remember that suctioning must only be undertaken when indicated, using safe and appropriate equipment, such as a Yanker sucker or suction catheter (Brinton & Fenton, 2015).

Patient positioning can greatly enhance airway patency, with both high and semi-Fowler's positions increasing chest expansion. Many acute respiratory patients also benefit from incentive spirometry, a patient-driven method of improving lung function and reducing the development of atelectasis. Incentive spirometry uses a specific breathing device designed to provide the patient with visual feedback so that they can quantify the depth of their breathing (Hess, 2016). Incentive spirometry is recommended to be used in conjunction with deep-breathing and coughing exercises, and is effective in managing asthma, COPD and respiratory infections as upper and lower respiratory secretions can be removed via effective coughing, while deep-breathing increases lung volumes and airway diameter, thus improving oxygenation (Hess, 2016; Scully, 2016).

Care of the acute asthmatic

As Wetzig, Blackwood and Currey (2016) discuss, primary management of the asthmatic patient should follow a tailored **asthma action plan** to prevent acute exacerbations, hospitalisation and respiratory arrest. When an acute event does occur, severity should be assessed and bronchodilators or beta2 agonists, such as salbutamol, administered as soon as possible, as these are considered first-line therapy (National Asthma Council Australia, 2016a; Wetzig, Blackwood & Currey, 2016). These can be administered via nebulisation or a metered dose inhaler (MDI) with a spacer, depending on the severity of the asthma. Nebulised mist treatments (NMT) are commonly prescribed for respiratory patients with severe or life-threatening severity, as they can be administered directly into the lungs (Williams & Hopper, 2015). Additionally, the moisture associated with nebulisation assists with clearance of pulmonary secretions (Scully, 2016), and intravenous administration of a beta2 agonist should only be used in patients where inhalation therapy may be considered ineffective (Chellel, 2010). Corticosteroids are recommended to commence within the first hour of an acute event. Oral corticosteroids such as prednisolone are preferred as they have been found to be as effective as intravenous corticosteroids during acute asthma in adults (National Asthma Council Australia, 2016a). In the care of the asthmatic patient, non-invasive ventilation strategies are preferable, as invasive ventilation treatments are more commonly associated with hyperinflation and bronchospasm, consequently increasing morbidity and mortality (Wetzig, Blackwood & Currey, 2016).

Asthma action plan – A written plan of instructions for ongoing management of asthma devised by the doctor and the patient, which also includes how to manage worsening asthma symptoms.

Care of the patient with an acute respiratory infection

Acute respiratory infections are categorised into upper respiratory tract infections (URTI) and lower respiratory tract infections (LRTI), and result from viruses, bacteria or fungi. URTIs include the common cold, bronchitis, sinusitis, pharyngitis and laryngitis, conditions that are often self-limiting and less acute than LRTIs. With LRTIs, the lungs are impacted and treatment is generally more complex. Pneumonia is a common LRTI requiring antibiotic therapy, oxygen therapy and intravenous fluid therapy (le May, 2015). With pneumonia, the patient can deteriorate rapidly, so nurses must be both attentive and observant. Furthermore, the choice of antibiotic therapy is dependent upon the type of respiratory condition, and a failure to correctly identify the illness can lead to inappropriate prescribing of antibiotics (Zoorob et al., 2012). It is also important for health professionals to understand that while antibiotic therapy may be beneficial, these medications contribute to the incidence of antimicrobial resistance (Zoorob et al., 2012).

The influenza virus significantly contributes to annual morbidity and mortality rates in Australia because of its highly contagious nature and ability to evolve over time. A range of symptoms manifest in cases of influenza, including chills, aches, loss of appetite, lethargy, cough and a sore throat. Pneumonia is a common complication of influenza, and in such occurrences antibiotic therapy generally is prescribed (Mathers, 2017). Clinicians and the public must understand that primary prevention is key when managing influenza, and that vaccines are widely available and generally extremely effective (Wetzig, Blackwood & Currey).

REFLECTIVE QUESTION

A patient with an acute exacerbation of COPD presents to the emergency department. Upon assessment, their oxygen saturations are 75 per cent on room air. Consider whether it is appropriate to provide supplemental oxygen to this patient, given that COPD patients are at greater risk of developing hypercapnic respiratory failure when administered supplemental oxygen therapy.

Patient education and discharge planning for the acute respiratory patient

Discharge planning – The process of developing a plan to maintain the patient's health status when they return home.

Patient education – Provision of information by health professionals to patients and their caregivers that will alter their health behaviours or improve their health status.

Nurses play an important role in providing **discharge planning** interventions and **patient education** for patients with an acute respiratory condition. Discharge planning and associated patient education can reduce readmission rates and the frequency of recurrent exacerbations in COPD patients. It is recommended that discharge planning commences within 24–48 hours of admission to the acute care environment (Yang et al., 2015).

The National Asthma Council Australia (2016b, p. 2) defines health literacy as an 'individual's capacity to obtain, process and understand basic health information and services they need to make appropriate health decisions'. It is important for nurses to assess the patient's health literacy prior to providing patient education/discharge planning, to enable the tailoring of these services to meet patients' specific needs. Poor health literacy is associated with a poor knowledge of medications, poor asthma control and incorrect inhaler technique (National Asthma Council Australia, 2016b).

Asthma

A written interim asthma action plan should be provided to the patient prior to discharge. Its purpose is to equip the patient with written instructions on how they can best manage their asthma following discharge until they are able to return to their usual GP for review (National Asthma Council Australia, 2016b) (Table 5.3).

Table 5.3   Summary of discharge planning and patient education requirements for patients with acute asthma

Discharge planning	Patient education
• Asthma action plan or interim asthma action plan • Ensure patient or carer can monitor and manage asthma at home • Provide a spacer if needed • Assess inhaler technique and adherence • Advise patient to make follow-up appointment with their GP • Consider referral to respiratory physician • Copy of discharge summary to be sent to patient's usual GP	• Correct technique for spacer or inhaler use • Current medications for asthma; relievers and preventers • General information about asthma • Asthma signs and symptoms

Source: National Asthma Council Australia (2016b).

The National Asthma Council Australia (2016b) recommends that an action plan be individualised for the patient and that it include medication dose, information and instructions for:

- oral corticosteroid course
- reliever in post-acute period and regular reliever regimen
- preventer
- what to do if symptoms get worse or recur.

COPD

Discharge planning for the patient following an acute exacerbation of COPD can be more complex due to the chronic nature of the disease. Discharge planning should therefore involve members of the multidisciplinary acute care team, the patient's regular general practitioner, the patient and their carer/family (Yang et al., 2015). As part of the discharge plan, a discharge pack – including the requirements in Table 5.4 – should be provided to the patient upon leaving the acute care setting.

Table 5.4 Summary of discharge planning and patient education requirements for acute exacerbations of COPD

Discharge planning	Patient education
• Pulmonary rehabilitation program referral • Assess social supports and domestic arrangements • Case conference with patient's GP • Plan for management of worsening symptoms • Arrange follow-up appointment with patient's GP	• General information about COPD • Spacer and inhaler use • Medications • Oxygen devices • Immunisations

Source: Yang et al. (2015).

Alison and colleagues (2017) recommend that patients with an acute exacerbation of COPD are referred to a pulmonary rehabilitation program prior to discharge, and that the program is commenced within two weeks of discharge. Outcomes from attendance of a pulmonary rehabilitation program for patients with COPD include increased exercise capacity, increased quality of life and a reduction in the occurrence of subsequent hospitalisations, mortality and adverse events (Alison et al., 2017).

Acute respiratory infection

It is important for the nurse to provide education on measures to prevent the spread of infection. This includes respiratory hygiene and cough etiquette, with an emphasis on these techniques while in the acute care setting in preparation for discharge. Topics such as covering the nose or mouth when coughing or sneezing; using tissues to contain respiratory secretions; correct disposal of tissues; hand hygiene following contact with respiratory secretions and contaminated surfaces; and keeping contaminated hands away from mucous membranes should be discussed with the patient (Koehler et al., 2010).

Deep breathing exercises and incentive spirometry should be demonstrated for the patient to assist in increasing vital capacity and pulmonary compliance, and these self-care behaviours should be continued for six to eight weeks following discharge (Carpenito, 2014; Farrell, 2017). Providing patient education on pathophysiology and the expected course of pneumonia may encourage the patient to comply with therapeutic regimens such as antibiotic therapy. The nurse needs to provide education on the correct use of antibiotics following discharge, instructing patients to take all doses that are prescribed for them, as antibiotic resistance can develop if medication is not taken consistently (Kulkarni & Dela Cruz, 2016). Discharge planning and education requirements are summarised in Table 5.5.

Table 5.5   Summary of discharge planning and patient education requirements for patients with an acute respiratory infection

Discharge planning	Patient education
• Advise to see GP if symptoms get worse or do not improve after three days of antibiotics • Arrange follow-up appointment with patient's GP • Continue deep breathing exercises for six to eight weeks • Antibiotics	• Pathophysiology and expected course of pneumonia • Measures to prevent spread of infection: respiratory hygiene and cough etiquette • Adequate hydration and nutrition • Quit smoking • Deep breathing exercises, incentive spirometry • Immunisations

Source: Carpenito (2014); Farrell (2017); Kulkarni and Dela Cruz (2016).

Patient-centred care and multidisciplinary collaboration

Patient-centred care (PCC) has many different definitions. The Nursing and Midwifery Board of Australia (2016) defines the principles of PCC as a collaborative and respectful partnership based on good communication, trust and understanding between the nurse and patient; the role of the family, community and the cultural and religious beliefs of the patient is also emphasised in PCC. The benefits of PCC are numerous: increased patient participation increases communication and leads to collaboration and shared decision-making between the patient and multidisciplinary health professionals (Delaney, 2017). These principles of PCC adapt the focus of clinical care to incorporate the needs of the patient, resulting in better patient experiences, decreased length of stay, decreased readmission rates and improved patient functional capacities (Delaney, 2017).

Cultural competence

There is an increasing need for nurses to provide culturally competent care. The continuing gap between the health status of minorities and other majority groups continues to be of concern, with communication barriers contributing to poorer health outcomes for minorities. In particular, morbidity and mortality from respiratory diseases among Aboriginal and

Torres Strait Islander people is higher than for other Australians across all age groups and regions; approximately 30 per cent of Aboriginal and Torres Strait Islander people report respiratory problems, with pneumonia or COPD being the most common causes of hospitalisation (Australian Health Ministers' Advisory Council, 2017; Australian Institute of Health and Welfare, 2014; National Asthma Council Australia, 2016b). Cultural diversity in patient groups is considerable, and this highlights the need for nurses to be culturally competent in the nursing care they provide to the diverse cultural groups for which they are responsible. An understanding of cultural beliefs and values of the patient is an essential component of providing PCC.

Some perceived barriers exist to providing culturally competent nursing care, and an increased awareness of these barriers can assist with the development of cultural competence in nursing practice. Barriers to providing culturally competent nursing care include diversity in patient populations, a lack of resources, and personal biases or prejudices (Hart & Mareno, 2013). The development of cultural competence in nursing practice is a process that involves education and reflection by the nurse. Reflection and self-examination of personal cultural beliefs and practices need to be explored to determine the influence these may have on nursing practice and the ability to provide culturally competent PCC (Elliott, Aitken & Chaboyer, 2011). It is important that the nurse respects others' beliefs and ideals, and does not let their own biases or prejudices influence others (Ignatavicius & Workman, 2013).

Hart and Mareno (2013) describe three principles of cultural competence: acknowledging the cultural differences of the patient and their family; being inclined to incorporate these beliefs and values into the management plan; and respecting and valuing the lifeways of differing cultures. In order to understand the values and beliefs of the patient, it is important for the nurse to build a positive therapeutic relationship with the patient and their family. This understanding will enable the translation of their values and beliefs into positive nursing interventions for the patient (Elliott, Aitken & Chaboyer, 2011). Douglas and colleagues (2014) agree, describing culturally competent nursing practice as nurses' knowledge about their own cultural beliefs and the impact these can have on patients, and the actions the nurse initiates to integrate culture into clinical practice.

Multidisciplinary collaboration

Multidisciplinary collaboration is described by Yeager (2005) as the education or knowledge generated from different professions working together to enable the provision of efficient patient-centred care. Furthermore, Yeager (2005) indicates the goal of collaboration within the **multidisciplinary team** being the development, delivery and evaluation of excellent PCC.

Patel (2016) refers to multidisciplinary collaboration as integrated respiratory care, indicating that it can enhance the patient's care experience, along with improving outcomes in long-term respiratory disease. Patel suggests that this model of care be considered for other acute respiratory conditions such as asthma, bronchiectasis, interstitial lung disease and respiratory failure. Vitacca and colleagues (2014) also conclude that multidisciplinary collaboration for treatment and care of those patients recovering from acute respiratory failure can reduce mortality and disability, and assist in preventing and managing crises (Yang et al., 2015). The multidisciplinary team for patients with acute respiratory conditions consists of many different health professionals, including but not limited to respiratory nurses, specialist physicians, physiotherapists, occupational therapists, social workers, pharmacists, dietitians and general practitioners (Yang et al., 2015).

Some examples of multidisciplinary collaboration in the care of a patient with acute respiratory conditions include physiotherapy and pharmacy. For example, collaboration with physiotherapists is essential in the management of bronchiectasis. Treatments to manage bronchiectasis include exercise, airway clearance manoeuvres, breathing exercises and the use of inhaled medications (Nicolson & Lee, 2017). As physiotherapists have an important role to play in a number of these treatments, including exercise programs, education of patients with airway clearance issues and breathing exercises, the nurse needs to collaborate with the physiotherapist to incorporate these recommendations into their nursing interventions.

Another example of multidisciplinary collaboration includes the role of the pharmacist in asthma management. Abdelnour and colleagues (2011) found that pharmacists, as part of the multidisciplinary team for the management of asthma, identified issues around medication adherence, side-effects, inhaler device use and asthma action plans. Through identification of these issues and multidisciplinary collaboration, the pharmacists could implement individual interventions around these issues to improve patient outcomes.

REFLECTIVE QUESTION

Consider the role of each of the members of the multidisciplinary team in caring for an acute asthmatic. As a nurse, consider your role in collaborating with each team member to provide safe, quality nursing care to your patient.

SUMMARY

Learning objective 1: Demonstrate understanding of the underlying pathophysiology, risk factors and incidence of common acute respiratory conditions.

The incidence of acute respiratory conditions ranges from very common (asthma and respiratory infections) to less common (acute respiratory distress syndrome). Some conditions, such as asthma, reduce alveoli ventilation through decreases in airway diameter, while pneumonia and acute respiratory distress syndrome trigger alveolar oedema and directly alter gas exchange. Most, if not all, respiratory conditions manifest symptoms such as dyspnoea and cough, and may ultimately result in acute respiratory failure.

Learning objective 2: Describe a comprehensive nursing assessment for the patient with common acute respiratory conditions.

Comprehensive respiratory nursing assessment can assist in guiding clinical management, determining treatment interventions and preventing the incidence of adverse events. A comprehensive respiratory assessment commences with a thorough patient history, incorporating physical examination techniques such as inspection, palpation, auscultation and percussion. Additional assessment investigations should be utilised to assist in the identification of the underlying pathophysiological cause to ensure enhanced patient outcomes.

Learning objective 3: Utilise comprehensive assessment findings to plan and develop evidenced-based management strategies.

Care planning and nursing management of an acutely ill respiratory patient should be based on the comprehensive respiratory assessment findings. Treatment interventions should continually be reassessed and altered accordingly. Common interventions for acute respiratory conditions include oxygen administration, secretion management, lung expansion techniques and medication administration. Management plans need to be individualised for each patient – for example, specific considerations in care of the acute asthmatic patient need to include a tailored asthma action plan, whereas care planning for an acute respiratory condition needs to consider inappropriate use of antibiotics.

Learning objective 4: Describe patient education and discharge planning interventions required to assist a person with acute respiratory conditions.

Nurses have an important role to play in facilitating discharge planning and patient education for acute respiratory patients. Patient education and discharge interventions should be tailored to each patient and their acute respiratory condition, taking into consideration the patient's health literacy so that individuals' needs are specifically met. Effective discharge planning can reduce readmission rates and the frequency of recurrent exacerbations for acute respiratory patients.

Learning objective 5: Understand the concepts of multidisciplinary collaboration, cultural awareness and patient-centred care in caring for patients with acute respiratory conditions.

Multidisciplinary collaboration and cultural awareness are essential components of patient-centred care. Increased participation of the patient and the emphasis of communication in patient-centred care lead to multidisciplinary collaboration and shared decision-making between the patient and the multidisciplinary team. Morbidity and mortality rates from respiratory diseases among Aboriginal and Torres Strait Islander people are higher than for other Australians across all age groups and regions, indicating that there is a growing need for nurses to be aware of cultural implications and develop cultural competence in their nursing practice.

REVIEW QUESTIONS

5.1 Describe three clinical manifestations that result from hypoxaemia.

5.2 Explain how comprehensive respiratory assessment guides the clinical management and treatment of a patient presenting with an acute lower respiratory infection.

5.3 Care plans are an important aspect of holistic respiratory care for the acutely ill asthmatic patient. Develop a care plan for a 22-year-old male suffering an acute exacerbation of asthma, and provide a rationale for each component of care.

5.4 Patient education and discharge planning are vital for acute respiratory conditions. Describe the patient education you would provide for Samantha, who has been admitted with community acquired pneumonia.

5.5 Explain the role of each member of the multidisciplinary team in the care of a patient with an acute respiratory condition.

RESEARCH TOPIC

Reflect on your cultural competence in nursing practice. What personal cultural beliefs and practices do you have, and how might these personal cultural beliefs and practices influence your nursing care for an Aboriginal patient with an acute respiratory condition?

FURTHER READING

Asthma Australia (2018). Website. Retrieved from https://www.asthmaaustralia.org.au.

Ferkol, T. & Schraufnagel, D. (2013). The global burden of respiratory disease. *Annals of the American Thoracic Society*, 11(3), 404–6.

National Australian Asthma Handbook (2016). Australia's national guidelines for asthma management. In *National Australian Asthma Handbook*. Retrieved from http://www.asthmahandbook.org.au.

REFERENCES

Abdelnour, M., Armour, C.L., Reddel, H.K. & Bosnic-Anticevich, S.Z. (2011). Multidisciplinary asthma care teams: The role of the specialist pharmacist. *Australian Pharmacist*, 30(8), 686.

Alison, J.A., McKeough, Z.J., Johnston, K., McNamara, R.J., Spencer, L.M., Jenkins, S.C., ... Holland, A.E. (2017). Australian and New Zealand pulmonary rehabilitation guidelines. *Respirology*, 22(4), 800–19.

Asha, S., Kenneally, J. & Hodge, A. (2015). Respiratory emergencies. In K. Curtis & C. Ramsden (eds), *Emergency and Trauma Care for Nurses and Paramedics*. Sydney: Elsevier, pp. 467–506.

Australian Bureau of Statistics (2012). Diseases of the respiratory system (J00-J99). Retrieved from http://www.abs.gov.au/ausstats/abs@.nsf/Lookup/by Subject/3303.0~2012~Main Features~Diseases of the Respiratory System (J00-J99)~10032.

Australian Health Ministers' Advisory Council (2017). *Aboriginal and Torres Strait Islander Health Performance Framework Report*. Canberra: AHMAC. Retrieved from https://www.pmc.gov.au/sites/default/files/publications/2017-health-performance-framework-report_0.pdf.

Australian Institute of Health and Welfare (AIHW) (2014). *Mortality from Asthma and COPD in Australia*. Cat. no. ACM 30. Canberra: AIHW. Retrieved from http://aihw.gov.au/WorkArea/DownloadAsset.aspx?id=60129548230.

Brinton, J. & Fenton, W. (2015). Clinical skills. In K. Curtis & C. Ramsden (eds), *Emergency and Trauma Care for Nurses and Paramedics*. Sydney: Elsevier, pp. 313–84.

Bullock, S. & Hales, M. (2013). *Principles of Pathophysiology*. Sydney: Pearson Australia.

Carpenito, L.J. (2014). *Nursing Care Plans* (6th ed.). Philadelphia, PA: Wolters Kluwer Health/Lippincott Williams & Wilkins.

Chellel, A. (2010). Respiratory assessment and care. In F. Creed & C. Spiers (eds), *Care of the Acutely Ill Adult*. Oxford: Oxford University Press, pp. 39–87.

Cone, K. (2016). Promoting oxygenation. In A. Perry, P. Potter & W. Ostendorf (eds), *Nursing Interventions and Clinical Skills* (6th ed.). St Louis, MO: Elsevier, pp. 356–99.

Copstead, L.E. & Banasik, J.L. (2013). *Pathophysiology*. St. Louis, MO: Elsevier.

Criner, G. (2013). Respiratory failure. In G. Criner & G. D'Alonzo (eds), *Critical Care Study Guide: Text and Review*. New York: Springer, pp. 200–21.

Delaney, L.J. (2017). Patient-centred care as an approach to improving health care in Australia. *Collegian*, 25(1), 119–23.

Douglas, M.K., Rosenkoetter, M., Pacquiao, D.F., Callister, L.C., Hattar-Pollara, M., Lauderdale, J., ... Purnell, L. (2014). Guidelines for implementing culturally competent nursing care. *Journal of Transcultural Nursing*, 25(2), 109–21.

Eisel, S.J. & Kent, B. (2017). Nursing assessment: Respiratory system. In D. Brown, H. Edwards, L. Seaton & T. Buckley (eds), *Lewin's Medical-Surgical Nursing: Assessment and Management of Clinical Problems*. Sydney: Elsevier, pp. 476–91.

Elliot, M. & Coventry, A. (2012). Critical care: The eight vital signs of patient monitoring. *British Journal of Nursing*, 21(10), 621–5.

Elliott, D., Aitken, L. & Chaboyer, W. (2011). *ACCCN's Critical Care Nursing* (2nd ed.). Sydney: Elsevier.

Farrell, M. (ed.) (2017). *Smeltzer & Bare's Textbook of Medical-surgical Nursing* (4th ed., Vol. 1). Sydney: Lippincott Williams & Wilkins.

Ferkol, T. & Schraufnagel, D. (2013). The global burden of respiratory disease. *Annals of the American Thoracic Society*, 11(3), 404–6.

Grossman, S. & Porth, C. (2014). *Porth's Pathophysiology: Concepts of Altered Health States*. Philadelphia, PA: Wolters Kluwer Health/Lippincott Williams & Wilkins.

Harle, I. & Dudgeon, D. (2012). Multidimensional assessment of dyspnoea. In S. Ahmedzai, D. Baldwin & D. Currow (eds), *Supportive Care in Respiratory Disease*. Oxford: Oxford University Press.

Hart, P.L. & Mareno, N. (2013). Cultural challenges and barriers through the voices of nurses. *Journal of Clinical Nursing*, 23, 2223–33.

Hess, D. (2016). Airway clearance and lung expansion therapy. In D. Hess, N. MacIntyre, W. Galvin & S. Mishoe (eds), *Respiratory Care: Principles and Practice* (3rd ed.). Burlington, MA: Jones & Bartlett Learning, pp. 352–79.

Ignatavicius, D.D. & Workman, L.M. (2013). *Medical-surgical Nursing* (7th ed.). St Louis, MO: Saunders-Elsevier.

Koehler, A., Baggoley, C., Christiansen, K., Coates, L., Collignon, P., Cooper, C. … Boardman, C. (2010). *Australian Guidelines for the Prevention and Control of Infection in Healthcare*. Canberra: National Health and Medical Research Council. Retrieved from https://www.nhmrc.gov.au/book/html-australian-guidelines-prevention-and-control-infection-healthcare-2010.

Kulkarni, H. & Dela Cruz, C. (2016). What is pneumonia? *American Journal of Respiratory and Critical Care Medicine*, 193(1), 1–11.

le May, A. (2015). *Adult Nursing at a Glance*. Chichester: Wiley Blackwell.

Lung Foundation Australia (2017). Pneumonia. Retrieved from http://lungfoundation.com.au/patient-support/other-lung-conditions/pneumonia.

Mathers, W. (2017). Nursing management: Upper respiratory. In D. Brown, H. Edwards, L. Seaton & T. Buckley (eds), *Lewis's Medical-Surgical Nursing: Assessment and Management of Clinical Problems* (4th ed.). Sydney: Elsevier, pp. 500–23.

Matthay, M. & Slutsky, A. (2016). Acute respiratory distress syndrome. In L. Goldman & A. Schafer (eds), *Goldman-Cecil Medicine* (25th ed.). Philadelphia, PA: Elsevier/Saunders, pp. 655–64.

McDonald, V. & Penola, D. (2015). Alterations of pulmonary function across the lifespan. In J. Craft & C. Gordon (eds), *Understanding Pathophysiology* (2nd ed.). Sydney: Elsevier, pp. 679–709.

National Asthma Council Australia (2016a). *Australian Asthma Handbook*. Version 1.2. Retrieved from http://www.asthmahandbook.org.au.

——(2016b). What is asthma? Retrieved from https://www.nationalasthma.org.au/understanding-asthma/what-is-asthma.

Nicolson, C. & Lee, A. (2017). *Bronchiectasis Toolbox*. Retrieved from http://bronchiectasis.com.au.

Nursing Council of New Zealand (NCNZ) ([2007] 2016). *Competencies for Registered Nurses*. Retrieved from http://www.nursingcouncil.org.nz/Nurses.

Nursing and Midwifery Board of Australia (NMBA) (2016). *Registered Nurse Standards for Practice*. Melbourne: Australian Health Practitioner Regulation Agency. Retrieved from http://www.nursingmidwiferyboard.gov.au/Codes-Guidelines-Statements/Professional-standards.aspx.

Patel, I. (2016). Integrated respiratory care. *Medicine*, 44(6), 398–99.

Pilcher, J. & Beasley, R. (2015). Acute use of oxygen therapy. *Australian Prescriber*, 38, 98–100.

Ringdal, M. & Gullick, J. (2016). Respiratory assessment and monitoring. In L. Aitken, A. Marshall & W. Chaboyer (eds), *ACCCN's Critical Care Nursing* (3rd ed.). Sydney: Elsevier, pp. 438–69.

Schoenwald, A. & Douglas, C. (2017). Undertaking a focused assessment: Physical assessment of body systems. In J. Crisp, C. Douglas, G. Rebeiro & D. Waters (eds), *Potter and Perry's Fundamentals of Nursing* (5th ed.). Sydney: Elsevier, pp. 578–621.

Schraufnagel, D. & Turino, G. (2010). The challenge. In D. Schraufnagel (ed.), *Breathing in America: Diseases, Process and Hope*. New York: American Thoracic Society, (pp. 259–82). Retrieved from https://www.thoracic.org/patients/patient-resources/breathing-in-america/resources/breathing-in-america.pdf.

Scully, N. (2016). Preserving oxygenation. In J. Crisp, C. Douglas, G. Rebeiro & D. Waters (eds), *Potter and Perry's Fundamentals of Nursing* (5th ed.). Sydney: Elsevier, pp. 1241–318.

Shelledy, D. & Peters, J. (2014). *Respiratory Care: Patient Assessment and Care Plan Development*. Burlington, VA: Jones & Bartlett Learning.

Smith, J. & Rushton, M. (2014). How to perform respiratory assessment. *Nursing Standard*, 30(7), 34–6.

Talley, N. & O'Connor, S. (2014). *Clinical Examination: A Systematic Guide to Physical Diagnosis* (7th ed.). Sydney: Elsevier.

VanMeter, K., Hubert, R.J. & Gould, B.E. (2014). *Gould's Pathophysiology for the Health Professions* (6th ed.). St Louis, MO: Elsevier/Saunders.

Vitacca, M., Paneroni, M., Peroni, R., Barbano, L., Dodaj, V., Piaggi, G., … Ceriana, P. (2014). Effects of a multidisciplinary care program on disability, autonomy, and nursing needs in subjects recovering from acute respiratory failure in a chronic ventilator facility. *Respiratory Care*, 59(12), 1863–71.

Walkey, A.J., Summer, R., Ho, V. & Alkana, P. (2012). Acute respiratory distress syndrome: Epidemiology and management approaches. *Clinical Epidemiology*, 4, 159–69.

Wetzig, S., Blackwood, B. & Currey, J. (2016). Respiratory alterations and management. In L. Aitken, A. Marshall & W. Chaboyer (eds), *ACCCN's Critical Care Nursing* (3rd ed.). Sydney: Elsevier, pp. 438–69.

Williams, L. & Hopper, P. (2015). *Understanding Medical Surgical Nursing* (5th ed.). Philadelphia, PA: F.A. Davis.

World Health Organization (2011). *Pulse Oximetry Training Manual*. Geneva: WHO. Retrieved from http://www.who.int/patientsafety/safesurgery/pulse_oximetry/who_ps_pulse_oximetry_training_manual_en.pdf.

Yang, I., Dabscheck, E., George, J., Jenkins, S., McDonald, C., McDonald, V., … Zwar, N. (2015). *COPD-X Plan: Australian and New Zealand Guidelines for the Management of Chronic Obstructive Pulmonary Disease*. Sydney: Lung Foundation and Thoracic Society of Australia and New Zealand. Retrieved from http://copdx.org.au.

Yeager, S. (2005). Interdisciplinary collaboration: The heart and soul of health care. *Critical Care Nursing Clinics of North America*, 17(2), 143–8.

Zoorob, R., Sidani, M., Fremont, R. & Kihlberg, C. (2012). Antibiotic use in acute upper respiratory tract infections. *American Family Physician*, 86(9), 817–22.

6 Acute cardiovascular conditions

Amali Hohol, Melissa Johnston,
Emma Luck and Grant Williams-Pritchard

LEARNING OBJECTIVES

At the completion of this chapter, you should be able to:

1   describe the pathophysiology of a range of acute cardiovascular conditions and identify risk factors that impact their prevalence and treatment
2   understand the common medical, interventional and surgical approaches to managing patients who are experiencing cardiovascular issues
3   define the role of acute cardiovascular nurse and the importance of critical thinking and evidence-based practice in the care of the acute cardiac patient
4   understand the importance of multidisciplinary collaboration and the role of the nurse in providing culturally competent person-centred care for patients with acute cardiovascular conditions
5   understand the nursing role in client education and discharge planning requirements for those with acute cardiovascular conditions.

Introduction

The World Health Organization (WHO, 2016) states that cardiovascular (CV) disease accounts for approximately 31 per cent of all annual global deaths, making it the leading cause of death worldwide. Acute CV conditions are commonly complex and multifaceted, and health professionals working within acute care areas are often required to make immediate and difficult clinical decisions to prevent loss of life (Tubaro et al., 2015). Clinicians must understand that many CV conditions are preventable, and that patient outcomes are highly dependent upon early diagnosis and appropriate treatment strategies (Tubaro et al., 2015). Nurses must therefore approach such situations with strong assessment techniques, appropriate evidence-based interventions and high levels of clinical competence to ensure positive patient outcomes (Humphreys & Cooper, 2011).

This chapter explores the underlying pathophysiology of a range of acute CV conditions, as an understanding of the pathophysiological alterations that occur in the presence of CV disease supports nurses to make sound cardiac care decisions based on a physiological rationale. A wide range of medical, interventional and surgical interventions can be used in the management of the acute cardiovascular patient, and several of these strategies will be explored. The nurse's role in caring for acutely ill cardiac patients will be explained, from the initial presentation phase through to discharge planning, highlighting the need for sound critical thinking skills and the application of evidence-based practice. To support the provision of holistic care, this chapter will also review the concepts of patient-centred care and cultural competence in the context of the acute CV patient.

Through the provision of evidence-based practice, nurses are supported in their ability to make clinically appropriate decisions for the acute CV patient. This ensures that nurses deliver high standards of nursing practice. Exploring the pathophysiology of acute CV conditions provides foundation knowledge and guides nursing interventions and treatment strategies. It is important to ensure that acute CV care delivery is safe, patient-centred, culturally appropriate and adheres to the legal and ethical frameworks which govern the nursing profession.

The following identifies the national competency standards for the registered nurse from the Nursing and Midwifery Board of Australia (NMBA) and the Nursing Council of New Zealand (NCNZ) that are addressed in this chapter.

Australian Registered Nurse Standards for Practice

Standard 1: Thinks critically and analyses nursing practice

Standard 2: Engages in therapeutic and professional relationships

Standard 3: Maintains the capability for practice

Standard 4: Comprehensively conducts assessments

Standard 5: Develops a plan for nursing practice

Standard 6: Provides safe, appropriate and responsive quality nursing practice

Standard 7: Evaluates outcomes to inform nursing practice

(NMBA, 2016)

NURSING STANDARDS

New Zealand: Competencies for Registered Nurses

Competency 1.1: Accepts responsibility for ensuring that his/her nursing practice and conduct meet the standards of the professional, ethical and relevant legislated requirements

Competency 1.2: Demonstrates the ability to apply the principles of the Treaty of Waitangi/ Te Tiriti o Waitangi to nursing practice

Competency 1.5: Practises nursing in a manner that the health consumer determines as being culturally safe

Competency 4.1: Collaborates and participates with colleagues and members of the health care team to facilitate and coordinate care

Competency 4.2: Recognises and values the roles and skills of all members of the health care team in the delivery of care

(NCNZ, [2007] 2016)

Pathophysiology and risk factors of acute cardiovascular conditions

Acute cardiovascular conditions – Affect the heart and blood vessels, and commonly have a rapid onset and short duration, and are life-threatening.

Acute cardiovascular conditions generally have a rapid onset and short duration, and are considered life-threatening (Mulryan, 2011). However, a patient with pre-existing chronic CV illness, such as heart failure, can suffer severe exacerbation of their disorder, which requires acute management (Argulian et al., 2012). Advances in acute cardiovascular care have resulted in improved treatment options, allowing for prolongation of patient life (Heras, Sionis & Price, 2015).

CV disease encompasses conditions that affect the heart and blood vessels. They often result in ischemia, a lack of blood supply to all or part of a tissue or organ. In an acute setting, CV disease may be life-threatening if the brain or heart are directly affected. **Atherosclerosis** and aneurysms are two of the most common disorders of the arterial circulation. While their pathogenesis may be chronic in nature, both can have acute exacerbations, producing a wide variety of manifestations, depending on the arteries affected. Diseases of the heart may affect any of its three layers (pericardium, myocardium and endocardium), and often result in decreased cardiac output (CO). As with arterial disorders, a decreased CO will reduce the blood supply to peripheral tissues and organs, thereby reducing their functional capacity.

Atherosclerosis – The development of atheromatous plaques, causing hardening and narrowing of the arteries.

Disorders of the arterial circulation

Atherosclerosis

Atherosclerosis is a form of blood vessel hardening that is characterised by the presence of atheromatous plaques in the tunica intima of medium and large-sized arteries (Grossman & Porth, 2014). These lesions consist of a diverse collection of cholesterol, calcium, smooth muscle cells and collagen fibres covered by a fibrous cap (Craft et al., 2015). Over time, the atherosclerotic plaques restrict blood flow and may cause ischemia. The ultimate consequences of atherosclerosis depend upon the arteries that are most affected, and may lead to myocardial infarction, cerebrovascular accidents or rupturing of aneurysms (Figure 6.1).

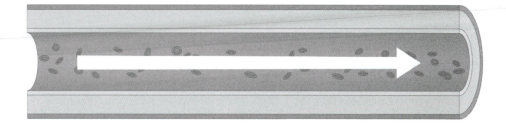

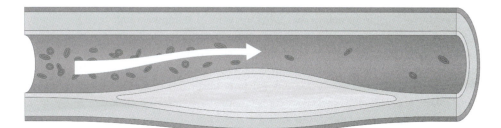

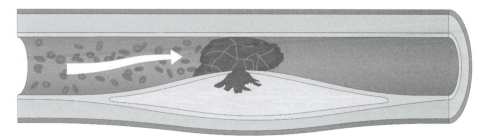

Figure 6.1   Stages of atherosclerosis

Aneurysms

An aneurysm is generally caused by the weakening of a blood vessel wall that results in localised dilation (VanMeter, Hubert & Gould, 2014). As the blood vessel expands and weakens, hypertension can exacerbate and accelerate the progression of the aneurysm. External structures, or tissue surrounding the aneurysm, may also be compressed as the vessel dilates (Grossman & Porth, 2014). As the arterial wall weakens, there is an increased risk of thrombus and emboli formation. Furthermore, blood flow to the distal artery may cease completely if the aneurysm is left untreated and ruptures. In this emergency situation, the lack of distal blood supply would be accompanied by a haemorrhage into nearby tissues (Grossman & Porth, 2014).

Diseases of the heart

Acute pericarditis

Acute pericarditis describes inflammation of the pericardium, which may be idiopathic (up to 90 per cent), or caused by a number of factors including infection, neoplasms and trauma (Doctor et al., 2017). The process of inflammation may lead to an accumulation of fluid in the pericardial cavity, known as a pericardial effusion (Grossman & Porth, 2014). With the pericardial cavity having a relatively small capacity, this increase in fluid can result in cardiac tamponade, a condition where the heart is compressed, making it difficult for the heart to relax and refill with blood (Grossman & Porth, 2014).

Acute coronary syndrome

The function of the myocardium is most often affected by decreases in blood supply to the coronary circulation caused by atherosclerosis, known as coronary artery disease (CAD) (Craft et al., 2015). **Acute coronary syndrome (ACS)** is an umbrella term used to describe a range of diseases that result in acute cardiac ischemia (unstable angina) or myocardial infarction (Lange & Hillis, 2012). ACS generally occurs when the fibrous cap of a previously formed plaque is dislodged, leading to **platelet aggregation** or thrombus formation (Lange & Hillis, 2012). On less common occasions, the occlusion may also be caused by coronary vasospasms, emboli or arteritis (Amsterdam et al., 2014). The subsequent degree of occlusion determines whether there is temporary injury or permanent death (infarction) of the myocardium. A transient or subtotal occlusion results in either unstable angina or non–ST-elevation myocardial infarction (NSTEMI). The distinguishing feature in this case is the elevation of cardiac biomarkers associated with NSTEMI due to the minimal necrosis of cardiac tissue (Grossman & Porth, 2014). With ST-elevation myocardial infarction (STEMI), however, there is complete occlusion of the artery resulting in transmural injury or infarction of the full myocardial thickness (Grossman & Porth, 2014). MI has many complications, including but not limited to cardiac arrhythmias, congestive heart failure and cardiogenic shock (Bangalore & Owlia, 2017).

Acute heart failure

Heart failure (HF) is characterised by the heart's inability to perfuse body tissues with a sufficient volume of blood under resting conditions. In the acute setting, there are two types of HF: newly arisen acute heart failure in a relatively healthy heart and acutely decompensated chronic heart failure (ADCHF) (Hummel et al., 2015). Newly arisen acute heart failure may be the consequence of previous cardiac events such as MI and cardiac tamponade (Newby, Grubb & Bradbury, 2014), while ADCHF is usually triggered by events such as arrhythmias and valvular dysfunction in diseased hearts (Hummel et al., 2015). In both conditions, the major manifestation is shortness of breath due to pulmonary oedema (Grossman & Porth, 2014).

Risk factors

There are several modifiable and non–modifiable risk factors common to many types of acute cardiovascular disease (CVD). Most risk factors listed are in relation to the chronic development of atherosclerosis and are outlined in Table 6.1.

Acute coronary syndrome (ACS) – The consequence of atherosclerotic plaque rupture or clot formation in the coronary arteries, which causes reduce blood flow to the myocardium.

Platelet aggregation – The adhesion of platelets to one another to create a thrombus at the site of vascular injury.

Table 6.1   Acute CV risk factors

Non-modifiable	Modifiable
• Age	• Smoking
• Gender	• High cholesterol
• Ethnicity	• Hypertension
• Family history	• Diabetes mellitus
• Social history	• Inactivity
	• Overweight and obese
	• Poor diet
	• Alcohol intake

Source: National Vascular Disease Prevention Alliance (2012).

Medical, interventional and surgical management of acute cardiovascular conditions

The management of acute CVD requires a differential diagnosis of the underlying patho-physiological process to determine the most effective treatment (Frachi & Angiolilo, 2015). With vascular occlusion resulting in myocardial ischemia or infarct, rapid reperfusion of the coronary vessels is required (Morrow, 2017; Topol & Teirstein, 2016). When the heart valve(s) are affected, they must be repaired or replaced to restore normal uni-directional cardiac blood flow (Morrow, 2017). If a conduction issue results in cardiac arrhythmia, the symptoms may either be medically managed or could warrant surgical intervention (Morrow, 2017). For acute CVD, pre-hospital delays are the largest contributor to poor prognosis, and the shorter the time between symptom onset and treatment, the less likely the patient is to experience long-term morbidity and mortality risks (Morrow, 2017).

Diagnosis

The diagnosis of acute cardiac abnormality will often utilise a combination of non-invasive and invasive tests or assessments. Although not an exhaustive list, the more common diagnostic tools include physical examination, cardiac markers, electrocardiogram (ECG), trans-esophageal echocardiogram (TOE), computerised tomography (CT) scan, and cerebral or cardiac angiogram (Crawford, 2010; Morrow, 2017). The selection of these diagnostic test(s) is predicated on the suspected origin and extent of vessel or tissue injury, and indicates whether medical, interventional or surgical treatment is most appropriate. Promptly diagnosing the underlying condition is paramount to the delivery of timely and effective treatment.

Medical management

Pharmacotherapy is effective in treating and managing a broad range of acute cardiac conditions. If the patient has ACS, then prescribed medications are intended to interrupt the process of platelet aggregation (Topol & Teirstein, 2016). When a blood vessel is damaged, platelets rush to the site to form a plug and mitigate endothelial damage; however, anti-platelet medications are used for the patient who has atherosclerosis to minimise exacerbation of the disease process. If the patient is experiencing abnormal cardiac conduction, resulting in arrhythmia or tachycardia, medication will be used to manage the heart rate. The most common medications to treat acute CVD include anti-hypertensives, anti-arrhythmics, anti-coagulants, anti-platelets, nitrates, opioids, statins and thrombolytics (Table 6.2).

Interventional management

The **interventional management** of acute CVD utilises both non-invasive and invasive techniques. Non-invasive intervention includes defibrillation and cardioversion, which are used to treat cardiac arrhythmias or tachycardias. The technique relies on the synchronised delivery of electrical shocks to the myocardium to restore normal sinus rhythm (Venes, 2013). The most common invasive technique is percutaneous coronary intervention (PCI), and this is the preferred treatment for STEMI as it aims

Interventional management – The use of cardiac specific non-invasive and invasive techniques used to manage acute cardiovascular conditions.

Table 6.2   Common medications used to treat acute CVD

Medication	Pharmacological action	Common examples
Anti-hypertensives	Manage elevated blood pressure and the complications associated with stroke, myocardial infarction and aneurysm (Black & Elliott, 2013).	• Angiotensin converting enzyme (ACE) inhibitor • Calcium channel blocker
Anti-arrhythmics (including beta-blockers)	Manage irregular heart rhythm and rate by affecting different phases of the cardiac action potential (Brahmajee & Baman, 2014).	• Metoprolol • Amiodarone • Verapamil • Digoxin
Anti-coagulants	Inhibit the coagulation of blood, but increase the risk of bleeding (Gaglia, Gurbel & Waksman, 2014).	• Heparin • Clexane
Anti-platelets	Decrease platelet aggregation, prevent thrombus formation (Kitchens, Kessler & Konkle, 2013), and used in the **primary prevention** and ongoing management of CV and cerebrovascular disease (Kitchens, Kessler & Konkle, 2013).	• Aspirin • Clopidogrel
Nitrates	Used for heart failure, hypertension and in the management of chest pain. Induce vasodilation, and can be administered via oral, sublingual, transdermal or intravenous injection (Bope & Kellerman, 2017).	• Isosorbide mononitrate • Glyceryl trinitrate
Opiates	Treat pain and distress, and reduce sympathetic nervous system activity. Additionally, opiates dilate peripheral blood vessels, thus reducing the workload on the heart (Keenan, 2011).	• Morphine
Statins	Used in the management of hypercholesterolemia (Xie & Zhou, 2017). Statins are effective in decreasing mortality for individuals with pre-existing CV, or those who are at high risk of developing CV.	• Atorvastatin • Simvastatin
Thrombolytics	Dissolve (lyse) blood clots and restore vascular patency by transforming plasminogen to plasmin. (Kitchens, Kessler & Konkle, 2013; Morrow, 2017). Thrombolytic medication is used to manage STEMI, stroke, pulmonary embolism and deep vein thrombosis (Kitchens, Kessler & Konkle, 2013). For acute CV presentation, primary thrombolysis is most effective when given within two to three hours of symptom onset, and is limited to a twelve-hour window for administration (Topol & Teirstein, 2016). **Secondary prevention** is then used to manage the patient, and prevent recurrence of coronary occlusion.	*First generation* • Streptokinase • Urokinase *Second generation* • Alteplase • Tenecteplase

Primary prevention – Implemented prior to disease onset, with the aim of protecting an individual against a specific condition.

Secondary prevention – Strategies implemented following disease onset, with the aim of minimising the impact of that disease on the individual.

to reperfuse the myocardium and restore normal coronary blood flow (Bahatt, 2013; Lüscher, 2016). The intervention uses angiography to visualise the stenotic vessel, so that the location and severity of the occlusion can be determined (Lüscher, 2016). A balloon angioplasty may then be performed by inserting a catheter through the groin and advancing towards the affected vessel. Once the balloon tip is in place, it is inflated, compressing the plaque against the vessel wall and restoring normal blood flow (Morrow, 2017). A stent may also be deployed to maintain vessel patency (Figure 6.2). In some instances, a drug-elucidating stent that is coated in medication to prevent clot reformation may be used. This technological advancement has revolution-ised the procedure (Lüscher, 2016).

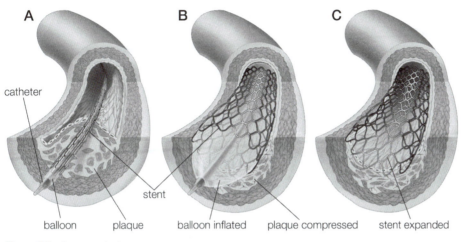

Figure 6.2   Stent angioplasty

Surgical management

The surgical management of acute CVD – where feasible – is used as a last resort, as this approach requires a large incision to directly access the damaged blood vessel or organ (Moorjani, Ohri & Wechsler, 2014). However, the benefits of surgical management are that bleeding due to hemorrhage may be controlled more effectively, and hemostatic agents can be applied to the site to accelerate clotting processes, preventing blood loss (Moorjani, Ohri & Wechsler, 2014). The detractions are an increased risk of post-operative infection and internal adhesions, and cosmetic considerations for the patient (Moorjani, Ohri & Wechsler, 2014). Common types of surgical intervention for acute CVD include CABG (coronary artery bypass graft), aneurysm repair and emergency embolectomy.

REFLECTIVE QUESTION

Consider the importance of pharmacological management in the treatment of ACS, and how this minimises the likelihood of potential myocardial ischemia and infarct.

SKILLS IN PRACTICE

A familiar cardiac tale …

Kylie is a 52-year-old female who lives in a rural area. She lives with her husband, Brian, and has two older children who have left home. Kylie is 167 cm tall and weighs 98 kg with a BMI of 35. She works as a receptionist for a solicitor and lives a sedentary lifestyle. Kylie currently smokes two packs of cigarettes per week and drinks two large glasses of red wine on most evenings. Kylie has been feeling fatigued for the past four days and was at home watching television when she experienced a sudden onset of epigastric pain around 2.00 pm. Initially, Kylie thought it was the takeaway she had eaten for lunch, so did not think much of it at the time. Later that afternoon, the pain had not subsided and started to intensify and radiate into her jaw and left shoulder. Kylie explained to her husband that the discomfort now felt like a crushing pain in her chest. Brian became increasingly concerned and took Kylie to the hospital at 5.00 pm that afternoon. Kylie has a family history of coronary heart disease, with her grandfather dying from a myocardial infarction at the age of 60. Jane, Kylie's mother, aged 72, also has a previous history of a myocardial infarction and paroxysmal atrial fibrillation, while her brother, Ben, who is 55, suffers from severe hypertension.

On arrival at the local emergency department, it is determined that Kylie is experiencing a STEMI. Kylie is administered thrombolysis which fails to resolve the ST-elevation and her chest pain continues to worsen. At 7.00 pm Kylie is flown to a larger hospital with interventional cardiac services and undergoes successful emergency PCI. Post-surgery, Kylie requires dual-antiplatelet therapy, beta-blockers and anti-hypertensives. Kylie is also referred to cardiac rehabilitation; however, the nearest service provider is 90 minutes away from her home.

QUESTION

What impact do you think residing in a rural area had on the management of Kylie's acute cardiovascular event, and how will it affect her ability to manage her cardiovascular health post discharge?

Care planning and nursing management of the acute cardiovascular patient

Acute CV nurses must possess high levels of clinical judgement, critical analysis and accountability. The skills of these nurses must allow them to interpret electrocardiograms, identify cardiac arrhythmias and maintain an individual's haemodynamic status under both stable and unstable conditions. Evidence-based practice (EBP) is the foundation of competent nursing care, so acute CV nurses must develop the expertise and knowledge to support patients through complicated clinical situations (Hamric et al., 2014). Therefore, acute CV nurses must understand the importance of basic and advanced life support, CV assessment, ECG interpretation and the general ongoing care of the patient.

Basic and advanced life support

Basic life support is a skill in which all health professionals should be proficient. Recognising that ventilation and chest compressions reduce the rate of deterioration and increase the likelihood of successful resuscitation during a cardiopulmonary arrest is imperative (Gregory & Quinn, 2010). Advanced life support (ALS) is the application of specialised treatments used to further support breathing and circulation in emergency situations. While not all nurses are required to have these skills, they should understand the principles of ALS. It is highly recommended that nurses working in cardiac units are ALS competent (Jevon, 2010).

Cardiovascular assessment

A comprehensive CV assessment should not occur until a primary survey has been completed, as the primary survey guides the identification of life-threatening conditions. Once the primary survey is complete and the patient is stabilised, a more detailed and focused cardiovascular assessment can occur (Jarvis & Eckhardt, 2016). Assessment of the CV system is a fundamental skill when caring for any patient with a CV condition, as adept assessment skills assist in the diagnosis and subsequent management of that individual (Younker, 2011). A CV assessment will commence with a comprehensive patient history, including a review of symptoms, family and social history (including a risk assessment for cardiovascular disease) and vital signs, prior to moving on to the physical examination.

Physical examination

Physical examination of the cardiovascular system follows the principles of inspection, palpation and auscultation. Percussion is generally not included in CV assessment. Assessment of the precordium should begin with inspection of the chest wall to identify any scars, deformities, location of the apex beat and unusual pulsations. The apex beat should be palpated at appropriately mid-clavicular line, fifth intercostal space. The clinician should take note of the characteristics of the beat, as it corresponds with the contraction of the left ventricle, and if abnormal can indicate a broad range of CV conditions (Talley & O'Connor, 2014). A hand should also be placed over the heart to assist in identifying the presence of abnormal impulses such as heaves or thrills (Talley & O'Connor, 2014). Both the bell and the diaphragm of the stethoscope should be used to auscultate the heart. The clinician should listen for each component of the cardiac cycle, the first and second heart sound, and any additional or abnormal sounds that may point to a cardiac murmur (Ranson & Braithwaite, 2017; Talley & O'Connor, 2014).

In addition to examining the precordium, the hands should be inspected for signs of blue discoloration, as this may indicate peripheral cyanosis and possible reduced cardiac output. In addition, capillary refill should be checked, as delayed (> 2 seconds) refill can also be a sign of reduced cardiac output (Ranson & Braithwaite, 2017). The radial pulse should be palpated to determine rate and rhythm, while the jugular venous pressure (JVP) of the patient should be observed, as this can estimate the patient's blood volume and cardiac function, recognising that in cases of elevated JVP the patient may be experiencing heart failure or tamponade (Talley & O'Connor, 2014).

ECG interpretation

The ability to interpret ECGs (electrocardiograms) is a valuable diagnostic skill, as it is important to understand that the ECG is the most significant assessment tool in the treatment of ACS (Kucia & Oldroyd, 2010a). Advanced CV nurses have the capacity to identify not only the key components of the hearts conduction system, but also rhythm abnormalities, conduction disturbances, electrolyte imbalances and myocardial ischemia and infarction (Ballestas et al., 2015). While ECG interpretation is generally considered an advanced skill of the registered nurse, all RNs should have the ability to determine when the characteristics of an ECG differ from the norm, and therefore recognise when to consult with other, more qualified health professionals (Scully, 2016).

General care

As outlined by Keenan (2011), the acute CV patient requires constant monitoring and management. Rest is crucial to reduce the myocardial workload, and large-bore intravenous access should be obtained in preparation for possible emergency situations. Continuous ECG monitoring should be initiated to ensure early detection and management of abnormalities (Kucia & Oldroyd, 2010b). Preferably, the acute CV patient will be admitted to a cardiac-specific unit, allowing closer monitoring than may be possible on a general medical or surgical ward (Keenan, 2011). Acute CV nurses need to be able to undertake rapid but accurate assessment, collect and analyse all relevant data, and engage high-level decision-making skills to prioritise their nursing care in complex and possibly life-threatening situations. Without the development of critical thinking, the CV nurse is likely to compromise patient safety (Shoulders, Follett & Eason, 2014).

REFLECTIVE QUESTION

Critical thinking is a learnt skill. Consider how a newly graduated nurse may critically analyse a complex, life-threatening situation in comparison to an advanced CV nurse and the impact that this may have on the safety of the patient.

Collaborative patient-centred nursing care

The concept of patient-centred care (PCC) has become a globally recognised approach to healthcare delivery. PCC ensures that the patient is treated with respect, provided with the opportunity to make autonomous decisions regarding their own treatment and strives to address both the emotional and physical needs of the individual. The PCC model guides not only nurses, but all members of the healthcare team (Kitson et al., 2012). To optimise the management of each individual patient, collaborative and culturally appropriate care is required. Members of differing healthcare disciplines bring their own skills and knowledge to each situation, but these often address only a specific part of the patient's acute care admission. It is important to understand that without a holistic multidisciplinary approach to treatment, PCC is not provided, and therefore patient outcomes can be diminished (Mueller et al., 2015).

Collaborative care

Collaborative care of the CV patient requires both cooperation and interaction between specialties to ensure that the mutual goals of the patient and the healthcare team are addressed successfully (Han et al., 2015). Multidisciplinary approaches to CVD in the acute care setting can result in not only enhanced patient outcomes, but also a reduction in the length of the hospital admission (Han et al., 2015). Multidisciplinary patient rounds should be implemented, and should include the patient and their family or carers. This approach enhances communication between health professionals and the patient and their family or carers, while acknowledging the individual contribution of each party to the continued care of the patient (Mitchell, Wilson & Aitkin, 2016).

While not every multidisciplinary team member will be required for every CV patient in the acute environment, it is important that each situation is assessed to determine which professional input is needed most (Christ & Mueller, 2016). For example, Morrow and colleagues (2012) outline how some CV patients within the acute care environment will be prescribed an increased number of medications, and therefore the expertise of a pharmacist is needed. The inclusion of pharmacists has seen a reduction in adverse drug events, shortened hospital stays and decreased mortality rates. A geriatrician may be included in the care of an 85-year-old acute HF patient, but would not be required in the care of a 60-year-old patient. In all cases, the development of the multidisciplinary team should be based on the patient's individual physical and emotional needs (Christ & Mueller, 2016).

Cultural competence

As Davidson and colleagues (2010) discuss, nurses must acknowledge that cultural diversity can impact treatment interventions and patient outcomes. Not only must health professionals acknowledge language barriers; they must also consider an individual's beliefs and practices. Similarly, nurses must acknowledge their own personal cultural beliefs and values, and not confuse these with the cultural needs of their patient (Webb & Kirov, 2014). A lack of cultural competence – particularly in the acute care environment – can heighten anxiety and worry in both the patient and their family. This consequently results in inadequate care provision by the healthcare team (Davidson et al., 2010; Thackrah & Thompson, 2013).

Nurses must possess cultural sensitivity skills when working in acute CV care environments, as often it is the nurse who supports the patient and their family through situations that may involve end-of-life decision-making. A failure to communicate in a culturally appropriate manner can result in distrust. Within the Australian healthcare environment, it is particularly important that nurses possess cultural competence, as 28 per cent of the population are immigrants (Northam et al., 2015). Furthermore, as the Australian Institute of Health and Welfare (AIHW, 2015) highlights, 27 per cent of Aboriginal and Torres Strait Islander adults suffer from CVD – it is currently the most significant contributor to mortality among this population, with approximately 3 per cent of all hospitalisations in this group resulting from CVD during 2013–14. Both hospitalisation and death rates due to cardiac conditions are higher for Aboriginal and Torres Strait Islander people, being 1.9 and 1.6 times greater respectively than those of other Australians (AIHW, 2016). However, health systems fail to effectively engage Aboriginal and Torres Strait Islander communities, which means considerable health inequalities continue to exist (Thackrah & Thompson, 2013). For this reason, Aboriginal and Torres Strait Islander cultural competence is a much-needed skill of the nurse working within acute cardiac environments, as building stronger relationships between patients and the healthcare system will result in greater service provision and enhanced patient outcomes (Thackrah & Thompson, 2013).

Patient education and discharge planning for the acute cardiovascular patient

Nurses have an important role to play in the education and discharge planning requirements for patients with acute CV conditions. One of the most significant roles the nurse has, which can impact and improve outcomes, is to educate patients about their cardiovascular condition and related self-care needs prior to discharge (London, 2016). Nurses have a unique opportunity through the development of the therapeutic relationship to provide pre-discharge education to patients. Eshah (2012) has found with ACS that this motivates patients to adhere to a healthy lifestyle following discharge. There are many barriers to patient education for nurses, including a lack of confidence, motivation, competence and skill. In order to provide **patient education**, nurses need to overcome these barriers by educating health professionals using a structured approach to improve knowledge, as this increases education encounters and improves patient outcomes (Sherman, 2016).

Patient education –
A fundamental aspect of nursing care and is the provision of health-related information to the patient, which allows patients to become more involved in the decision-making process.

Patient education

Education provided to patients with acute CV conditions needs to be individualised to meet each patient's particular needs. Information may need to be repeated over various timeframes, as the information needs of patients may change, especially for those who have suffered a stroke (National Stroke Foundation, 2010). Information should be provided in a language and format that can be understood easily while considering cultural and linguistic barriers that may affect information comprehension. Provision of information and education is not only very important for acute cardiovascular patients; it is also vital for their families and carers (Chew et al., 2016). The National Stroke Foundation (2010) recommends that stroke patients and their families or carers should be provided with routine follow-up opportunities for clarification or reinforcement of the information provided to them.

Identification of risk factors for a future cardiovascular event needs to be assessed to guide the education provided. Modification of a patient's lifestyle and risk factor reduction are the focus of secondary prevention in stroke and acute coronary syndromes, in particular myocardial infarction (Eshah, 2012; National Stroke Foundation, 2010). Secondary prevention strategies are critically important for reducing the occurrence of new vascular events for those patients who survive to discharge from hospital with an acute cardiovascular condition (Chew et al., 2016; National Stroke Foundation, 2010). Chew and colleagues (2016) list these strategies as including:

* adoption of healthy lifestyle behaviours
* intensive risk factor modification
* adherence to prescribed medications.

Nurses can assist patients to adopt these strategies through patient education, specifically lifestyle advice and medication information (Table 6.3). The lifestyle advice should cover topics such as smoking cessation, physical exercise, nutrition and moderation of alcohol intake (Chew et al., 2016; National Stroke Foundation, 2010).

Table 6.3   Examples of patient education goals and resources

Education topic	Goals	Possible resources available
Smoking cessation	• Quit smoking • Avoid second-hand smoke	• Quitline • Specialised smoking cessation program • Nicotine replacement therapy
Nutrition	• Limit saturated fatty acid intake • Limit salt intake	• Dietitian
Moderate alcohol intake	• Consume a low-risk amount of alcohol, no more than two standard drinks per day	• Brief interventions, referral to GP • Clinics or agencies with expertise in addiction
Regular physical activity	• 30 minutes of moderate-intensity physical activity on most if not all days of the week	• Structured rehabilitative physical activity program • Cardiac rehabilitation program

Weight management	• Waist measurement:
	  Men <94 cm
	  Women <80 cm
	• Body Mass Index range 18.5–24.9 kg/m²
		• Cardiac rehabilitation program

Source: National Heart Foundation of Australia and Cardiac Society of Australia and New Zealand (2012); National Stroke Foundation (2010).

Discharge planning

Lifestyle advice and goals discussed with the patient should be documented clearly in the discharge plan, as well as all additional information resources given to the patient. This constitutes an important part of the discharge plan, and provides a summary for the patient, their family or carer, and all treating health professionals in continuing care (Chew et al., 2016; National Stroke Foundation, 2010). Acute cardiovascular patients should be referred to a cardiac rehabilitation program prior to discharge (Chew et al., 2016). A cardiac rehabilitation program involves comprehensive health behaviour interventions targeting risk factor modification, including physical activity, dietary modification, lipid control and smoking cessation, in conjunction with psychological counselling delivered in the outpatient setting (Martin et al., 2012). Hall, Murphy and Scanlon (2016) identify that cardiac rehabilitation begins prior to discharge and has four phases. The first phase begins in hospital with the identification of **modifiable risk factors** and the nurse's role in providing education. Participation in cardiac rehabilitation is associated with a decreased risk of mortality and resource use with a decrease in all-cause mortality of 15–28 per cent reported (Martin et al., 2012; Sage, 2013). This highlights the importance of referral and participation in a cardiac rehabilitation program following discharge for those following an acute cardiovascular event.

Modifiable risk factors – Those factors that can be changed through adopting healthy lifestyle behaviours.

Patients with a diagnosis of acute coronary syndrome require a chest pain management plan to be established prior to discharge, and this should be communicated to the patient and documented in the discharge plan (Chew et al., 2016). A chest pain management plan entails guidance for the patient on the use of prescribed medicines to manage acute or worsening of symptoms such as chest pain and to understand what to do, such as call for an ambulance or present to the emergency department for acute care (Chew et al., 2016). For those patients with a diagnosis of stroke, a comprehensive discharge plan developed in collaboration with the patient, family or carer and multidisciplinary team needs to be considered to ensure safe discharge (National Stroke Foundation, 2010). Stroke patients should be assessed prior to discharge to determine the level of support needed, including home visits, aids and community services (National Stroke Foundation, 2010).

REFLECTIVE QUESTION

Education of the cardiovascular patient positively impacts the likelihood of future CV events. Consider the difficulties you might face trying to educate a patient who smokes but is unwilling to quit, and is unwilling to engage with you.

SUMMARY

Learning objective 1: Describe the pathophysiology of a range of acute cardiovascular conditions, and identify risk factors that impact their prevalence and treatment.

CV disease affects the heart and blood vessels. Disorders of the circulation include atherosclerosis, which can lead to ACS and stroke. Aneurysms, if unstable and rupture, can result in significant haemorrhage. Acute pericarditis and acute heart failure are examples of heart disease, and often lead to a reduction in cardiac output, resulting in a systemic decrease in organ and tissue perfusion. Acute CV conditions have a range of modifiable and non-modifiable risk factors, including but not limited to age, ethnicity, smoking, hypertension and obesity.

Learning objective 2: Understand the common medical, interventional and surgical approaches to managing patients who are experiencing cardiovascular issues.

Prompt medical, surgical and interventional management of the patient who is experiencing an acute CV event is paramount to decreasing the likelihood of morbidity and mortality. While a range of treatment approaches may be used, the accurate diagnosis of the underlying cardiac condition predicates which option is best for each individual on a case-by-case basis. International advancements in biomedical technology are further revolutionising both non-invasive and invasive techniques, ultimately augmenting patient survival rates.

Learning objective 3: Define the role of acute cardiovascular nurse and the importance of critical thinking and evidence-based practice in the care of the acute cardiac patient.

The role of the CV nurse is complex and multifaceted. CV nurses must have a range of clinical skills that allow them to provide high-quality care to their patients. In addition to the general care of the patient, the CV nurse must understand basic and advanced life support, CV-specific assessment skills, ECG interpretation and pharmacology knowledge. The CV nurse appreciates how EBP influences healthcare and can use EBP in conjunction with critical thinking to guide their nursing practice.

Learning objective 4: Understand the importance of multidisciplinary collaboration and the role of the nurse in providing culturally competent person-centred care for patients with acute cardiovascular conditions.

The provision of holistic cardiovascular nursing care must utilise a collaborative framework. Input from a range of health specialties ensures that care is tailored to the patient, and therefore aligns with the concept of PCC. Care provision must be culturally appropriate. Not only must the cultural needs of immigrants be considered, but nurses need to possess the cultural sensitivity to build therapeutic relationships with Aboriginal and Torres Strait Islander peoples. Through cultural competence, the cardiovascular nurse can achieve better patient outcomes.

Learning objective 5: Understand the nursing role in client education and discharge planning requirements for those with acute cardiovascular conditions.

Providing appropriate education to the CV patient about their condition is paramount for reducing further acute events. Education must be patient specific and inclusive of the patient's family and carers, and cover a range of topics aimed at adopting a healthy lifestyle, risk modification and medication adherence. Discharge planning should ensure that the patient is referred to the relevant services prior to leaving the acute setting.

REVIEW QUESTIONS

6.1 Describe the pathogenesis of acute pericarditis and how it may lead to new onset acute heart failure.

6.2 Discuss the medical, interventional and surgical approaches that are most commonly being used to manage and treat acute CVD.

6.3 Explain the importance of advanced nursing skills in the care of the CV patient.

6.4 Identify barriers to cultural competence that can result in sub-optimal patient care when discussing self-management behaviours with the cardiovascular patient.

6.5 Describe the patient education and discharge planning requirements for a client who has been diagnosed with a myocardial infarction.

RESEARCH TOPIC

According to the AIHW (2017), 63 per cent of Australians are overweight or obese, making excess weight the second highest contributor to disease burden. In Australia, the rates of obesity and overweight continue to rise. What impact does this have currently on the prevalence of acute cardiovascular conditions and healthcare resources, and what potential effect will this have in the future?

FURTHER READING

Karras, C., Donlan, S. M., Aitchison, R., Aitchison, P., Wang, E. & Kharasch, M. (2013). Acute coronary syndromes. *Disease-a-Month*, 59(5), 202–9.

Morrow, D.A. (ed.) (2017). *Myocardial Infarction: A Companion to Braunwald's Heart Disease*. St Louis, MO: Elsevier.

Ponikowski, P., Voors, A.A., Anker, S.D., Bueno, H., Cleland, J.G., Coats, A.J., ... Jessup, M. (2015). 2016 ESC Guidelines for the diagnosis and treatment of acute and chronic heart failure. *European Heart Journal*, 37(27), 2129–200.

Tubaro, M., Vranckx, P., Price, S. & Vrints, C. (eds) (2015). *The ESC Textbook of Intensive and Acute Cardiovascular Care*. Oxford: Oxford University Press.

Venes, D. (2013). *Taber's Cyclopedic Medical Dictionary* (22nd ed.). Philadelphia, PA: F.A. Davis Company.

REFERENCES

Amsterdam, E.A., Wenger, N.K., Brindis, R.G., Casey, D.E., Ganiats, T.G., Holmes, D.R., ... Yancy, C.W. (2014). 2014 AHA/ACC guideline for the management of patients with non-ST-elevation acute coronary syndromes: A report of the American college of cardiology/American heart association task force on practice guidelines. *Circulation*, 130(25), 2354–94.

Argulian, E., Herzog, E., Aziz, E. & Kukin, M. (2012). Pathway for the management of acute heart failure. In E. Herzog (ed.), *The Cardiac Survival Guide*. Philadelphia, PA: Lippincott Williams & Wilkins, pp. 91–9.

Australian Institute of Health and Welfare (AIHW) (2015). Cardiovascular disease, diabetes and chronic kidney disease: Australian facts. Retrieved from http://www.aihw.gov.au/WorkArea/DownloadAsset.aspx?id=60129553626.

—— (2016). *Better Cardiac Care Measures for Aboriginal and Torres Strait Islander People: Second National Report*. Cat. no. IHW 169. Canberra: AIHW. Retrieved from http://www.aihw.gov.au/WorkArea/DownloadAsset.aspx?id=60129557605.

—— (2017). Overweight and obesity. Retrieved from http://www.aihw.gov.au/overweight-and-obesity.

Bahatt, D.L. (2013). Timely PCI for STEMI: Still the treatment of choice. *The New England Journal of Medicine*, 12(4), 1446–7.

Ballestas, H., Bekken, N., Davis, J., Hill, K., Kline, C., Knauff, C., Leonard, T. & Richards, N. (2015). *ECG Strip Ease: An Arrhythmia Interpretation Workbook*. Philadelphia, PA: Wolters Kluwer.

Bangalore, S. & Owlia, M. (2017). *Non-ST-elevation Myocardial Infarction*. Retrieved from http://bestpractice.bmj.com/best-practice/monograph/150/follow-up/complications.html.

Black, H.R. & Elliott, W.J. (eds). (2013). *Hypertension: A Companion to Braunwald's Heart Disease*. Philadelphia, PA: Elsevier/Saunders.

Bope, E.T. & Kellerman, R.D. (2017). *Conn's Current Therapy 2017*. Philadelphia, PA: Elsevier.

Brahmajee, K.N. & Baman, T.S. (eds) (2014). *Inpatient Cardiovascular Medicine*. Hoboken, NJ: John Wiley & Sons.

Chew, D.P., Scott, I.A., Cullen, L., French, J.K., Briffa, T.G., Tideman, P.A., ... Aylward, P.E.G. (2016). National Heart Foundation of Australia & Cardiac Society of Australia and New Zealand: Australian Clinical Guidelines for the Management of Acute Coronary Syndromes. *Heart, Lung and Circulation*, 25(9), 895–951.

Christ, M. & Mueller, C. (2016). Call to action: Initiation of multidisciplinary care for acute heart failure begins in the Emergency Department. *European Heart Journal*, 5(2), 141–9.

Craft, J., Gordon, C.D., Huether, S.E., McCance, K.L., Brashers, V.L. & Rote, N.S. (2015). *Understanding Pathophysiology* (2nd ed.). Sydney: Mosby/Elsevier.

Crawford, M.H. (ed.) (2010). *Cardiology*. Philadelphia, PA: Mosby/Elsevier.

Davidson, P., Gholizadeh, L., Haghshenas, A., Rotem, A., DiGiacomo, M., Eisenbruch, M. & Salamonson, Y. (2010). A review of the cultural competence view of cardiac rehabilitation. *Journal of Clinical Nursing*, 19(9/10), 1335–42.

Doctor, N.S., Shah, A.B., Coplan, N. & Kronzon, I. (2017). Acute pericarditis. *Progress in Cardiovascular Diseases*, 59(4), 349–59.

Eshah, N.F. (2012). Predischarge education improves adherence to a healthy lifestyle among Jordanian patients with acute coronary syndrome. *Nursing and Health Sciences*, 15, 273–9.

Frachi, F. & Angiolilo, D.J. (2015). Novel antiplatelet agents in acute coronary syndrome. *Nature Reviews Cardiology*, 12(1), 30–47.

Gaglia, M.A., Gurbel, P.A. & Waksman, R. (eds) (2014). *Antiplatelet Therapy in Cardiovascular Disease*. Chichester: John Wiley & Sons.

Gregory, P. & Quinn, T. (2010). Out-of-hospital cardiac arrest and automated external defibrillator. In A. Kucia & T. Quinn (eds), *Acute Cardiac Care: A Practical Guide for Nurses*. Chichester: Blackwell, pp. 81–98.

Grossman, S. & Porth, C. (2014). *Porth's Pathophysiology: Concepts of Altered Health States*. Philadelphia, PA: Wolters Kluwer Health/Lippincott Williams & Wilkins.

Hall, C., Murphy, M. & Scanlon, A. (2016). Cardiac rehabilitation in the acute care setting: Integrative review. *Australian Critical Care*, 30(2), 99–106.

Hamric, A., Hanson, C., Tracy, M. & O'Grady, E. (2014). *Advanced Practice Nursing: An Integrative Approach* (5th ed.). St Louis, MO: Elsevier.

Han, K.T., Park, E.C., Kim, S.J., Kim, W., Hahm, M.I., Jang, S.I. & Lee, S.G. (2015). Effective strategy for improving health care outcomes: Multidisciplinary care in cerebral infarction patients. *Health Policy*, 119(8), 1039–45.

Heras, M., Sionis, A. & Price, S. (2015). Training and certification in acute cardiac care. In M. Tubaro, P. Vranckx, S. Price & C. Vrints (eds), *The ESC Textbook of Intensive and Acute Cardiovascular Care* (2nd ed.). Oxford: Oxford University Press, pp. 5–12.

Hummel, A., Empen, K., Dörr, M. & Felix, S.B. (2015). De novo acute heart failure and acutely decompensated chronic heart failure. *Deutsches Arzteblatt International*, 112(17), 298–310.

Humphreys, M. & Cooper, L. (2011). Emergency cardiac care. In M. Humphreys (ed.), *Nursing the Cardiac Patient*. Chichester: Wiley-Blackwell, pp. 156–77.

Jarvis, C. & Eckhardt, E. (2016). General survey, measurement and vital signs. In C. Jarvis (ed.), *Jarvis's Physical Examination and Health Assessment* (2nd ed.). Sydney: Elsevier, pp. 101–32.

Jevon, P. (2010). *Advanced Cardiac Life Support*. Chichester: John Wiley & Sons.

Keenan, J. (2011). Therapeutic interventions in acute coronary syndromes. In M. Humphreys (ed.), *Nursing the Cardiac Patient*. Chichester: Wiley-Blackwell, pp. 97–111.

Kitchens, C.S., Kessler, C.M. & Konkle, B.A. (2013). *Consultative Haemostasis and Thrombosis*. St Louis, MO: Elsevier Saunders.

Kitson, A., Marshall, A., Bassett, K. & Zeitz, K. (2013). What are the core elements of patient-centred care? A narrative review and synthesis of the literature from health policy, medicine and nursing. *Journal of Advanced Nursing*, 69(1), 4–15.

Kucia, A. & Oldroyd, C. (2010a). Electrocardiogram interpretation. In A. Kucia & T. Quinn (eds), *Acute Cardiac Care*. Chichester: Blackwell, pp. 81–98.

—— (2010b). Cardiac monitoring. In A. Kucia & T. Quinn (eds), *Acute Cardiac Care*. Chichester: Blackwell, pp. 99–108.

Lange, R.A. & Hillis, L.D. (2012). Acute coronary syndrome: Unstable angina and non-ST elevation myocardial infarction. In L. Goldman & A. Schafer (eds), *Goldman's Cecil Medicine* (25th ed.). Philadelphia, PA: Elsevier/Saunders, pp. 432–41.

London, F. (2016). *No Time to Teach: The Essence of Patient and Family Education for Health Care Providers* (2nd ed.). Atlanta, GA: Pritchett & Hull.

Lüscher, T.F. (2016). The management of acute coronary syndromes: Towards optimal treatment of STEMI and non-STEMI. *European Heart Journal*, 37(3), 203–5.

Martin, B.J., Hauer, T., Arena, R., Austford, L.D., Galbraith, P.D., Lewin, A.M., … Aggarwal, S.G. (2012). Cardiac rehabilitation attendance and outcomes in coronary artery disease patients. *Circulation*, 126, 677–87.

Mitchell, M. Wilson, D. & Aitken, L. (2016). Family and cultural care of the critically ill patient. In L. Aitken, A. Marshall, & W. Chaboyer (eds), *ACCN's Critical Care Nursing* (3rd ed.). Sydney: Elsevier, pp. 193–230.

Moorjani, N., Ohri, S.K. & Wechsler, A.S. (eds) (2014). *Cardiac Surgery: Recent Advances and Techniques*. Boca Raton, FL: Taylor & Francis.

Morrow, D.A. (ed.) (2017). *Myocardial Infarction: A Companion to Braunwald's Heart Disease*. St Louis, MO: Elsevier.

Morrow, D.A., Fang, J.C., Fintel, D.J., Granger, C.B., Katz, J.N., Kushner, F.G., … Page, R.L. (2012). Evolution of critical care cardiology: Transformation of the cardiovascular intensive care unit and the emerging need for new medical staffing and training models. *Circulation*, 126(11), 1408–28.

Mueller, C., Christ, M., Cowie, M., Cullen, L., Maisel, A.S., Masip, J., … DiSomma, S. (2015). European Society of Cardiology – Acute Cardiovascular Care Association position paper on acute heart failure: A call for interdisciplinary care. *European Heart Journal: Acute Cardiovascular Care*, 6(1), 81–6.

Mulryan, C. (2011). *Acute Illness Management*. London: Sage.

National Heart Foundation of Australia and Cardiac Society of Australia and New Zealand (2012). *Reducing Risk in Heart Disease: An Expert Guide to Clinical Practice for Secondary Prevention of Coronary Heart Disease*. Retrieved from https:// heartfoundation.org.au/images/uploads/publications/Reducing-risk-in-heart-disease.pdf.

National Stroke Foundation (2010). *Clinical Guidelines for Stroke Management*. Retrieved from https://informme.org.au/guidelines/clinical-guidelines-for-stroke-management-2010.

National Vascular Disease Prevention Alliance (2012). *Absolute Cardiovascular Disease Risk*. Retrieved from https://www.heartfoundation.org.au/images/uploads/ publications/Absolute-CVD-Risk-Full-Guidelines.pdf.

Newby, D.E., Grubb, N.R. & Bradbury, A. (2014). Cardiovascular disease. In B. Walker, N. Colledge, S. Ralston, & I. Penman (eds), *Davidson's Principles and Practice of Medicine* (22nd ed.). New York: Elsevier, pp. 525–641.

Northam, H.L., Hercelinskyj, G., Grealish, L. & Mak, A.S. (2015). Developing graduate student competency in providing culturally sensitive end of life care in critical care environments: A pilot study of a teaching innovation. *Australian Critical Care*, 28(4), 189–95.

Nursing Council of New Zealand (NCNZ) ([2007] 2016). *Competencies for Registered Nurses*. Retrieved from http://www.nursingcouncil.org.nz/Nurses.

Nursing and Midwifery Board of Australia (NMBA) (2016). *Registered Nurse Standards for Practice*. Melbourne: Nursing & Midwifery Board of Australia. Retrieved from http:// www.nursingmidwiferyboard.gov.au/Codes-Guidelines-Statements/Professional-standards.aspx.

Ranson, M. & Braithwaite, W. (2017). Cardiovascular assessment. In H. Abbott & M. Ranson (eds), *Clinical Examination Skills for Health Professionals* (2nd ed.). Glasgow: M&K Publishing.

Sage, S. (2013). Maximising the benefits of cardiac rehabilitation. *British Journal of Cardiac Nursing*, 8(8), 371–4.

Scully, N. (2016). Preserving oxygenation. In J. Crisp, C. Douglas, G. Rebeiro & D. Waters (eds), *Potter and Perry's Fundamentals of Nursing* (5th ed.). Sydney: Elsevier, pp. 1241–1318.

Sherman, J.R. (2016). An initiative to improve patient education by clinical nurses. *MEDSURG Nursing*, 25(5), 297–333.

Shoulders, B., Follett, C. & Eason, J. (2014). Enhanced critical thinking in clinical practice: Implications for critical and acute care nurses. *Dimensions of Critical Care Nursing*, 33(4), 207–14.

Talley, N. & O'Connor, S. (2014). *Clinical Examination: A Systematic Guide to Physical Diagnosis*. Sydney: Elsevier.

Thackrah, R.D. & Thompson, S.C. (2013). Refining the concept of cultural competence: Building on decades of progress. *The Medical Journal of Australia*, 199(1), 35–8.

Topol, E.J. & Teirstein, P.S. (eds) (2016). *Textbook of Interventional Cardiology*. Philadelphia, PA: Elsevier/ Saunders.

Tubaro, M., Vranckx, P., Price, S. & Vrints, C. (eds) (2015). *The ESC Textbook of Intensive and Acute Cardiovascular Care*. Oxford: Oxford University Press.

VanMeter, K., Hubert, R.J. & Gould, B.E. (2014). *Gould's Pathophysiology for the Health Professions*. St Louis, MO: Elsevier/Saunders.

Venes, D. (2013). *Taber's Cyclopedic Medical Dictionary* (22nd ed.). Philadelphia, PA: F.A. Davis Company.

Webb, M. & Kirov, E. (2014). *Clinical Cases: Nursing Care Case Studies*. Sydney: Elsevier.

World Health Organization (WHO) (2016). Cardiovascular diseases (CVDs). Retrieved from http://www.who.int/mediacentre/factsheets/fs317/en.

Xie, S.Q. & Zhou, J.R. (2017). Effect of statins and the clinical nursing characteristics in patients with acute myocardial infarction. *Pakistan Journal of Pharmaceutical Sciences*, 30(5), 1843–9.

Younker, J. (2011). Assessment of the cardiovascular system. In M. Humphreys (ed.), *Nursing the Cardiac Patient*. Chichester: Blackwell, pp. 19–35.

Acute renal conditions

Melissa Arnold-Chamney, Sharon Latimer,
Matthew Barton and Janet Kelly

LEARNING OBJECTIVES

At the completion of this chapter, you should be able to:

1 define acute kidney injuries (AKI); identify underlying pathophysiology, risk factors and presentations associated with an AKI
2 describe nursing assessment and management strategies for the individual with an AKI
3 understand the concepts of patient-centred care and health education in relation to AKI
4 identify and discuss the nurse's role in the coordination and collaborative management of individuals with AKI.

Introduction

The renal system is composed collectively of the kidneys, ureters, urinary bladder and urethra. Together, the kidneys receive approximately one-quarter of the body's cardiac output, which is necessary to perform their primary function of filtration. However, the renal system – or, more specifically, the kidneys – performs seven important homeostatic functions:

1 regulation of fluid, electrolyte and calcium balance
2 regulation of acid–base balance
3 excretion of metabolic wastes
4 regulation of blood pressure
5 regulation of vitamin D production
6 regulation of red blood cell production
7 **gluconeogenesis**.

Glucogenesis – A metabolic pathway that results in the generation of glucose.

Acute kidney injury (AKI) can occur to anyone within the community or hospital setting, and AKI not only causes interruption to the seven homeostatic functions of the kidneys but can also impact other major body organs. This chapter considers the pathophysiology of the kidneys, causes, types and clinical features of AKI and, crucially, the nurse's role in the prevention and early detection of this life-threatening illness.

NURSING STANDARDS

The following identifies the national competency standards for the registered nurse from the Nursing and Midwifery Board of Australia (NMBA) and the Nursing Council of New Zealand (NCNZ) that are addressed in this chapter.

Australian Registered Nurse Standards for Practice

The content of this chapter will be linked to six of the seven standards. Standard 1 in particular considers using the best evidence for safe practice and respects cultures and responds to the role of family and community that underpin the health of Aboriginal and Torres Strait Islander peoples and other cultures.

Standard 1: Thinks critically and analyses nursing practice

Standard 2: Engages in therapeutic and professional relationships

Standard 4: Comprehensively conducts assessments

Standard 5: Develops a plan for nursing practice

Standard 6: Provides safe, appropriate and responsive quality nursing practice

Standard 7: Evaluates outcomes to inform nursing practice

(NMBA, 2016)

New Zealand: Competencies for Registered Nurses

Competency 1.1: Accepts responsibility for ensuring that his/her nursing practice and conduct meet the standards of the professional, ethical and relevant legislated requirements

Competency 1.2: Demonstrates the ability to apply the principles of the Treaty of Waitangi/ Te Tiriti o Waitangi to nursing practice

Competency 1.5: Practises nursing in a manner that the health consumer determines as being culturally safe

Understanding acute kidney injuries

This section will define **acute kidney injuries (AKI)**, the underlying pathophysiology including the risk factors and clinical presentations that a person with AKI may have. AKI, formerly known as acute renal failure (ARF), is defined as sudden harm or injury to the kidneys (Kidney Health Australia, 2017). As suggested by the name, the signs and symptoms of AKI usually occur over a short period. The importance of maintaining accurate, comprehensive and timely documentation is critical within AKI as any changes in the patient's condition will need to be acted upon quickly to prevent the need for renal replacement therapy (RRT).

Acute kidney injury (AKI) – An abrupt impairment to the kidneys.

Although anyone can be affected by AKI, older people, those living in remote areas, those who are socioeconomically disadvantaged and Aboriginal and Torres Strait Islander people have higher hospitalisation or death rates than other Australians. AKI hospitalisation and death rates of Aboriginal and Torres Strait Islander people are at least twice those of other Australians, and AKI hospitalisation rates in the 85 years and over age group are at least four times those in the 65–74 years age group (AIHW, 2015).

Defining acute renal conditions

AKI is when an abrupt impairment occurs to the kidneys and an abrupt decline in glomerular filtration rate (GFR) occurs from the individual's baseline. This results in retention of metabolic nitrogenous wastes (creatinine and BUN) and the loss of the kidney's homeostatic regulation of body fluids, acid-base and electrolytes (Mehta et al., 2007). AKI can be with or without anuria/oliguria; it will often be short-term and kidney function returns. However, long-term kidney function can vary from nil, partial or full recovery. Unfortunately, permanent damage can occur and the person may eventually require RRT. All patients admitted as an emergency, regardless of specialty, should have their electrolytes checked routinely on admission and appropriately thereafter, as this will prevent the insidious and unrecognised onset of AKI (Stewart, 2009).

Understanding pathophysiology and risk factors for AKI

AKI has replaced the term 'acute renal failure', which reflected a whole spectrum of renal injury, ranging from patients with minor alterations in their blood chemistry to those dependent on dialysis. Over recent decades, in excess of 30 different definitions have been proposed to define AKI; consequently, its exact incidence isn't clear due to this lack of consensus on its definition (Finlay et al., 2017). Nevertheless, AKI is frequent and affects 25–67 per cent of critically ill patients and independently elicits a 30–60 per cent mortality rate, even after normalisation for illness severity (White et al., 2013).

In 2002, the Risk, Injury, Failure, Loss of function and End-stage kidney disease (RIFLE) criteria were developed to ensure that an accepted definition of AKI existed (Table 7.1). The RIFLE criteria consist of three graded levels (risk, injury and failure) of kidney injury, which is incumbent upon the magnitude of serum creatinine and urine output changes, with two outcome measures (loss and ESKD) (Palevsky et al., 2013).

Table 7.1   The RIFLE criteria for AKI

	GFR criteria	Urine output criteria
Risk	1.5 fold increase in creatinine or >25% decrease in GFR	UO < 0.5 mL/kg/h for 6 h
Injury	2 fold increase in creatinine or >50% decrease in GFR	UO < 0.5 mL/kg/h for 12 h
Failure	3 fold increase in creatinine or >75% decrease in GFR or ≥ 4 mg/dL creatinine or acute rise ≥ 0.5 mg/dL of creatinine	UO < 0.3 mL/kg/h for 24 h or anuria for 12 h
Loss	Complete loss of kidney function > 4 weeks	
ESKD	End-stage kidney disease (> 3months)	

Note: As GFR and/or UO worsens, the patient's grading moves from risk to failure. GFR: glomerular filtration rate; UO: urine output; ESKD: end-stage kidney disease.

Source: Adapted from Bellomo, Kellum and Ronco (2012).

In 2004, the Acute Kidney Injury Network (AKIN) proposed some amendments. AKIN required that at least two values of serum creatinine (SCr) be taken within a 48-hour period, but did not consider eGFR, whereas RIFLE does. Kidney Disease: Improving Global Outcomes (KDIGO) criteria were merged with RIFLE and AKIN criteria, with the aim of achieving an earlier diagnosis of AKI (Palevsky et al., 2013). Within these criteria lies the inference that small rises in SCr and short periods of oliguria should be acted upon. With all of them, the implication is that progression down the criteria is associated with increased lengths of stay in both ICU and hospital wards, an increased chance of mortality and less chance of renal recovery (Lopes et al., 2008).

Depending on the aetiology and when the patient seeks medical intervention, the clinical manifestations from the AKI may be diverse. Nonetheless, the most widely accepted diagnostic criteria for AKI is:

A sudden (<48 hours) reduction in kidney function, with an absolute increase in serum creatinine of more than or equal to 26.4 μmol/l, an increase in serum creatinine of more than or equal to 50% (from baseline), and or a fall in urine output less than 0.5 ml/kg per hour for at least six hours.

(Mehta et al., 2007)

Clinical course of AKI

There are four phases: initiating, oliguric, diuretic and recovery. The initiating phase commences when the kidneys are injured and can last for several hours or days. The second phase is the oliguric phase, which can last from one to two weeks. As kidney function improves, the patient enters the diuretic phase. Lastly, the recovery phase commences, which can take up to one year (Thomas, 2014).

Urine output during AKI

- Anuria – no urine output
- Oliguria <400 ml/day
- Non-oliguria >400 ml/day
- Polyuria – normal or high urine output

Risk factors

A number of factors can increase an individual's risk of AKI. These include pre-existing chronic kidney disease (CKD), advanced age, diabetes, hypertension, medications that are **nephrotoxic** (aminoglycosides, non-steroidal anti-inflammatory drugs [NSAIDs]), and obesity (Chawla et al., 2014; Sharfuddin & Molitoris, 2011). Those at most risk of AKI are older patients with numerous comorbidities (Lewington, Cerda & Mehta, 2013).

Nephrotoxic – A substance that can result in kidney damage.

Renal hypoxia, sepsis and nephrotoxic drugs most frequently cause AKI. Urinary tract obstruction is also frequent, especially among elderly men and patients with malignancy; therefore, these aetiologies must be excluded if the cause of AKI is unclear (Harty, 2014). As the cause of AKI is often multifactorial, a key goal when assessing a patient with AKI is to identify its aetiological classification.

Incidence and cost

Worldwide, the incidence of AKI is rising, with a recent report suggesting that 20 per cent of acutely ill, hospitalised adults experience this disease (Susantitaphong et al., 2013). However, the exact incidence of AKI is unknown, with more research needed in this area (AIHW, 2015). In Australia, for the period 2000–13, hospital admissions for AKI more than doubled (8050 to 18 010), representing 1.6 per cent of all hospitalisations (AIHW, 2015). AKI affects patients, nurses and healthcare systems. For patients, there is a strong association between AKI and increased morbidity and mortality (Lewington, Cerdá & Mehta, 2013). Males experience AKI at a rate 40 per cent higher than females, and in 2012 more than 5000 deaths were recorded in Australia from this disease (AIHW, 2015). These figures rise dramatically for people living in remote parts of Australia, compared with those living in metropolitan cities (AIHW, 2015). AKI increases nurses' workloads because this patient group in Australia has an average length of stay of 11.4 days – twice the average hospital admission (5.6 days) (AIHW, 2015). AKI also results in a rising economic burden for healthcare organisations; however, an accurate estimate of these costs has not been determined (AIHW, 2015).

Clinical features and diagnosis of AKI

Clinical features of AKI are produced by the rapid deterioration of renal function, which includes reduced urinary output (oliguria to anuria), accumulation of nitrogenous wastes, shortness of breath, hyperkalaemia, oedema and fatigue (Kidney Health Australia, 2017). AKI has a number of causative factors (which fall into three main groupings – see below), including hypovolaemia (e.g. post major surgery, myocardial infarction or a motor vehicle accident), direct kidney tissue damage because of medications or infections, blockages within the renal system such as kidney stones (nephrolithitis) or an enlarged prostate (Barasch, Zager & Bonventre, 2017).

Diagnosis

Early detection of AKI is vital so that rapid and appropriate treatment can be instigated. To confirm a diagnosis of AKI, a comprehensive patient history, physical and blood examination must be undertaken. Sudden rises in the patient's serum creatinine and/or reduced urine output is diagnostic of AKI (Lewington, Cerdá & Mehta, 2013). According to the Kidney Disease: Improving Global Outcomes (KDIGO) (2012) clinical practice guidelines, AKI is diagnosed when there is a ≥0.3 mg/dl increase in serum creatinine within 48 hours, or a 50 per cent increase in serum creatinine above the baseline within seven days, or the urine output is <0.5 ml/kg/hr for six hours.

Aetiology

The aetiologies for AKI are heterogeneous; therefore, they are commonly grouped based on the location of renal injury: pre-renal causes, intra-renal causes and post-renal causes.

Frequently, AKI is a short-term condition with one of three possible outcomes:

1 a return to normal kidney function
2 a reduction in kidney function without the need for dialysis (removing water and waste products from the blood by artificial means)
3 a permanent reduction in kidney function requiring dialysis (Kidney Health Australia, 2017).

However, in some instances AKI can result in mild chronic kidney disease (CKD) or severe damage to the kidneys, with the patient requiring long-term dialysis (AIHW, 2015).

Pathophysiology

Renal hypoperfusion, sepsis or nephrotoxic drugs (Table 7.2) most frequently cause AKI.

Table 7.2   AKI causes

Pre-renal	Intra-renal	Post-renal
• Body fluid depletion (excessive fluid losses, reduced intake) • Haemorrhage • Heart failure • Sepsis • Drugs (e.g. diuretics) • Cardiogenic shock • Cirrhosis (hepatorenal syndrome) • Renal artery stenosis	• Acute tubular necrosis • Hypertension • Rhabdomyolysis • Interstitial nephritis • Acute glomerulonephritis • Drugs (NSAIDs, aminoglycosides) • Pyelonephritis	• Bladder outflow obstruction (e.g. benign prostatic hypertrophy or malignancy) • Neurogenic bladder • Pelvic or abdominal malignancy • Kidney stones • Retroperitoneal fibrosis

Source: Perlman, Heung and Ix (2014).

Urinary tract obstruction is common, especially in elderly men and patients with malignancy, and must always be excluded if the cause of AKI is unclear. In hospitalised patients, the cause is often multifactorial. A small proportion of patients with AKI have intrinsic renal disease, such as acute interstitial nephritis or glomerulonephritis that requires urgent specialist assessment and therapy. One of the key goals when assessing a patient with AKI is to rapidly identify and reverse the cause, and obtain prompt nephrology input.

- *Pre-renal causes* are the result of impaired renal perfusion, despite the kidney's ability to auto-regulate and maintain its blood flow and GRF. Reduced renal perfusion can occur when there has been: (1) increased fluid loss (haemorrhage, dehydration, burns, GIT dysfunction); (2) low fluid intake; and/or (3) low effective circulating volume (sepsis, heart failure, shock, hepatorenal syndrome) (Perlman, Heung & Ix, 2014).

- *Intra-renal causes* are due to diseases that initially affect the nephrons intrinsically. These diseases can be further divided into acute tubular necrosis (ATN) (ischaemia and neph-rotoxic injury) and inflammatory diseases (e.g. glomerulonephritis, drug-induced, vasculitis).

- *Post-renal causes* result from mechanical obstruction of the urinary outflow tract (retroperitoneal fibrosis, lymphoma, tumour, prostate hyperplasia, strictures, renal calculi, ascending urinary infection (including pyelonephritis) and urinary retention). Subsequently, renal injury results from increased intra-tubular pressure yielding tubular ischaemia and atrophy. Evidence also suggests that injury results from an influx of monocytes and macrophages.

Regardless of the origin of aetiology – pre-renal, intra-renal or post-renal – all forms of AKI, if unmanaged, will result in ATN, and the severity of renal injury and the timing of medical intervention will determine whether the AKI is irreversible (Perlman, Heung & Ix, 2014). Patients with pre-renal causes of AKI will first develop azotaemia, due to their reduced GFR. If therapeutic intervention is timely and sufficient, the azotaemia can typically be reversed before manifesting into ATN (Perlman, Heung & Ix, 2014). If not, AKI will worsen and the patient's urinary output will diminish along with their kidneys' excretory function, with common symptoms of fatigue and malaise present (Kidney Health Australia, 2017).

As the fluid and electrolyte balance becomes affected, patients may exhibit dyspnoea, orthopnoea, shortness of breath, peripheral oedema and hyperkalaemia, while the build-up of nitrogenous wastes and lack of acid–base balance will cause altered levels of consciousness and potential coma (Tögel & Westenfelder, 2014). Patients with an intra-renal cause – which may be vascular, glomerular, tubular or interstitial in origin – will have a degree of necrosis to their nephrons. These necrotic cells may accumulate in the nephrons' tubules, leading to granular casts in the patient's urine and an increase in tubular pressure, subsequently reducing GFR and leading to oliguria, azotemia, hyperkalemia and metabolic acidosis (Kidney Health Australia, 2017). Finally, an obstruction to the urinary outflow of the kidney, which typifies the post-renal causes, will result in an increase in renal tubular pressure, altering the pressure gradient between the glomerulus and the renal tubules and subsequently reducing the patient's GFR. This may cause an increase in reabsorption of urea relative to creatinine, altering the BUN-to-creatinine ratio; like the other two AKI causes, this will cause oliguria and azotemia (Kidney Health Australia, 2017).

REFLECTIVE QUESTION

Explain the different types of AKI and some causes of each in relation to pre-renal, intra-renal and post-renal AKI.

SKILLS IN PRACTICE

Jasper Pittard

Jasper is a 36-year-old Aboriginal man married to Arabella. Jasper and Arabella are farmers, living in a regional area with their two young children. Jasper suffered extensive leg injuries in a motorbike accident involving a kangaroo and barbed wire fence. He was not found for some hours and suffered extensive blood loss. Arabella went looking for him and found him barely conscious. He was retrieved via the Royal Flying Doctor service and sent to an metropolitan acute trauma hospital. Arabella was unable to accompany him on the plane and followed by road the next day. Their two children stayed with Jasper's mother and sister on a neighbouring farm. Due to the blood loss from the accident, Jasper ended up with pre-renal AKI.

While in hospital, Jasper found that some of the nurses appeared hesitant to talk to him as an Aboriginal man. A number of staff were surprised that he was a farmer who was working, and many people made judgements about his literacy level and priorities. He felt very lonely until his wife arrived, as it was his first time in hospital and his uncle had previously been admitted for cardiac issues and died in this same hospital. There was one nurse who had previously worked in rural and remote areas in Australia who recognised his need for family contact and assisted him with this. Jasper's mobile phone survived the impact but went flat, and needed charging. The nurse located a charger. She also provided him with a second urine bottle so that he did not have to ask for this, as he was uncomfortable asking female nurses for it. The nurse asked whether Jasper wanted to see the Aboriginal Liaison Officer (ALO) and he did. She also asked the ALO to come to handover to discuss culturally responsive ways to ensure privacy and dignity for Jasper. Nurses needed to ensure that they made sufficient time and space for Jasper to ask them any questions that he or his family may have about his renal illness, and to provide him with sufficient information for his ongoing self-management.

After fifteen days in hospital, Jasper was discharged home. He was still in a lot of pain from his initial injury, including broken ribs, and wanted to get back to working on the farm as much as possible. He therefore took large amounts of ibuprofen for pain relief and developed intra-renal AKI, which meant that he needed to return to the metropolitan hospital a week after his original discharge for further treatment and short-term haemodialysis (HD).

QUESTIONS

- What are the key elements of the clinical management of an individual presenting to an emergency department of a metropolitan hospital with an AKI?
- What information does Jasper need in order to stay well after discharge?

Management of clients with renal conditions

The management will depend on the type of AKI, as it is the underlying issue that requires treatment. This may include correction of the primary disorder, such as removing the nephrotoxic insult or removing the obstruction. Other AKI causes include septicaemia, burns, trauma or even poisonous animals and plants. Management also includes correction of fluid and electrolyte disorders, prevention of infection, maintenance of optimum nutrition and treatment of systemic effects of uraemia. The provision of education and support to the patient and family is also crucial (Thornburg & Gray-Vickrey, 2016). AKI that has developed because of a pre-renal cause in the community will often respond to fluid replacement and temporary withdrawal of drugs that adversely affect kidney function (Thornburg & Gray-Vickrey, 2016).

Treatment for each identified condition

- Identify and treat any infection.
- Optimise fluid balance.
- Cease or limit the use of nephrotoxic medications.
- Monitor creatinine, calcium, glucose, phosphate, potassium and sodium on a daily basis.
- Check weight daily.
- Undertake daily urinalysis.
- Treat acute complications.
- Remove any urinary tract obstruction urgently.
- Provide a nephrologist referral and possible RRT intervention.

Fluid imbalance

The risk of fluid imbalance is high in patients with reduced kidney function; however, oliguria present in AKI may also be an indicator of blockage in the urinary system. Therefore, urine output should be measured accurately in all AKI patients (Rahman, Shad & Smith, 2012). Nurses play a pivotal role in determining whether a patient is hypovolaemic or hypervolaemic via the maintenance of accurate fluid balance charting, as volume homeostasis and electrolyte rebalance are critical in the management of AKI patients (Severs, Rookmaaker & Hoorn, 2015). Nursing staff need to be alert to a patient's urine output, which is likely to be reduced to <0.5 ml/kg/h if their blood pressure is reduced.

For pre-renal AKI, fluid resuscitation is imperative to restore renal perfusion and prevention of intrinsic AKI. Signs and symptoms of fluid overload must be closely monitored, as should vital signs. Cardiovascular response needs monitoring in relation to increasing the intravascular volume, as an increase in both central venous pressure and blood pressure should occur. Pulmonary oedema is a severe complication, often due to the mismanagement of intravenous fluid administration to patients who are anuric or oliguric (Mahon, Jenkins & Burnapp, 2013).

Hyperkalaemia

Hyperkalaemia is defined as a serum potassium >5.0 mmol/L; this can cause severe cardiac alterations and is often a fatal complication of AKI. Potassium is freely filtered by the glomerulus and 90–95 per cent is reabsorbed in the proximal tubule and loop of Henle. Urinary excretion of potassium begins in the distal convoluted tubule and is further regulated by the distal nephron and collecting duct (Giebisch & Wingo, 2013). A loss of nephron function therefore results in potassium retention. With AKI, there is a rapid decrease in GFR and tubular flow, often accompanied by a hyper-catabolic state, tissue injury and a high acute potassium level. Acute hyperkalaemia with a serum potassium >6 mmol/L and/or evidence of ECG changes requires immediate attention, such as cardiac monitoring and acute medical interventions. If not resolved, emergency RRT will be necessary. Acute management goals are to induce potassium transport into the intracellular space and remove potassium from the body to quickly restore the normal electrophysiology of the cell membrane and prevent cardiac arrhythmia (Kovesdy, 2014). This can be provided by giving intravenous insulin and dextrose, which help to move the potassium back to the intracellular compartment. Oral or rectal potassium is a slower acting treatment that can be used to stabilise potassium. The most efficient treatment is RRT.

Uraemia

Uraemic toxins will accumulate quickly, and symptoms can include nausea, vomiting, hiccups, increased bleeding, infection risk, neurological problems, irritability, confusion and twitching (Thomas, 2014).

Nutrition

AKI patients are usually unwell, and their metabolism can be under great stress, which requires extra calories and protein. One of the leading factors in the mortality of AKI patients is their protein calorie malnutrition. The main aims of nutritional support are to prevent protein energy wasting, repair tissue damage, preserve organ function, maintain fluid and biochemistry balance, and enhance recovery (Murphy & Byrne, 2010).

Mental health

People with mental health conditions can be at an increased risk of AKI for several reasons, and nurses need to be aware of depressed patients who are withdrawn and at risk of dehydration. In addition, lithium, which is used to help treat some mental health conditions, can cause AKI if a patient's lithium levels are elevated. Patients with mental health issues may not seek medical help during episodes of illness (Hulse & Davies, 2015).

Renal and urogenital assessment

Tests used to provide information about renal conditions include blood and urine tests and imaging processes.

Interpretation of diagnostic tests: Urine tests

Urine tests can reveal indicators of kidney disease, urinary tract infections and other renal processes.

Creatinine clearance test

Urine is collected and refrigerated over a 24-hour period and the level of creatinine excreted is measured. The comparison of this with serum creatinine indicates the volume of blood filtered by the kidneys each minute (National Kidney Foundation, 2016).

Urinalysis

Urinalysis – Indicates urinary issues, including urinary tract infections, diabetes and kidney disease. The test involves checking the appearance, odour, concentration and content of the urine.

On admission, a baseline **urinalysis** should be taken for all patients and repeated daily thereafter for patients at risk of AKI or who have AKI. On admission, a midstream urine specimen should be taken for microscopy and culture. A urinalysis identifies indicators of urinary tract infections, diabetes and kidney disease.

Normal urine is clear and pale yellow, with a urinoid odour. The odour and colour can be intensified in concentrated urine. There are numerous causes of change to smell, including ketoacidosis, which causes a strong fruity smell, and infection, causing a pungent smell (Strasinger & Di Lorenzo, 2014).

It is useful to undertake a urinalysis for the following in relation to AKI:

- *Specific gravity (SG)*. Measures concentration of solutes in urine. Low SG may be due to renal failure, excessive fluid intake, acute glomerulonephritis and acute tubular necrosis. High SG may be due to dehydration, but can also be an indicator of heart or liver failure.
- *Haematuria*. The presence of blood in the urine may indicate kidney damage, trauma, infections or renal calculi.
- *Protein*. Normally not detected, but elevated levels (proteinuria) indicate kidney dysfunction or disease, injury or inflammation to the bladder or urinary tract.
- *Leukocytes*. White cells present in the urine are associated with urinary tract infection.
- *Nitrates*. Formed by the breakdown of urinary nitrates, suggesting a bacterial infection such as *E. coli*, *Staphylococcus* or *Kliebsiella*.
- *pH*. Normal urine is acidic with a pH range of 4.5 to 8. (Note that urine becomes alkaline over time, so a fresh sample must be used for testing accuracy.)

(Strasinger & Di Lorenzo, 2014)

Interpretation of diagnostic tests: Blood tests

Several blood tests are used to diagnose renal conditions.

Serum creatinine

Creatinine is a waste product from the normal breakdown of muscle tissue and is cleared through the kidneys. Elevated creatinine levels (above 1.2 in women and 1.4 in men) are an early sign of poor kidney function. Serum creatinine will increase as kidney function decreases, with a rise occurring within 48 hours of clinical presentation indicative of AKI (Bellomo, Kellum & Ronco, 2012; Rahman, Shad & Smith, 2012).

Blood urea nitrogen (BUN)

The kidneys excrete nitrogen, which is a waste product of consumed proteins. Normal BUN is 7–20, with an elevated BUN indicating decreasing kidney function (National Kidney Foundation, 2016).

Glomerular filtration rate (GFR)

Measures the effectiveness of kidney filtration of wastes and excess fluids from the blood. Normal GFR value is >90 but varies depending on age, gender and body size. A GFR <60 is a sign of kidney dysfunction. Treatment such as dialysis or kidney transplant will be required for GFR <15 (Chadwick & Macnab, 2015; National Kidney Foundation, 2016).

Potassium

Potassium is present in all cells, and is the most abundant cation in the body. Hyperkalaemia (raised potassium) is often a fatal AKI complication due to the kidney being unable to excrete potassium effectively when the patient is oliguric or anuric (Thomas, 2014).

Imaging

Imaging techniques used for renal conditions include ultrasound, CT scans and x-rays.

Ultrasound

May determine abnormalities in size or position of the kidneys as well as diagnosing obstructions such as stones and tumours (Rhaman, Shad & Smith, 2012).

CT scan

The contrast dye assists in diagnosing obstructions and structural abnormalities within the kidneys (Chadwick & Macnab, 2015).

X-ray

Chest x-ray can confirm pulmonary oedema and abdominal x-ray can confirm renal calculi.

Nursing assessment and management

This section describes nursing assessment and management strategies for the individual with AKI. All nurses should be able to recognise AKI when it occurs. Through prevention or early detection, nurses can help to reduce the morbidity and mortality associated with AKI, thus improving patients' quality of life and reducing the financial impact of AKI on the healthcare system (Hulse & Davies, 2015). The National Institute for Health and Care Excellence (NICE, 2013) recommends that all hospital patients should have their clinical observations recorded regularly using an early warning-style system. This aids identification of patients at risk of AKI due to their deteriorating clinical condition.

Aspects to consider during nursing assessment

- What are their current clinical observations compared with baseline observations?
- Have there been any recent physical changes or genito-urinary issues that may lead to possible obstruction?
- Have any recent studies been undertaken using contrast medium, which is nephrotoxic?
- Does the client or any member of their family have a history of CKD?
- Are there any comorbid chronic health issues (e.g. diabetes mellitus, liver failure, hypertension)?
- What medications does the client take, including over the counter and herbal preparations?

(Mahon, Jenkins & Burnapp, 2013)

Specifically, the NICE guidelines (2013) assist nurses in the prevention and management of patients with AKI through:

- ongoing assessment and monitoring of individual patients for their AKI risk
- educating patients and their carers about maintaining hydration
- educating patients and their carers about managing AKI risk factors such as hypertension and cardiovascular disease
- avoiding nephrotoxic medications
- maintaining a healthy weight and good nutrition
- monitoring patients' urine output
- as appropriate, maintaining contact with relevant members of the multidisciplinary team, such as specialist medical officers.

REFLECTIVE QUESTION

Explain how the therapeutic intervention for pre-renal AKI management may be contraindicated for intra-renal and post-renal AKI.

Care planning

A number of different therapies can be considered for the treatment of renal conditions, including the following.

Renal replacement therapy

Renal replacement therapy (RRT) can be instigated for fluid overload, which is unresponsive to diuretics, severe metabolic acidosis or hyperkalaemia, symptomatic uraemia (e.g. bleeding, pruritus, pericarditis) and continued biochemical deterioration and oliguria or anuria despite other treatments. There are a number of different therapy options: **haemodialysis (HD)**, continuous renal replacement therapy (CRRT), sustained low-efficiency dialysis (SLED) and **peritoneal dialysis (PD)**. Not all therapeutic options may be available or suitable for the patient's haemodynamic state or comorbid conditions, so the doctor's preference is critical (Murphy & Byrne, 2010).

Insertion and care of access for HD

If a patient with AKI requires HD, CRRT or SLED, they almost certainly will have a non-tunnelled temporary haemodialysis catheter (NTHC) inserted. These catheters have two separate tubes: one carries blood from the patient to the HD machine; the other returns blood to the patient. Nursing staff must be aware that this access is for RRT use only to minimise infection and clotting risks.

Catheter insertion

Insertion of a NTHC is a core procedure of nephrology practice. This procedure is undertaken via percutaneous placement under local anaesthesia, and should include ultrasound guidance into the selected vein and be secured with a stitch. 2D imaging ultrasound guidance should be undertaken whether the situation is elective or an emergency (NICE, 2002). Ultrasound is used to assess vein size and patency prior to venous puncture, and ultrasound guidance during venepuncture minimises the incidence of venous access-related complications, decreases the procedure time and increases the rate of initial technical success.

The life of a NTHC differs with insertion site; in general, internal jugular and subclavian vein catheters are suitable for one to three weeks of use, whereas femoral catheters are suitable for one HD session in ambulatory patients and three to seven days for bed-bound patients (Dugué et al., 2012). Subclavian NTHC should be avoided in people at risk of progressing to chronic kidney disease stage 4 to 5 due to the risk of venous stenosis, which compromises future permanent access options (Mahon, Jenkins & Burnapp, 2013).

Confirmation of the catheter tip position must be documented using fluoroscopy or chest film prior to use of the catheter. While urgent HD may be life-saving, mechanical and infectious complications related to the insertion of a NTHC can prove fatal (Clark & Barsuk, 2014; Vats, 2012).

Renal replacement therapy (RRT) – Undertaken for both acute and permanent kidney damage. If kidney damage is permanent, then without RRT the person will die.

Haemodialysis (HD) – Purifies the blood of the patient whose kidneys are not functioning.

Peritoneal dialysis (PD) – Uses the person's peritoneum as the membrane for fluid and electrolyte/waste product removal.

Catheter care

A sterile transparent semi-permeable dressing or sterile gauze can be used as line dressings. Gauze dressings are recommended for patients with bleeding or diaphoresis, but must be changed every 48 hours. Transparent dressings allow for visualisation of the access site and should be changed after seven days (O'Grady et al., 2011). At the end of each HD session, the NTHC must be flushed with saline and an anti-coagulant agent in accordance with hospital policy, to maintain the patency of the catheter. It is imperative to remove the anticoagulant 'lock' from the catheter prior to the next HD session (Mahon, Jenkins & Burnapp, 2013).

Patient-centred care

In Australia, acute care services aim to provide equal quality medical care for all people, *regardless* of culture, religion, race or gender, to ensure that all citizens receive a good basic standard of care. However, not all patients come to acute care with the same resources, understanding and experiences. It is therefore vital that nurses and multidisciplinary health professionals also provide care that is *regardful* of individual patients and their specific situations. This is particularly important when patients are part of a minority, vulnerable or culturally different group to mainstream Australia, such as Aboriginal and Torres Strait Islander people, refugees, migrants, people from rural and remote locations, people with disability, or people with an intellectual disability or mental illness. **Cultural safety** is an important consideration when providing care to these groups.

Cultural safety – Care is culturally safe if it is perceived to be so by the person receiving the care.

Fundamentals of care: Cultural safety

Nurses can undertake particular actions to provide quality cultural as well as clinical care (Best, 2014; Taylor & Guerin, 2014). They can begin by asking patients and their family members whether they have any specific needs or concerns. This may identify the need for interpreters, cultural support, same-gendered care, accommodation or transport assistance, telephone access, particular food avoidance, more detailed or clearer explanations, and more opportunities for two-way discussions about their care and options. The way the healthcare system is structured and the roles of each health carer may be confusing, and need further explanation. Nurses can access detailed information on how to provide culturally safe care via CATSINaM (2018).

For Jasper (see Skills in Practice above), many of these needs may arise. He may also be concerned about how he will be treated by both staff and other patients. He may have family members who had negative experiences in hospital, or were very ill and died. He may wish to discuss his condition and care options with other members of his family and/or his primary health carers, and nurses can help to arrange this, as well as to provide Jasper with appropriate written and visual resources.

It is important to ask every patient whether they are of Aboriginal or Torres Strait Islander descent, even if they do not 'appear' to be Aboriginal. This is necessary in order to meet individual patients' needs, and to ensure population-based health impacts and improvements can be measured and responded to.

Health promotion and patient education

Health literacy is more than reading health information: it refers to 'the cognitive and social skills which determine the motivation and ability of individuals to gain access to, understand and use information in ways which promote and maintain good health' (WHO, 2018). Increasing patients' access and use of health information is a way to improve their engagement in their care (WHO, 2018).

Nurses play a vital role in health promotion and patient education. Patients with AKI require emotional support as well as education, and nurses must comprehensively assess the patient and family's AKI knowledge and understanding. Remember that the patient may have decreased concentration levels, fatigue or even nausea due to uraemia, and this can affect their ability to focus (Hulse & Davies, 2015). Learning new health information can also be intimidating for some patients. Therefore, prior to the delivery of any patient education, nurses should consider the following adult learning factors (Russell, 2006):

- the patient's motivation to learn
- the fact that patients learn better when an education session is underpinned by mutual respect, trust and effective communication
- the patient's prior knowledge and experiences on the topic
- the patient's knowledge gap, which should be identified through the use of careful questioning
- an awareness that new patient learning should be built on prior knowledge and experiences.

Identifying the patient's and nurse's preferred learning style (visual, auditory, kinaesthetic) allows for learning to be planned and delivered in a variety of ways (listening, doing, saying), improving the learning and the associated experience. Throughout the education session, nurses should check for learning through strategies such as the 'teach-back method', and gently correct any misunderstanding of the information (Tamura-Lis, 2013). The provision of resources such as pamphlets allows the patient to reinforce their learning at a later time.

Barriers

A number of barriers to patient learning exist such as a lack of time, confidence and motivation (Russell, 2006). By considering these barriers, nurses can then implement strategies to optimise the learning opportunity (Russell, 2006). For example, a patient may lack the confidence to administer a new medication. Dividing the education session into short sections may be less intimidating for the patient, and can increase their confidence and willingness to engage (Russell, 2006).

Preparation

Preparation for the education session is paramount. Nurses should consider the patient, environmental and individual factors that can impact the education session, and implement strategies to minimise their impact (Russell, 2006):

- *Patient factors* include culture, first language, gender, age, illness, literacy, sensory barriers (hearing, visual), need for an interpreter.
- *Environmental factors* include lighting, noise, temperature, privacy, preparation of resources.
- *Individual factors* include comfort, pain, pace/speed of session, time of session (morning or afternoon), opportunity for reinforcement/application of knowledge.

REFLECTIVE QUESTIONS

- As a nurse, what do you consider to be important aspects to consider when looking after someone from a different culture from your own for yourself and your patients?
- Based on the normal function of the nephron, explain how the clinical manifestations of AKI appear.

The nurse's role and the importance of collaboration with MDT in the delivery of person-centred care

Nurses are pivotal to ensuring patient-centred care occurs, as they are present on the wards day and night, have ongoing contact with patients and family members, and interact with the many different multidisciplinary team members involved in patient care. Nurses advocate for patients, and are a key component in communication and overall coordination of care. The best situation for comprehensive person-centred care is when nurses and multidisciplinary team members work together, complementing each other's skills, knowledge and resources.

The nursing care of AKI is challenging and multifaceted, as the patient can be critically ill and requires constant monitoring since most organs can be affected. It is therefore vital that nurses understand what AKI is, and have a good comprehension of its management in order to deliver holistic care to the patient concerned (Murphy & Byrne, 2010). 'The commitment of nurses to implementing proven strategies for the prevention of AKI … is a critical link to ensuring optimal patient outcomes' (Lambert et al., 2017, p. 17). Nurse leaders are pivotal to ensuring the multidisciplinary healthcare team provides a coordinated approach to care for patients with AKI, and Lambert and colleagues (2017) state that standardised evidence-based approaches to care that involve the multidisciplinary team could have the potential to reduce AKI incidence (Lambert et al., 2017). Care for people with AKI requires the provision of ongoing education for nurses and continual collaboration with the multidisciplinary team to effectively manage the AKI patient (Murphy & Byrne, 2010).

Discharge planning

Patient education needs to include information about medication; ways to prevent AKI from occurring again; managing comorbid conditions such as diabetes and hypertension; not taking over the counter medication without consulting with a GP or nephrologist; and the need to inform any healthcare provider that they have had AKI, as contrast medium can be nephrotoxic. Patients also require dietary information and must understand the importance of any dietary restrictions imposed. They should be aware of signs and symptoms that can occur, who to contact and the telephone numbers of the renal ward. It is imperative that they have a follow-up review with a nephrologist. This appointment time should be given to the patient upon discharge. Additional discharge-planning considerations for patients returning to rural and remote settings are listed in Table 7.3.

Table 7.3 Additional discharge-planning considerations for patients returning to rural and remote settings

Aspect	Factors	Considerations
Health literacy	Do the patient, their family members and primary carers understand their diagnosis, treatment and ongoing care requirements?	Further explanations, with supportive written material and diagrams, website links. Interpreters required?
		Same information shared between tertiary hospitals and primary care.
Discharge/transfer of care	Primary carers – doctor, remote area nurse and/ or Aboriginal health professional contacted	Names, contact details, transfer of care information sent (record date how information is exchanged – fax, phone, letter, email).
	Family contacted	Family is aware the patient is being discharged/ transferred (may have intermittent phones, limited mobile reception).
	Detailed discharge information shared with patient (nursing, allied health discharge plan, discharge summary)	Contents of discharge/ transfer of care information discussed with patient and a copy given to them in case they require medical treatment in another location on the way home.
Travel home	Safe return to home via car, bus, plane or combination	Distance, road condition, season (very hot, wet), time of day/night, accompanied or alone, cost, financial assistance, phone coverage.
Follow-up care	Contact person at city hospital	A contact person they can ring if they have difficulties.
	Healthcare organisations available in the location	GP surgery, local hospital, Aboriginal health service, fly in services (Royal Flying Doctor Service or outreach).
	Allied health	Availability, waiting lists and frequency of pharmacist, physiotherapy, occupational therapy and social work services.

(cont.)

Table 7.3   (cont.)

Aspect	Factors	Considerations
	Pharmacy supplies	Time required getting in new supplies (days or weeks). Consider extending discharge medication to three weeks' supply.
	Renal follow-up appointment	Return to city or outreach options.
		Transport and accommodation support.

Source: Adapted from Kelly et al. (2016).

SUMMARY

Learning objective 1: Define acute kidney injuries (AKI); identify underlying pathophysiology, risk factors and presentations associated with an AKI.

AKI is a condition where an abrupt injury occurs to the kidneys. Often it will be short-term and kidney function will return. Nurses need to be able to identify underlying pathophysiology, risk factors and presentation for pre-renal, intra-renal and post-renal injury.

Learning objective 2: Describe nursing assessment and management strategies for the individual with an AKI.

The nurse's role includes individualised assessment and management of the person with AKI. Nurses undertake a variety of roles, including coordination of care, identifying early signs of deterioration, possible RRT and supporting the individual throughout care delivery.

Learning objective 3: Understand the concepts of patient-centred care and health education in relation to AKI.

As with all individuals, patient-centred care is integral to the management of AKI. It incorporates strategies relating to not only the patient but also their family and the multidisciplinary healthcare team. Through well-developed and seamlessly executed care coordination, the individual needs of the patient will be met.

Learning objective 4: Identify and discuss the nurse's role in the coordination and collaborative management of individuals with AKI.

Nurses collaborate with healthcare team members to form a partnership and negotiate the provision of rapid, holistic, appropriate physical and psychological care to individuals with AKI.

REVIEW QUESTIONS

7.1 How would you initially assess a patient for potential AKI when they arrive on the ward/ at the clinic?

7.2 Explain the three classifications of AKI and provide three causes for each classification.

7.3 What are the signs and symptoms of AKI?

7.4 What urine, blood and imaging tests would be appropriate to determine AKI?

7.5 How could you provide culturally safe care for a newly arrived refugee AKI patient?

RESEARCH TOPIC

Read the following article on renal patient journey mapping processes.

Kelly, J., Wilden, C., Herman, K., Martin, G., Russell, C. & Brown, S. (2016). Bottling knowledge and sharing it: Using patient journey mapping to build evidence and improve Aboriginal renal patient care. *Renal Society of Australasia Journal*, 12(2), 48–55.

Using either the case studies in the above article or someone you have looked after, consider which factors might affect a person's discharge planning, journey home and follow-up care. Identify how you as a nurse could ensure that the needs of the patient and their family are met. Critically reflect upon three aspects of care that could have improved the healthcare experiences and outcomes for this patient and other Aboriginal patients in the future.

FURTHER READING

Kelly, J., Wilden, C., Chamney, M., Martin, G., Herman, K. & Russell, C. (2016). Improving cultural and clinical competency and safety of renal nurse education. *Renal Society of Australasia Journal*, 12(3), 106–12.

Kelly, J., Wilden, C., Herman, K., Martin, G., Russell, C. & Brown, S. (2016). Bottling knowledge and sharing it: Using patient journey mapping to build evidence and improve Aboriginal renal patient care. *Renal Society of Australasia Journal*, 12(2), 48–55.

Kidney Health Australia (2018). Acute kidney injury. Retrieved from http://kidney.org.au/your-kidneys/detect/acute-kidney-injury.

London Acute Kidney Injury Network (2018). Website. Retrieved from http://www.londonaki.net/index.html.

Mahon, A., Jenkins, K. & Burnapp, L. (2013). *Oxford Handbook of Renal Nursing*. Oxford: Oxford University Press.

Palmer, J. (2017). Climate change and kidney disease: The deadly new link. Sydney *Morning Herald Good Weekend*, 3 May. Retrieved from http://www.smh.com.au/good-weekend/climate-change-and-kidney-disease-the-deadly-new-link-20170503-gvxzjz.html.

Smith, J. (2016). *Australia's Rural, Remote and Indigenous Health* (3rd ed.). Sydney: Elsevier.

REFERENCES

Australian Institute of Health and Welfare (AIHW) (2015). *Acute Kidney Injury in Australia: A First National Snapshot*. Canberra: AIHW.

Barasch, J., Zager, R. & Bonventre, J. V. (2017). Acute kidney injury: A problem of definition. *The Lancet*, 389(10071), 779–81.

Bellomo, R., Kellum, J.A. & Ronco, C. (2012). Acute kidney injury. *The Lancet*, 380(9843), 756–66.

Best, O. (2014). The cultural safety journey: An Australian nursing context. In O. Best & B. Fredericks (eds) *Yatdjuligin: Aboriginal and Torres Strait Islander Nursing and Midwifery Care*. Melbourne: Cambridge University Press.

CATSINaM (2018). *Cultural Safety Statement*. Retrieved from http://www.catsinam.org.au/static/uploads/files/cultural-safety-endorsed-march-2014-wfginzphsxbz.pdf.

Chadwick, L. & Macnab, R. (2015). Laboratory tests of renal function. *Anaesthesia & Intensive Care Medicine*, 16(6), 257–61.

Chawla, L.S., Eggers, P.W., Star, R.A. & Kimmel, P.L. (2014). Acute kidney injury and chronic kidney disease as interconnected syndromes. *New England Journal of Medicine*, 371(1), 58–66.

Clark, E.G. & Barsuk, J.H. (2014). Temporary hemodialysis catheters: Recent advances. *Kidney International*, 86(5), 888–95.

Dugué, A., Levesque, S., Fischer, M., Souweine, S., Mira, J., Megarbane, B., Daubin, C., du Cheyron, D. & Parienti, J. (2012). Vascular access sites for acute renal replacement in intensive care units. *Clinical Journal of the American Society of Nephrology*, 7(1), 70–7.

Finlay, S., Asderakis, A., Ilham, A., Elker, D., Chapman, D. & Ablorsu, E. (2017). The role of nutritional assessment and early enteral nutrition for combined pancreas and kidney transplant candidates. *Clinical Nutrition ESPEN*, 17, 22–7.

Giebisch, G.H. & Wingo, C.S. (2013). Renal potassium homeostasis: A short historical perspective. *Seminars in Nephrology*, 33, 209–14.

Harty, J. (2014). Prevention and management of acute kidney injury. *Ulster Medical Journal*, 83(3), 149–57.

Hulse, C. & Davies, A. (2015) Acute kidney injury: Prevention and recognition. *Nursing Times*, 111(30–31), 12–15.

Kelly, J., Wilden, C., Herman, K., Martin, G., Russell, C. & Brown, S. (2016). Bottling knowledge and sharing it: Using patient journey mapping to build evidence and improve Aboriginal renal patient care. *Renal Society of Australasia Journal*, 12(2), 48–55.

Kidney Disease: Improving Global Outcomes (KDIGO) (2012). Acute Kidney Injury Work Group. KDIGO clinical practice guideline for acute kidney injury. *Kidney International*, 2, 1–138.

Kidney Health Australia (2017). Acute kidney injury. Retrieved from http://kidney.org.au/your-kidneys/detect/acute-kidney-injury.

Kovesdy, C.P. (2014). Management of hyperkalaemia in chronic kidney disease. *National Review of Nephrology*, 10(11), 653–62.

Lambert, P., Chaisson, K., Horton, S., Petrin, C., Marshall, E., Bowden, S., Scott, L., Conley, S., Stender, J., Kent, G., Hopkins, E., Smith, B., Kelloway, A., Roy, N., Homsted, B., Downs, C., Ross, C. & Brown, J. (2017). Reducing acute kidney injury due to contrast material: How nurses can improve patient safety. *Critical Care Nursing*, 37(1), 13–26.

Lewington, A.J., Cerda, J. & Mehta, R.L. (2013). Raising awareness of acute kidney injury: A global perspective of a silent killer. *Kidney International*, 84(3), 457–67.

Lopes, J.A., Fernandes, P., Jorge, S., Gonçalves, S., Alvarez, A., Costa e Silva, Z. et al. (2008). Acute kidney injury in intensive care unit patients: A comparison between the RIFLE and the Acute Kidney Injury Network classifications. *Critical Care*, 12(4), R110.

Mahon, A., Jenkins, K. & Burnapp, L. (2013). *Oxford Handbook of Renal Nursing*. Oxford: Oxford University Press.

Mehta, R.L., Kellum, J.A., Shah, S.V., Molitoris, B.A., Ronco, C., Warnock, D.G. & Levin, A. (2007). Acute Kidney Injury Network: Report of an initiative to improve outcomes in acute kidney injury. *Critical Care*, 11(2), R31.

Murphy, F. & Byrne, G. (2010). The role of the nurse in the management of acute kidney injury. *British Journal of Nursing*, 19(3), 146–52.

National Institute for Health and Care Excellence (NICE) (2013). *Acute Kidney Injury: Prevention, Detection and Management of AKI Up to the Point of Renal Replacement Therapy*. London: NICE. Retrieved from https://www.nice.org.uk/guidance/cg169.

National Kidney Foundation (2016). Tests to measure kidney function damage and detect abnormalities. Retrieved from: https://www.kidney.org/atoz/content/kidneytests.

Nursing Council of New Zealand (NCNZ) ([2007] 2016). *Competencies for Registered Nurses*. Retrieved from http://www.nursingcouncil.org.nz/Nurses.

Nursing and Midwifery Board of Australia (NMBA) (2016). *Registered Nurse Standards for Practice*. Melbourne: Nursing & Midwifery Board of Australia. Retrieved from

http://www.nursingmidwiferyboard.gov.au/Codes-Guidelines-Statements/
Professional-standards.aspx.

O'Grady, N.P., Alexander, M., Burns, L.A., Dellinger, E.P., Garland, J., Heard, S.O. et al.
(2011). Guidelines for the prevention of intravascular catheter-related infections.
*Clinical Infectious Diseases: An Official Publication of the Infectious Diseases
Society of America*, 52(9), e162–e193.

Palevsky, P.M., Liu, K.D., Brophy, P.D., Chawla, L.S., Parikh, C.R., Thakar, C.V., Tolwani, A.J.,
Waikar, S.S. & Weisbord, S.D. (2013). KDOQI US commentary on the 2012 KDIGO
clinical practice guideline for acute kidney injury. *American Journal of Kidney
Diseases*, 61(5), 649–72.

Perlman, R., Heung, M. & Ix, J. (2014). Renal disease. In G. Hammer & S. McPhee (eds),
Pathophysiology of Disease: An Introduction to Clinical Medicine. New York:
McGraw Hill, pp. 455–82.

Rahman, M., Shad, F. & Smith, M.C. (2012). Acute kidney injury: A guide to diagnosis and
management. *American Family Physician*, 86(7), 631–9.

Russell, S. (2006). An overview of adult-learning processes. *Urologic Nursing*, 26(5), 349–
52, 370.

Severs, D., Rookmaaker, M.B. & Hoorn, E.J. (2015). Intravenous solutions in the care of
patients with volume depletion and electrolyte abnormalities. *American Journal of
Kidney Disease*, 66(1), 147–53.

Sharfuddin, A.A. & Molitoris, B.A. (2011). Pathophysiology of ischemic acute kidney injury.
National Review of Nephrology, 7(4), 189–200.

Stewart, J.A. (2009). Adding insult to injury: Care of patients with acute kidney injury.
British Journal of Hospital Medicine (London), 70(7), 372–3.

Strasinger, S.K. & Di Lorenzo, M.S. (2014), *Urinalysis and Body Fluids* (6th ed.).
Philadelphia, PA: F.A. Davis Company.

Susantitaphong, P., Cruz, D.N., Cerda, J., Abulfaraj, M., Alqahtani, F., Koulouridis, I. et al.
(2013). World incidence of AKI: A meta-analysis. *Clinical Journal of the American
Society of Nephrology*, 8(9), 1482–93.

Tamura-Lis, W. (2013). Teach-back for quality education and patient safety. *Urologic Nursing*,
33(6), 267–98.

Taylor, K. & Guerin, P. (2014). *Health Care and Indigenous Australians: Cultural Safety in
Practice*. Sydney: Palgrave Macmillan.

Thomas N. (ed.) (2014). *Renal Nursing* (4th ed.). Chichester: Wiley Blackwell.

Thornburg, B. & Gray-Vickrey, P. (2016). Acute kidney injury: Limiting the damage. *Nursing*,
46(6), 24–34.

Tögel, F. & Westenfelder, C. (2014). Recent advances in the understanding of acute kidney
injury. *F1000Prime Reports*, 6, 83.

Vats, H.S. (2012). Complications of catheters: Tunneled and nontunneled. *Advanced
Chronic Kidney Disease*, 19(3), 188–94.

White, L., Hassoun, H., Bihorac, A., Moore, L., Sailors, M., McKinley, A., Valdivia, A. &
Moore, F. (2013). Acute kidney injury (AKI) is surprisingly common and a powerful
predictor of mortality in surgical sepsis. *Journal of Trauma and Acute Care Surgery*,
75(3), 1–16.

World Health Organization (WHO) (2018). Health promotion. Retrieved from
http://www.who.int/topics/health_promotion/en.

Acute neurological conditions

8

Amali Hohol, Leeanne Ford,
Julia Gilbert, Ronak Reshamwala
and Michael Todorovic

LEARNING OBJECTIVES

At the completion of this chapter, you should be able to:

1   define acute neurological conditions and understand their prevalence, underlying pathophysiology and risk factors
2   describe nursing assessment and management strategies for the individual with an acute neurological condition
3   understand the concepts of patient-centred care in coordinated care approaches
4   explain the role of the nurse in discharge planning for the patient with an acute neurological condition
5   understand advanced nursing practice in relation to acute neurological conditions.

Introduction

Neurological conditions are diseases or conditions affecting the central and peripheral nervous system, caused by illness or injury and resulting in physical and/or psychological symptoms. Neurological conditions are a primary contributor to disability, are often incurable and worsen over time. For these reasons, neurological conditions are considered a significant global and economic public health burden (Gaskin et al., 2017). Acute neurological disorders are not specific to a certain demographic, and can impact people of all ages, irrespective of gender or ethnicity. The patient presenting with an acute neurological condition represents a unique nursing challenge, with the condition often impacting the person's quality of life. This impact can be significantly greater if disability is acquired at a young age.

The complexity of care associated with acute neurological conditions indicates a need for skilled healthcare providers to ensure the best possible patient outcomes. It is important that clinicians understand that rapid assessment and management of the acutely ill neurological patient is vital for achieving this (Creed, 2010). This chapter identifies the underlying pathophysiology, prevalence and risk factors of a range of acute neurological disorders. The key components of neurological assessment will be explained, and the management and treatment strategies for each neurological condition will be explored briefly. Coordinated, patient-centred care is fundamental to achieving the best patient outcomes, and this topic will also be discussed, along with the role of the nurse in the discharge planning process. The chapter will close by examining advanced nursing practice in the care of acutely unwell neurological patients.

It is imperative that nurses caring for the patient with an acute neurological condition has the capability to evaluate their practice based on pre-determined goals, plans and outcomes. It is also necessary that nurses review and revise their practice accordingly to ensure that the patient is supported to meet expected goals and outcomes. In the provision of best practice, registered nurses must also ensure that they accurately document and communicate their care priorities to other nurses and interdisciplinary healthcare professionals, as well as to the patient and their family or carers. This facilitates nurses to deliver high standards of nursing care.

NURSING STANDARDS

The following identifies the national competency standards for the registered nurse from the Nursing and Midwifery Board of Australia (NMBA) and the Nursing Council of New Zealand (NCNZ) that are addressed in this chapter.

Australian Registered Nurse Standards for Practice

Standard 1: Thinks critically and analyses nursing practice

Standard 2: Engages in therapeutic and professional relationships

Standard 3: Maintains the capability for practice

Standard 4: Comprehensively conducts assessments

Standard 5: Develops a plan for nursing practice

Standard 6: Provides safe, appropriate and responsive quality nursing practice

Standard 7: Evaluates outcomes to inform nursing practice

(NMBA, 2016b)

New Zealand: Competencies for Registered Nurses

Competency 1.4: Promotes an environment that enables health consumer safety, independence, quality of life, and health

Competency 1.5: Practises nursing in a manner that the health consumer determines as being culturally safe

Competency 2.1: Provides planned nursing care to achieve identified outcomes

Competency 2.2: Undertakes a comprehensive and accurate nursing assessment of health consumers in a variety of settings

Competency 2.3: Ensures documentation is accurate and maintains confidentiality of information

Competency 3.1: Establishes, maintains and concludes therapeutic interpersonal relationships with health consumers

Competency 3.2: Practises nursing in a negotiated partnership with the health consumer where and when possible

Competency 4.1: Collaborates and participates with colleagues and members of the health care team to facilitate and coordinate care

Competency 4.2: Recognises and values the roles and skills of all members of the health care team in the delivery of care

(NCNZ, [2007] 2016)

Pathophysiology, prevalence and risk factors associated with acute neurological conditions

The nervous system is a fast-acting communication network of nerve fibres and neurons that allow the body to monitor and interact with its environment. Structurally, the nervous system can be divided into the **central nervous system (CNS)** and the **peripheral nervous system (PNS)**. The CNS comprises the brain and spinal cord and processes, and coordinates sensory input and motor function, while the PNS is responsible for the transmission of signals to and from the CNS and comprises the spinal and cranial nerves (Chamberlain & Kuzmiuk, 2016). The cranial cavity houses the brain (Figure 8.1), which is covered by membranes, fluid and the skull bones. Brain tissues are protected by the cranial bones, cranial meninges and the cerebrospinal fluid. The following acute neurological conditions arise from dysfunction relating to these anatomical systems and structures.

Central nervous system (CNS) – Comprises the spinal cord and brain, and controls most bodily functions.

Peripheral nervous system (PNS) – Comprises the spinal and cranial nerves, which provides sensory and motor feedback to the CNS.

Cerebrovascular disorders

Cerebrovascular accident (stroke) is one of the leading causes of death and disability in Australia, reported to affect over 470 000 people in 2012 (Stroke Foundation, 2013b). Stroke is considered an impairment of neurological function, with sudden onset, that lasts for more than 24 hours. Pathophysiologically, a stroke is an interruption to the brain's blood supply, resulting in reduced oxygenation to brain tissue, subsequently resulting in brain cell damage or death (Kerr, 2012).

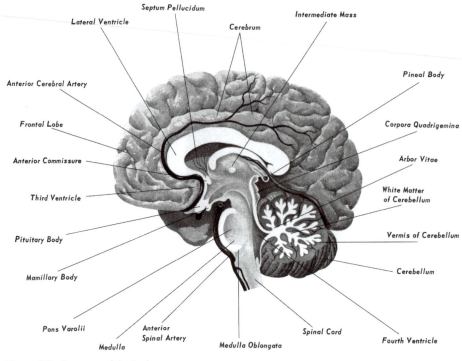

Figure 8.1   Anatomy of the brain

There are two main types of stroke: ischemic and haemorrhagic. **Ischemic strokes** are caused by an occlusion or substantial stenosis vessel that supplies blood to the brain. These blockages can be due to a thrombus (blood clot) formed secondary to a disrupted fatty plaque (atherosclerosis) or an embolism (vessel-blocking material) that may include part of a thrombus, fat globule or gas bubble (Iwasaki et al., 2011; Johnston & Connolly, 2015). Non-modifiable risk factors for stroke include age, gender (more prevalent in males) and a family history of stroke, while modifiable risk factors include hypertension, hypercholesterolemia, smoking, obesity and overweight, poor diet and excessive alcohol intake (Stroke Foundation, 2017).

Haemorrhagic strokes are less common than ischemic strokes; however, they are associated with a greater rate of morbidity and mortality (Feigin et al., 2015). They are caused by a ruptured cerebral vessel, resulting in intra-cerebral, sub-arachnoid and intra-ventricular bleeding. The cerebrovascular changes that underlie most intra-cerebral haemorrhages are commonly due to chronic hypertension or the deposition of beta-amyloid plaques in medium/small-sized cerebral arteries (Johnston & Connolly, 2015).

Transient ischemic attacks (TIAs) result from a temporary disruption of cerebral blood flow. TIAs may be caused by partial blood vessel occlusion, or by vessel spasm or narrowing. As the occlusion is only temporary, neurological deficits will resolve within 24 hours of onset and leave no permanent neurological dysfunction (Johnston & Connolly, 2015). Often, TIAs are warnings that a stroke is developing.

Spinal cord trauma

In Australia, approximately 362 cases of new **spinal cord injury (SCI)** are reported each year (Johnston & Connolly, 2015). SCI is more prevalent in males (84 per cent) than females (16 per cent), with most injuries occurring between the ages of 15 and 24. As the

National Spinal Cord Injury Statistical Center (2016) explains, 80 per cent of SCI incidents are the result of traumatic injury, and may be caused by:

- motor vehicle accidents (46 per cent)
- falls (28 per cent)
- being hit or struck by an object (9 per cent)
- water-related incidents (9 per cent)
- other causes, including sport (8 per cent).

Trauma to the spinal cord results from damage to the vertebral column (Figure 8.2). SCIs occur either from primary or secondary injury. **Primary injury** is due to the initial mechanical trauma, which causes direct tissue destruction, and generally immediate permanent damage (Chamberlain & McGloin, 2016). Primary vertebral injuries occur due to acceleration, deceleration or demolition forces upon impact, and consequently cause compression, traction or shearing of tissues. In cases where a vertebral fracture has occurred, compression and damage to nerve fibres are due to bone fragments or connective tissues. Additionally, hyperextension, hyperflexion, vertical compression or rotation can damage the bones, ligaments, joints and neural tissue of the vertebral column (Boss & Heuther, 2014).

Primary injury – The initial insult, occurring at the time of the event.

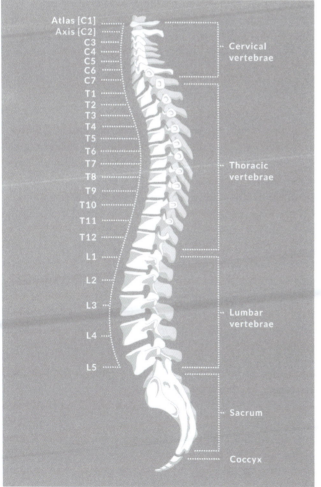

Figure 8.2   The spinal column

Secondary SCI is the result of vascular, cellular and biochemical reactions, which commence shortly after the initial injury and can continue for weeks (Boss & Heuther, 2014). In **secondary injury**, nerve fibres swell and disintegrate, and are related to mechanisms including ischemia, hypoxia, oedema, cellular and molecular inflammatory injury and cell death. Ischemia is the most common post-SCI event, and within hours spinal cord blood flow is reduced. Oedema will develop at the site of injury and disperse into the surrounding areas. Hypoxia may occur if airway maintenance and ventilation have been compromised and regulatory chemicals and free radicals, which may be harmful to the spinal cord, can be released secondary to the activation of immunity mechanisms (Chamberlain & McGloin, 2016). Most adult injuries occur at the cervical vertebrae or between the last few thoracic vertebra and the beginning of the lumbar vertebrae. Neurological dysfunction associated with SCI is directly related to the vertebrae involved (Johnston & Connolly, 2015).

Secondary injury – The activation of mechanisms of the body in response to the primary injury.

Traumatic brain injury (TBI)

Traumatic brain injury (TBI) is considered a serious form of head injury. In 2004–05, the incidence of TBI was 150 per 100 000 population. Falls are the most common cause of TBI (35 per cent), followed by motor vehicle/traffic accidents (17 per cent), being struck against/by an object (16.5 per cent) and assaults (10 per cent) (Chamberlain & McGloin, 2016). TBIs are classified into focal brain injuries and diffuse axonal injuries. Focal head injuries include both blunt (closed) trauma, whereby the injury does not expose the brain to the external environment, and penetrating (open) trauma, which occurs when the injury penetrates the dura and exposes the cranial contents to the exterior environment (Johnston & Connolly, 2015).

Traumatic brain injury (TBI) – Brain dysfunction due to an outside force.

Focal brain injury

Focal brain injuries generally produce contusions, whereby brain tissue is injured without breaking the inner pia mater (Johnston & Connolly, 2015). The brain is floating in the cerebrospinal fluid of the cranial cavity, and when impacted it tries to keep moving forward due to its inertia, even when the skull comes to a sudden stop. This causes the brain to strike against the inside of the skull at the site of injury, resulting in a coup injury (Johnston & Connolly, 2015). However, if the brain ricochets after this first strike and moves in the opposite direction to hit the opposing end of the skull, it is considered a contrecoup injury (Salzar et al., 2017).

If brain trauma causes rupture of the vasculature inside the cranial cavity, the resulting extravasation of the blood is known as intra-cranial haemorrhage. The risk of haemorrhage is increased in the presence of hypertension, anti-coagulation therapy, excessive alcohol intake and drug abuse (Caceres & Goldstein, 2012). Depending on the site of the ruptured vessel, the blood may pool at different sites and cause the following types of haemorrhages as outlined by Johnston and Connolly (2015):

- *Extradural (or Epidural) haemorrhage*. Bleeding occurs exterior to the dura mater, and blood pools between the meninges and the skull.
- *Subdural haemorrhage*. Bleeding starts in the subdural space, between dura mater and arachnoid layer.
- *Subarachnoid haemorrhage*. Bleeding into the subarachnoid space results from an injured or defective blood vessel.

- *Intra-cerebral haemorrhage*. Bleeding occurs directly in the brain parenchyma as a result of localised injury.

Contusions and bleeding of the brain often cause oedema, which develops in and around damaged tissue, and contributes to raised **intra-cranial pressure (ICP)** and brain tissue compression. Compressed brain tissue can be forced into the ventricles, or downward to the spinal cord, which is generally fatal (Johnston & Connolly, 2015).

Intra-cranial pressure (ICP) – The pressure inside the skull. Normally this comprises the brain and cerebrospinal fluid.

Diffuse axonal Injury

Diffuse axonal injury results from shaking, shearing and inertial forces and cause shearing of axons and associated neuroglia, and haemorrhagic contusions (Chamberlain & McGloin, 2016). Following traumatic mechanisms, the brain cells simultaneously send action potentials, causing mass electrical discharges and releasing glutamate, a neurotransmitter. This causes alterations to the ion flow of potassium and calcium ion channels, affecting mitochondria function and resulting in a subsequent energy crisis. Cells are unable to restore their electrolyte balance and neurons become functionally impaired (Johnston & Connolly, 2015).

Infections and inflammation

There are two main infections that affect the CNS: meningitis and encephalitis. Meningitis relates to the meninges, while encephalitis affects the brain parenchyma (Chamberlain & McGloin, 2016). Statistically, while viral meningitis is not reported in Australia, approximately one in 100 000 persons is diagnosed with bacterial meningitis (Boss & Heuther, 2014). Encephalitis is most often caused by the herpes simplex virus (HSV) and has an annual incidence of one in 250 000 to 500 000 (Chamberlain & McGloin, 2016).

Meningitis

The bacteria that often cause meningitis are found in the nasopharynx prior to becoming blood borne. The bacteria induce an inflammatory response in the meninges, cerebrospinal fluid (CSF) and ventricles, causing neutrophils to travel to the subarachnoid space (Boss & Heuther, 2014). This reaction creates a thickening of the CSF, which disrupts the normal flow of CSF around the brain and spinal cord and results in hydrocephalus (fluid accumulation in the brain). This is further compounded by purulent exudate collecting at the base of the brain, and around the cranial and spinal nerves. The cells of the meninges become oedematous and increase ICP, while small to medium subarachnoid blood vessels become engorged, interfering with normal cerebral circulation and potentially causing thrombosis (Johnston & Connolly, 2015).

Encephalitis

Viruses, such as HSV, acquire access to the CNS via the bloodstream, olfactory bulb or cricoid plexus. The infection causes significant cell degeneration, while oedema, necrosis and haemorrhage may also develop. These factors increase ICP and may eventuate into brain herniation (Boss & Heuther, 2014). In addition, interference with the blood–brain barrier can cause septic shock, disseminated intravascular coagulopathy and multi-organ failure (Chamberlain & McGloin, 2016).

Nursing assessment and management of acute neurological conditions

Acute neurological conditions generally worsen prior to the patient becoming stable. Neurological symptoms can fluctuate, and an improvement in symptoms does not indicate an improvement in the patient's condition (Wijdicks, 2016). The clinical manifestations of acute neurological conditions are related directly to the underlying pathophysiology. While the signs and symptoms of neurological dysfunction are clear, they can be difficult to interpret as they are often non-specific, thus challenging even the most experienced health professional (Wijdicks, 2016). For this reason, careful, systematic assessment of the patient with an acute neurological condition is required.

Nursing assessment of the patient with an acute neurological condition

Neurological assessment of the patient initially occurs as part of the primary survey. The patient's level of consciousness (LOC) is determined, and alterations to airway, breathing and circulation can indicate neurological changes that warrant further investigation. Following the primary survey, and once the patient is considered stable, a comprehensive assessment of the patient's neurological function can occur (Schoenwald & Douglas, 2016). Neurological assessment should include assessing the LOC, health history, physical examination, vital signs and diagnostic testing.

Assessing level of consciousness

Initially, the neurological assessment should commence with a simple determination of the patient's LOC. Two common assessments of LOC include AVPU (alert, responds to voice, responds to pain, unconscious) and the Glasgow Coma Scale (GCS). It is recommended that the AVPU be used in emergency situations to rapidly determine patient deterioration, while the GCS provides a more comprehensive assessment of consciousness. The GCS is divided into three components: eye opening, best verbal response and best motor response. It is imperative that these components be correctly assessed to ensure accurate assessment (Creed, 2010).

Health history

A patient history begins with identifying the primary symptom/s, associated factors, and onset and duration of the symptoms. The clinician should determine whether symptom onset was rapid or gradual, whether an injury was involved, the injury mechanism and whether symptoms are improving or worsening (Goolsby & Grubb, 2011). Onset can be a significant detail, as acute symptom onset (within minutes to an hour) can indicate a vascular problem (i.e. stroke or subarachnoid haemorrhage), while symptoms that occur over hours to days might signal an inflammatory disorder such as meningitis. Table 8.1 provides a comprehensive list of acute neurological conditions and their associated symptoms.

Table 8.1   Assessable components of the physical neurological examination

Function	Assessable components
Mental status	Level of consciousness (LOC), orientation, memory, knowledge, attention span, concentration, language and abstract thoughts.
Cranial nerves	Each of the 12 pairs of cranial nerves should be tested.
Motor function	Assess muscle size and tone. Observe and check for tremor, involuntary movements, rigidity, atrophy, asymmetric strength, spasticity, flaccidity and fasciculations. Coordination should be tested, as the inability to coordinate movements can indicate cerebellar dysfunction.
Reflexes	In all extremities, check deep tendon reflexes. Specialised reflex manoeuvres may reveal abnormalities. Diminished, asymmetrical or absent reflexes are clinically relevant.

Source: Goolsby and Grubb (2011); Maher (2016).

The general history of the patient should be discussed and include a review of all body systems, as neurological conditions often impact other systems. The past medical and surgical history should be conferred and include any conditions that may potentially contribute to neurological impairment, such as hypertension (Goolsby & Grubb, 2011). A medication history should be included, ensuring both previous and current medications are identified, as certain drugs can cause neurological alterations. A family history will identify any inherited neurological conditions, and a social history may uncover lifestyle factors, such as alcoholism and/or illicit drug use, which are linked to neurological illness (Talley & O'Connor, 2014).

Physical examination

The physical assessment then progresses to the general inspection. A systematic and meticulous general inspection may reveal signs not detected when the cranial nerves are assessed. The whole head should be examined for injury or scarring, while the skin should be inspected for lesions (Talley & O'Connor, 2014). The functioning of the central and peripheral nervous system should then be determined. Examining the CNS entails testing higher functions such as gait, speech, mental status, sensory function and motor function. Assessment of the PNS will provide information on the cranial nerves and reflexes (Maher, 2016). The specific characteristics of each component of the physical neurological examination are provided in Table 8.1. In addition, the nurse should have an understanding of the clinical manifestations of acute neurological conditions and what these may indicate. The signs and symptoms of acute neurological dysfunction are outlined in Table 8.2.

Table 8.2   Symptoms of acute neurological conditions

Neurological condition/issue	Associated clinical manifestations
Stroke	Fluctuating LOC/GCS, facial paralysis, hemiparesis, hemiplegia, hemianaesthesia, aphasia, anosognosia, homonymous hemianopsia, contralateral sensory and motor limb deficits, urinary incontinence, sensory loss, apraxia, cognitive impairment, personality change, contralateral/bilateral weakness, dysarthria, dysphagia, ataxia, vertigo, nausea, vomiting, visual disturbances
Spinal cord injury	Symptoms are directly related to the level and severity of injury. The higher the injury the more significant the symptoms.
Diffuse axonal injury	Decreased LOC, increased ICP, decortication, decerebration, cerebral oedema
Focal injury	Focal alterations, seizures, other symptoms consistent with haemorrhage
Epidural haemorrhage	Fluctuating LOC, headache, nausea, vomiting, focal abnormalities
Subdural haemorrhage	Symptoms consistent with raised ICP
Subarachnoid haemorrhage	Sudden severe headache, altered LOC, nausea, vomiting, photophobia
Intra-cerebral haemorrhage	Neurological deficits, headache, nausea, vomiting, reduced LOC, hypertension
Meningitis	Fever, severe headache, nausea, vomiting, nuchal rigidity, decreased LOC, photophobia
Encephalitis	Generally, presentation is non-specific, and onset may include fever, headache, nausea, vomiting. As the condition progresses, any neurological symptom may occur.
Increased intra-cranial pressure	Altered LOC, Cushing's triad, altered body temperature, altered pupillary response, decreased motor function, decortication, decerebration, headache, vomiting

Sources: Laskowski-Jones (2011a, 2011b); Lewis et al. (2017); Zomorodi (2017).

Vital signs

Vital signs are significant indicators of neurological dysfunction. Specific alterations to vital signs can signal that the patient's condition is deteriorating. However, nurses must understand that alterations of physiological status are generally late signs (Creed, 2010). The Cushing's triad is one example of when vital signs can indicate declining neurological function. In such events, the blood pressure will increase and the pulse pressure (the difference between the systolic and diastolic blood pressure) will widen. Bradycardia will result due to pressure on the brain stem and/or cerebral ischemia, and alterations to respirations will occur due to the level of brain stem involved. These three clinical manifestations are consistent with rising intra–cranial pressure (Creed, 2010).

Diagnostic testing

A range of diagnostic tests may be warranted in the assessment of the patient with an acute neurological condition. The most common are detailed in Table 8.3.

Table 8.3 Diagnostic tests for assessment of acute neurological conditions

Diagnostic study	Rationale
Magnetic resonance imaging (MRI)	Can be used with or without contrast to assist in the diagnosis of occult lesions.
Computerised tomography (CT)	Screens for expanding mass lesions such as those seen with subdural or epidural haematomas and haemorrhagic stroke. Without contrast, CT may evidence an embolic stroke. CT can also signal hydrocephalus.
Plain skull films (x-ray)	May detect extra-cranial abnormalities, including skull fractures or lesions.
Lumbar puncture (LP)	An invasive procedure that tests characteristics of cerebrospinal fluid. LP is useful in the detection of meningitis.
Laboratory studies	Full blood counts, erythrocyte sedimentation rate and metabolic profiles can assist in the identification of infection and metabolic abnormalities associated with neurological dysfunction.

Source: Goolsby and Grubb (2011); Talley and O'Connor (2014).

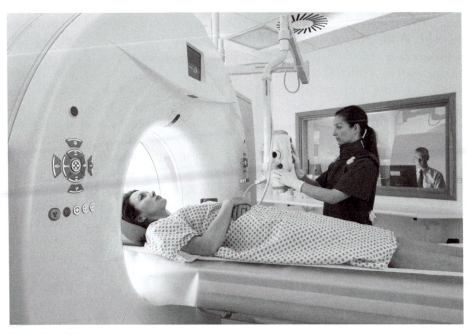

Figure 8.3   CT scanner

Nursing management of stroke

In cases of ischaemic stroke, it is necessary to determine whether the patient requires thrombolysis, a pharmacotherapy that dissolves all clots in the body. This treatment has a narrow administration window, with administration required within three hours of symptom onset (Creed, 2010). If the patient does not require thrombolysis, then conservative management is suggested. For haemorrhagic stroke, management and interventions will be determined by the associated symptoms and prevention of haemorrhagic expansion. In some cases, surgical endovascular removal of the haematoma may be required (Creed, 2010). For both ischemic and haemorrhagic strokes, nursing care during the acute phase includes the prevention of secondary injury, airway protection, maintaining haemodynamic stability (Chamberlain & McGloin, 2016).

Nursing management of spinal cord injury

The initial management of SCI involves spinal cord decompression, management of neurogenic shock and management of respiratory failure (Chamberlain & McGloin, 2016). Neurogenic shock is the loss of vasomotor tone, and clinical manifestations include hypotension, bradycardia and warm extremities that are associated with high thoracic injury. Neurogenic shock, once identified, must be treated immediately to maintain blood pressure; this is usually achieved through the administration of crystalloid solutions (Laskowski-Jones, 2011a). Free water infusions must be avoided as these can lead to the development of oedema around the spinal cord. Atropine may be administered if bradycardic and cardiac output becomes compromised (Chamberlain & McGloin, 2016). Many patients with SCI experience respiratory difficulties; therefore, intubation may be required. Once stable, care should focus on reducing complications in other body systems and supporting the patient in dealing with potential disability.

Nursing management of traumatic brain injury

The key management strategy in the care of the TBI patient is to prevent secondary injury. Treatment strategies are aimed at reducing ischemia by maintaining adequate cerebral blood flow (CBF) and reducing oxygen consumption (Chamberlain & McGloin, 2016). Nursing priorities include stabilising vital signs and reducing ICP. ICP monitoring should be established early, and the administration of hyperosmolar therapy, such as Mannitol or hypertonic saline infusions, may be initiated to decrease ICP by reducing brain volume (Ropper, 2012). It is fundamental that nurses continually reassess neurological functioning and rapidly respond to hypotension, as this contributes to the development of secondary injury. In the presence of hypotension, aggressive fluid management may be required to maintain CBF, and vasopressors may be prescribed; however, if cerebral ischemia is not evident, this intervention should be avoided (Urden, Stacy & Lough, 2013). TBI may also require sedation and mechanical ventilation to manipulate respiratory function. As Chamberlain and McGloin (2016) outline, inducing hyperventilation can reduce elevated ICP, but this strategy should be used with caution. If an intra-cranial haemorrhage is present, it is also important to control hypertension as elevated blood pressure can increase the size of the haematoma. When managing hypertension, it is also important to not reduce blood pressure too far, as this may also reduce cerebral perfusion (Caceres & Goldstein, 2012).

Management of the patient with infection

For the patient with acute meningitis, nursing management should focus on temperature control and pain management. Positioning of the head to reduce discomfort is important. Administration of analgesics such as codeine allows for pain relief without sedation. Fever can increase cerebral oedema and irritation of the cerebral cortex, resulting in seizures. Elevated temperature can be treated with aspirin or cooling blankets. Clinicians should avoid rapidly reducing the patient's temperature as this can induce shivering, causing a rebound increase in temperature. If fever is present, it is also necessary to remember that fluid loss could ensue, so careful fluid management should be undertaken (Lewis et al., 2017). The nursing management of encephalitis requires airway protection and defence from secondary injury such as cerebral oedema. The acute encephalitic patient may require aggressive airway, ventilation, sedation, seizure and haemodynamic support (Chamberlain & McGloin, 2016).

REFLECTIVE QUESTION

When considering the complexity of the nurse's role in the care of the acutely ill neurological patient, give thought to how neurological dysfunction impacts other body systems and how nurses can best manage potential complications.

SKILLS IN PRACTICE

Alcohol-fuelled assault and a subdural haematoma

Ben Smith is a 55-year-old male who, while out at the pub with some mates one evening, is physically assaulted by a stranger. During the assault, Ben sustains several blows to the body, including the left side of his head. Ben's mates manage to stop the assault and the assailant is escorted off the premises by security. Initially, Ben is shaken, but feels fine and decides to catch an Uber home to his wife, Nicole. Ben is somewhat intoxicated and goes straight to bed.

Several hours later, Ben develops a severe headache, which wakes him from his sleep. This is accompanied by nausea and vomiting. Concerned, Nicole calls for an ambulance and Ben is taken to the local hospital. On arrival, Ben struggles to remember the month and date, and when asked to explain the assault earlier that night he is unable to recall the details, often becoming confused. Upon assessment, it is noted that Ben is intermittently slurring his speech, he complains of feeling dizzy and his GCS fluctuates between 13 and 15 (Eyes = 3–4, Verbal = 4–5, Motor = 6). Ben has a history of atrial fibrillation and is currently prescribed an anti-coagulant.

Ben is ordered an urgent non-contrast head CT showing a significant acute sub-arachnoid haematoma, and a coagulation profile indicates that he is hypercoagulated. Ben is immediately taken to the operating theatre for an emergency surgical evacuation of the haematoma. Following a successful operation, he is transferred to the neurologic intensive care unit for ongoing assessment, monitoring and intervention.

QUESTION
Consider how Ben's presentation could initially be mistaken for alcohol intoxication. What strategies should be implemented during the assessment process to ensure a misdiagnosis does not occur?

Coordinated, patient-centred care for the patient with an acute neurological condition

Disability caused by neurologic dysfunction can have an impact on all domains of a person's life. Many acute neurological conditions have substantial physical, cognitive, emotional and behavioural consequences. Interventions therefore require the discipline-specific knowledge and skills of a range of medical, nursing and allied health specialties to ensure that a coordinated, multidisciplinary approach to care is provided. Health professionals must acknowledge that the use of a patient-centred care (PCC) framework when working in multidisciplinary teams ensures the patient's individual care needs will be met (Ferguson et al., 2013). Coordinated, multidisciplinary PCC places the patient and their family and/ or carers at the centre of their care, and recognises that that these individuals are integral members of the healthcare team. It therefore results in holistic care provision and increased levels of patient satisfaction.

Cultural competence and PCC

It is impossible to provide quality PCC without consideration of the cultural needs of the patient and their family. For multidisciplinary teams to provide culturally competent care, clinicians must have a thorough understanding of what culture is and how it impacts their patients (Kamrul, Malin & Ramsden, 2014). Contemporary culturally competent healthcare practice concentrates on communication, understanding of cross-cultural and social issues, and the recognition that all cultures have their own health beliefs (Epner & Baile, 2012). This new approach to culturally competent PCC avoids making assumptions about the patient and ensures that healthcare providers develop the skills necessary to provide quality patient care. Therefore, to ensure quality collaborative care is provided to the patient, all members of the multidisciplinary team must provide PCC within the patient's cultural context (Kamrul, Malin & Ramsden, 2014).

Rehabilitation

Rehabilitation – A treatment method that facilitates the process of recovery from injury, illness or disease; it is is aimed at restoring normal functioning.

Rehabilitation in the acute setting requires a coordinated, multidisciplinary effort to manage differing neurological conditions. The purpose of rehabilitation is to enhance the patient's quality of life through maximising their physical, cognitive, social and psychological functioning (Bhalerao et al., 2016). Multidisciplinary rehabilitation supports patients to achieve their highest level of independence and to participate in society. Using a team-based approach makes interventions more effective. For health practitioners to provide patient-centred holistic rehabilitation, they must recognise that rehabilitation requirements will evolve over time, and that interventions will require constant revision to ensure that the needs of the patient are adequately met through all stages of the individual's illness and recovery (Graham, 2012).

Collaborative care and rehabilitation of the stroke patient

Clinical evidence clearly indicates that stroke patient outcomes are greatly increased when care is managed by a multidisciplinary team. Compared with traditional care, coordinated stroke care reduces mortality risk, dependency and the need for specialised care (Clarke, 2013). Integrated care pathways have been demonstrated to be effective multidisciplinary care plans that guide stroke management. These pathways are often carried out by the stroke team. Integrated care pathways determine how care should be provided and coordinated. Standards of care are informed by evidence and best practice, despite being unique to the facility or service in which they are developed (Aziz et al., 2017). Integrated care pathways include a specific timeline over which goals, expected progress, investigations and treatment are anticipated to be met. The use of integrated care pathways in the management of the stroke patient encourages multidisciplinary teams to regularly evaluate their clinical practices to ensure that quality, well-coordinated care is provided (Aziz et al., 2017).

Irrespective of the considerable advances that have been made in the management of acute stroke, a high number of stroke victims suffer significant physical and functional impairment. Despite a stroke being an acute condition, it can often have long-term consequences for the patient (Aziz et al., 2017). Clinicians must understand that timely rehabilitation is fundamental to the management of the stroke patient, so the process of rehabilitation should commence as soon as any impairment is identified (Bhalero et al., 2016). Coordinated stroke rehabilitation will generally consist of a stroke team, which includes physiotherapists, occupational therapists, speech and language therapists, social workers, nurses and stroke physicians, to ensure that the holistic needs of the patient are addressed (Clarke, 2013).

Collaborative care and the rehabilitation of the TBI patient

The functional deficits resulting from TBI can vary from minor to major activity impairments and, like most acute neurological conditions, TBI can impact the overall wellbeing of the patient. Treatment therefore requires a coordinated multidisciplinary approach. The multidisciplinary model of TBI rehabilitation ensures that the patient and their family are the most important part of the healthcare team (Eapen et al., 2015).

The multidisciplinary team involved in the rehabilitation of the TBI patient will likely include physicians, nurses, neuropsychologists, social workers, speech and language pathologists, occupational therapists and physical therapists. The expertise of other health disciplines may be required in some cases, as the rehabilitation requirements of the TBI patient can be highly complex (Zampolini, 2011). Rehabilitative intervention for TBI patients needs to be implemented in a timely way to maximise cognitive function, reduce the length of hospitalisation and minimise the costs associated with care. Early rehabilitation is also important, as it can impact the patient's long-term quality of life (Eapen et al., 2015).

The rehabilitation process needs to be unique for each individual. This process is often long, and challenges a person's physical, emotional, social, spiritual and cognitive wellbeing. Yet rehabilitation has been shown to improve patient outcomes when early referrals are made to members of the multidisciplinary team (Wagner et al., 2003). Frequently, the TBI patient experiences a loss of strength and movement, and a deficit in balance and coordination. Chronic pain can also be a debilitating effect of a TBI (Johnson, 2010). Physiotherapists and the pain team can provide interventions to maximise function and maintain safety for the patient, both before and after discharge from the acute care setting.

Cognitive problems experienced after a TBI can include deficits in the ability to concentrate, remember and make appropriate judgements; language ability can also be affected (Johnson, 2010). The patient may have a deficit in their ability to regulate emotions, and can frequently experience mood swings, impulsivity and irritability. Post-traumatic stress disorder (PTSD) and personality changes are reported in people who have experienced a TBI (Johnson, 2010). Referrals to psychologists and group therapies can assist with coping mechanisms and therapies to help manage this.

Consider how best the multidisciplinary team might support a patient from a non-English speaking background who has a diagnosis of meningitis. In contemplating this, give thought to the multidisciplinary team members who may be required in this patient's management and their contribution to quality patient outcomes.

Discharge planning for the acute neurologic patient

Effective discharge planning ensures that the neurologic patient's healthcare needs are met after they have left the acute setting. This process also makes certain that there is a continuity of care provision. Successful discharge planning requires high levels of coordinated decision-making by the patient, their family and the multidisciplinary team. The transition from the acute setting to the community, or an alternate care environment, should be smooth and avoid disruption of the progress already achieved. This is particularly important in patients with neurological dysfunction, as generally the patient will have highly complicated care needs.

Discharge planning should be patient centred, so the process of discharge should be individualised. However, while the care requirements of each patient will differ, the steps involved in the discharge process are generally the same. Discharge planning commences on the day of admission to the acute care environment, and while a variety of health disciplines will be involved, it is often nurses who coordinate and drive the process. Nurses must assess each neurological patient carefully to determine potential special requirements, rehabilitation needs and predicted patient outcomes. Once these factors have been identified, discharge planning can be refined and tailored to the patient (Hickey, 2013).

Discharge planning for the stroke patient

Safe discharge from the acute setting is a multifaceted process for the stroke patient. Again, patients and their families should be involved in the discharge planning process, and have input regarding when discharge is to occur and what ongoing support services will be required. Clinicians must consider the impact that reintegration into the community will have for both the patient and their family, and this requires consideration of physical, psychological, financial and social factors (Stroke Foundation, 2013a).

Health professionals should be aware of early supported discharge (ESD) services, which enable stroke victims to transition from the acute environment into the home setting with ongoing rehabilitation more quickly than in the past. ESDs have several benefits, including reduced length of stay, reduced admission to institutional care and lower rates of long-term dependency. As the Stroke Foundation (2013a) outlines, ESD services have the following features:

- They consist of a stroke and multidisciplinary team.
- They plan and facilitate coordinated discharge planning from the acute care setting to the home, with the addition of rehabilitation services.
- They target mild to moderate stroke patients.
- They have well-established links to the acute healthcare service.

- They monitor the severity of stroke dependency, activities of daily living, patient satisfaction, length of stay and readmission rates using standardised assessments.

Healthcare providers have a responsibility to ensure that the patient and their family have been provided with appropriate information and education on their diagnosis, medications and management plan (Kerr, 2012). The minimum activities required before discharge, in order to ensure a safe transition, include:

- pre-discharge needs assessment by the multidisciplinary team (including assessment of clinical, functional, physical, social, informational and spiritual needs)
- communication and referral to a general practitioner, primary healthcare team, and other necessary services
- organisation of all medications and associated requirements
- organisation of specialist treatment and assessments
- carer training, as required
- a post-discharge care plan
- provision of information about support services (Stroke Foundation, 2013a).

Discharge planning for the patient with a TBI

The patient with a TBI may find the process of discharge quite difficult, as the impact of their injury may not be clearly evident until they are within their personal environment (Abrahamson et al., 2016). Discharge planning processes vary for TBI patients, depending on whether they are discharged from the acute care setting directly home, or discharged to a long-term care facility. If the patient is to be discharged home, various steps must first be undertaken, including home visits to ascertain whether home modifications are required and meetings with family and carers to discuss ongoing support and care requirements (Ownsworth & Fleming, 2014).

For many TBI patients and their families, discharge home is an exciting yet challenging milestone. Family members can experience feelings of concern about their ability to cope with the newly acquired care responsibilities. For the patient, discharge home is a significant transition period. Often, in the first few weeks, the patient will experience positive emotions regarding this transition. Over time, though, these emotions may be replaced by negative feelings of anger, frustration and anxiety, as it is in the home environment that the patient becomes more aware of their physical, cognitive and behavioural limitations (Ownsworth & Fleming, 2014). It is therefore imperative that discharge processes prepare the TBI patient for their return home. Healthcare providers must understand the care needs of the patient and their family, which requires effective coordination between services and also necessitates the involvement of the patient and their family in decision-making processes, and adapting these processes as required (Abrahamson et al., 2016).

Advanced nursing practice in the care of acute neurological disorders

Advancement in the treatment modalities of acute neurologic illness has resulted in a current focus on curative, rather than supportive, management – especially in patients who have suffered a stroke or significant brain trauma. Consequently, mortality rates have reduced.

Improvement in the medical management of patients with acute neurological conditions has meant that the nursing management of these patients has also evolved (Livesay, 2012). Neurologic intensive care units (ICUs) have become highly specialised, increasing the need for nurses with specialisation in neurology.

Nurses who practise at an advanced level will have a significant degree of professional knowledge, clinical reasoning and clinical judgement. Their clinical practice is guided by research and best available evidence, making them leaders in the nursing profession. Advanced level nurses generally work in a specialist area and ensure that their work is both safe and effective (NMBA, 2016a). It is important that neurologic nurses practising at an advanced level not only develop their expertise, but also ensure that they maintain the required level of knowledge and skill required by changing standards of care.

Research indicates that patient outcomes are improved when the health professionals caring for them have specialised knowledge and experience. Neurological nursing is multi-faceted, and therefore nurses must have a thorough understanding of how patients respond to acute neurological events. The care delivered must be based not only on an ability to think critically, drawing on a strong knowledge base, but also the best available evidence (Alexander, 2012). The specific needs of the neurologic patient demand that the neuro-logic nurse must have the required attributes to provide them with the best possible care. For example, with advanced stroke-management skills, it is vital to understand that their care priorities post-acute stroke must focus on the prevention of a secondary brain injury, ensuring airway patency and pre-empting complications (Theofanidis & Gibbon, 2016).

Clinical nurse specialists in neurologic ICUs have an important and complex role to play. In the acute care setting, clinical nurse specialists are integral to care coordination and the development of policies, guidelines and clinical pathways. The clinical nurse specialist works in and between multidisciplinary teams to ensure high-quality patient outcomes. Furthermore, they assume the role of coach, teacher and mentor, leading the development of future specialised neurologic nurses (Livesay, 2012).

REFLECTIVE QUESTION

Consider how a nurse with advanced practice skills may care for a patient with an acute neurological condition, in contrast to a new graduate nurse. What are the implications of this for patient outcomes?

SUMMARY

Learning objective 1: Define acute neurological conditions and understand their prevalence, underlying pathophysiology and risk factors.

There are a range of acute neurological conditions with differing underlying pathophysiological processes. Strokes are either ischemic or haemorrhagic in nature. Spinal cord trauma results in damage to the vertebral column from either primary or secondary injury. While primary injury can cause immediate permanent damage, secondary injury is complex and multifaceted. Traumatic brain injury can be caused by blunt force trauma or penetrative trauma, and produce focal or diffuse axonal injury.

Learning objective 2: Describe nursing assessment and management strategies for the individual with an acute neurological conditions.

Assessment of the patient with an acute neurological condition must be comprehensive and systematic. Careful assessment of the patient's LOC is required, in addition to their airway, breathing and circulation. Assessment should also include assessment of LOC, health history, physical examination, vital signs and diagnostic testing. The management of each acute neurological condition differs; however, primary interventions should be aimed at minimising secondary injury and further complications.

Learning objective 3: Understand the concepts of patient-centred care in coordinated care approaches.

Holistic care of the patient with an acute neurological condition must be collaborative and include healthcare provided from a range of disciplines. Integrated pathways provide a means to providing specialised and individualised care that addresses the comprehensive needs of the patient, while ensuring that standards of care are informed by the best available evidence. It is also important to acknowledge that acute neurological care must be both patient centred and culturally appropriate to ensure the best patient outcomes.

Learning objective 4: Explain the role of the nurse in discharge planning for the patient with an acute neurological condition.

Discharge planning for the patient with an acute neurological condition should commence as early as possible, and consider the physical, psychological, financial and social factors affecting the patient and their family. Clinicians must ensure that discharge from the acute setting is safe, from both a physical and psychological point of view, as many patients not only have physical impairment, but may find reintegration into the community a significant challenge.

Learning objective 5: Understand advanced nursing practice in relation to acute neurological conditions.

Contemporary developments in the management of acute neurological treatments and interventions have indicated a need for advanced practising acute neurological nurses. Nurses with well-developed neurological skills have a complex role, and are required to contribute to the development of policy, guidelines and clinical pathways. It is necessary to remember that nurses with advanced practice skills contribute to improved patient outcomes.

REVIEW QUESTIONS

8.1 Describe the pathogenesis of meningitis and describe how this condition interrupts normal cerebral blood flow.

8.2 Explain the importance of monitoring physiological status in the acute neurologic patient.

8.3 Identify which multidisciplinary team members would be involved in the management of a patient with a traumatic brain injury.

8.4 Why is it necessary for healthcare professionals to address issues related to community reintegration for the patient with an acute neurological condition?

8.5 How do acute neurological nurses with advanced practice skills improve patient outcomes?

RESEARCH TOPIC

Research the benefits and risks of hyperosmolar therapy in the management of raised ICP and explain how this intervention impacts patient outcomes.

FURTHER READING

da Paixão Oliveira, D., Umberto Pereira, C. & da Paixão Freitas, Z. (2016). Neurological evaluation about nursing knowledge of the patient with traumatic brain injury. *Journal of Nursing UFPE*, 10(5), 4249–54.

McCoy, K. & Harriet, C. (2016). Neurological integrated care pathway. *Australasian Journal of Neuroscience*, 26(1), 38–43.

Miller, S., Silverman, E. & Hoffman-Ruddy, B. (2017). Assessment of airway defenses in the neurologically impaired patient. *MEDSURG Nursing*, 26(2), 113–18.

Shah, S. (2017). Neurological assessment. *Nursing Standard*, 12(22), 49–54.

Woodward, S. & Mestecky, A. (eds) (2011). *Neuroscience Nursing: Evidence-based Theory and Practice*. Chichester: John Wiley & Sons.

REFERENCES

Abrahamson, V., Jensen, J., Springett, K. & Sakel, M. (2016). Experiences of patients with traumatic brain injury and their carers during transition from in-patient rehabilitation to the community: A qualitative study. *Disability and Rehabilitation*, 39(17), 1683–94.

Alexander, S.A. (ed.) (2012). *Evidence-based Nursing Care for Stroke and Neurovascular Conditions*. Oxford: Wiley-Blackwell.

Aziz, A.F.A., Nordin, N.A.M., Ali, M.F., Aziz, N.A.A., Sulong, S. & Aljunid, S.M. (2017). The integrated care pathway for post stroke patients (iCaPPS): A shared care approach between stakeholders in areas with limited access to specialist stroke care services. *BMC Health Services Research*, 17(35), 171–11.

Bhalerao, G., Shah, H., Bedekar, N. & Dabadghav, R. (2016). Perspective of neuro therapeutic approaches preferred for stroke rehabilitation by physiotherapists. *Indian Journal of Physiotherapy & Occupational Therapy*, 10(1), 47–50.

Boss, B. & Heuther, S. (2014). Disorders of the central and peripheral nervous systems and the neuromuscular junction. In K. McCance & S. Heuther (eds), *Pathophysiology: The Biologic Basics for Disease in Adults and Children* (7th ed.). St Louise, MO: Elsevier, pp. 581–640.

Caceres, J. & Goldstein, J. (2012). Intracranial haemorrhage. *Emergency Medicine Clinics in North America*, 30(3), 771–94.

Chamberlain, D. & Kuzmuik, L. (2016). Neurological assessment and monitoring. In L. Aitken, A. Marshall & W. Chaboyer (eds), *ACCCN's Critical Care Nursing* (3rd ed.). Sydney: Elsevier, pp. 511–45.

Chamberlain, D. & McGloin, E. (2016). Neurological alterations and management. In L. Aitken, A. Marshall & W. Chaboyer (eds), *ACCCN's Critical Care Nursing* (3rd ed.). Sydney: Elsevier, pp. 546–83.

Clarke, D.J. (2013). The role of multidisciplinary team care in stroke rehabilitation. *Progress in Neurology & Psychiatry*, 17(4), 5–8.

Creed, F. (2010). Neurological care. In F. Creed & C. Spiers (eds), *Care of the Acutely Ill Adult: An Essential Guide for Nurses*. Oxford: Oxford University Press, pp. 106–42.

Eapen, B., Allred, D., O'Rourke, J. & Cifu, D. (2015). Rehabilitation of moderate to severe traumatic brain injury. *Seminars in Neurology*, 35(1), 1–3.

Epner, D. & Baile, W. (2012). Patient-centered care: The key to cultural competence. *Annals of Oncology*, 23(3), 33–42.

Feigin, V.L., Krishnamurthi, R.V., Parmar, P., Norrving, B., Mensah, G.A., Bennett, D.A., … Davis, S. (2015). Update on the global burden of ischemic and hemorrhagic stroke in 1990–2013: The GBD 2013 study. *Neuroepidemiology*, 45(3), 161–76.

Ferguson, L.M., Ward, H., Card, S., Sheppard, S. & McMurtry, J. (2013). Putting the 'patient' back into patient-centred care: An education perspective. *Nurse Education in Practice*, 13(4), 283–7.

Gaskin, J. Gomes, J., Darshan, S. & Krewski, D. (2017). Burden of neurological conditions in Canada. *NeuroToxicology*, 61, 2–10.

Goolsby, M. & Grubb, L. (eds) (2011). *Advanced Assessment: Interpreting Findings and Formulating Differential Diagnoses*. Philadelphia, PA: F.A. Davis Company.

Graham, L. (2012). Organization of rehabilitation services. In M. Barnes & D. Good (eds), *Handbook of Clinical Neurology* (Vol. 110). Sydney: Elsevier, pp. 113–20.

Hickey, V. (2013). *The Clinical Practice of Neurological and Neurosurgical Nursing* (7th ed.). Sydney: Lippincott Williams & Wilkins.

Iwasaki, Y.-K., Nishida, K., Kato, T. & Nattel, S. (2011). Atrial fibrillation pathophysiology. *Circulation*, 124(20), 2264–74.

Johnson, G. (2010). Anger and depression. In *Traumatic Brain Injury Survival Guide*. Retrieved from http://www.tbiguide.com/angerdepress.html.

Johnston, A. & Connolly, F. (2015). Alterations of neurological functions across the life span. In J. Craft & C. Gordon (eds), *Understanding Pathophysiology* (2nd ed.). Sydney: Elsevier, pp. 185–240.

Kamrul, R., Malin, G. & Ramsden, R. (2014). Beauty of patient-centred care within a cultural context. *Canadian Family Physician*, 60(4), 313–15.

Kerr, P. (2012). Stroke rehabilitation and discharge planning. *Nursing Standard*, 27(1), 35–9.

Laskowski-Jones, L. (2011a). Nursing management: Peripheral and spinal cord problems. In D. Brown & H. Edwards (eds), *Lewis's Medical-surgical Nursing: Assessment and Management of Clinical Problems* (3rd ed.). Sydney: Elsevier, pp. 7020–164.

—— (2011b). Nursing management: Acute intracranial problems. In, D. Brown & H. Edwards (eds), *Lewis's Medical-surgical Nursing: Assessment and Management of Clinical Problems* (3rd ed.). Sydney: Elsevier, pp. 6574–7163.

Lewis, S., Burcher, L., Heitkemper, M. & Harding, M (2017). *Medical-surgical Nursing: Assessment and Management of Clinical Problems.* St Louis, MO: Elsevier.

Livesay, S. (2012). Neurologic problems. In J. Foster & S. Prevost (eds), *Advanced Practice Nursing of Adults in Acute Care.* Philadelphia, PA: F.A. Davis Company, pp. 184–238.

Maher, A. (2016). Neurological assessment. *International Journal of Orthopaedic and Trauma Nursing,* 22, 44–53.

National Spinal Cord Injury Statistical Center (2016). *Spinal cord injury facts and figures at a glance.* Retrieved from https://www.nscisc.uab.edu/Public/Facts%202016.pdf.

Nursing Council of New Zealand (NCNZ) ([2007] 2016). *Competencies for Registered Nurses.* Retrieved from http://www.nursingcouncil.org.nz/Nurses.

Nursing and Midwifery Board of Australia (NMBA) (2016a). Advanced nursing practice and speciality areas within nursing. Retrieved from http://www.nursingmidwiferyboard .gov.au/Codes-Guidelines-Statements/FAQ/fact-sheet-advanced-nursing-practice- and-specialty-areas.aspx.

—— (2016b). *Registered Nurse Standards for Practice.* Melbourne: Nursing & Midwifery Board of Australia. Retrieved from http://www.nursingmidwiferyboard.gov.au/ Codes-Guidelines-Statements/Professional-standards/registered-nurse-standards- for-practice.aspx.

Ownsworth, T. & Fleming, J. (2014). Community adjustment and re-engagement. In H. Levin, D. Shum & R. Chan (eds), *Understanding Traumatic Brain Injury: Current Research and Future Directions.* Oxford: Oxford University Press, pp. 235–54.

Ropper, A. (2012). Hyperosmolar therapy for raised intracranial pressure. *The New England Journal of Medicine,* 367(8), 746–52.

Salzar, R.S., Treichler, D., Wardlaw, A., Weiss, G. & Jacques., G. (2017). Experimental investigation of cavitation as a possible damage mechanism in blast-induced traumatic brain injury in post-mortem human subject heads. *Journal of Neurotrauma,* 34(8), 1589–602.

Schoenwald, A. & Douglas, C. (2016). Undertaking a focused assessment: Physical assessment of body systems. In J. Crisp, C. Douglas, G. Reberio & D. Waters (eds), *Potter and Perry's Fundamentals of Nursing* (5th ed.). Sydney: Elsevier, pp. 578–621.

Stroke Foundation (2013a). *Rehabilitation Stroke Services Framework.* Retrieved from https://strokefoundation.org.au/-/media/6676A175BD6F494F89034430FEE708C2 .ashx?la=en

—— (2013b). Economic impact of stroke in Australia. Retrieved from https:// strokefoundation.org.au/What-we-do/Research/Economic-impact-of-stroke-in- Australia.

—— (2017). Stroke risk factors. Retrieved from https://strokefoundation.org.au/About- Stroke/Preventing-stroke/Stroke-risk-factors.

Talley, N. & O'Connor, S. (2014). *Clinical Examination: A Systematic Guide to Physical Diagnosis.* Sydney: Elsevier.

Theofanidis, D. & Gibbon, B. (2016). Exploring the experiences of nurses and doctors involved in stroke care: A qualitative study. *Journal of Clinical Nursing,* 25(13–14), 1999–2007.

Urden, L., Stacy, K. & Lough, M. (2013). *Critical Care Nursing: Diagnosis and Management* (7th ed.). St Louis, MO: Elsevier.

Wagner, A., Fabio, T., Zafonte, R., Goldberg, G., Marion, D. & Peitzman, A. (2003). Physical medicine and rehabilitation consultation: Relationships with acute functional outcome, length of stay, and discharge planning after traumatic brain injury. *American Journal Physical Medicine & Rehabilitation*, 82(7), 526–36.

Wijdicks, E. (2016). *The Practice of Emergency and Critical Care Neurology*. New York: Oxford University Press.

Zampolini, M. (2011). Rehabilitation of traumatic brain injury in Italy: A multi-centred study. *Brain Injury*, 26(1), 27–35.

Zomorodi, M. (2017). Nursing management: The patient with a stroke. In D. Brown, H. Edwards, L. Seaton & T. Buckley (eds), *Lewis's Medical-surgical Nursing: Assessment and Management of Clinical Problems* (4th ed.). Sydney: Elsevier, pp. 1436–59.

9

Acute gastrointestinal conditions

Amali Hohol and Lyndal Taylor

LEARNING OBJECTIVES

At the completion of this chapter, you should be able to:

1 understand the underlying pathophysiology of a range of gastrointestinal conditions, their prevalence, associated risk factors and clinical manifestations
2 explain how to undertake a comprehensive gastrointestinal assessment
3 identify and discuss common evidence-based management strategies for acute gastrointestinal disorders
4 explore the relevance of quality patient education and outcome-focused discharge planning with acute gastrointestinal conditions
5 understand the importance of working in collaboration with other healthcare professionals to ensure patient-centred and culturally competent care is provided.

Introduction

Up to 62 per cent of acutely ill patients will exhibit symptoms of gastrointestinal (GI) dysfunction during an acute care admission (Blaser et al., 2012). Unfortunately, the presence of GI dysfunction has been linked to poor clinical outcomes, and an increase in the rate of morbidity and mortality (Blaser et al., 2012; Soenen et al., 2016). Early signs of GI dysfunction are often not evident (Martin, 2007). Therefore, timely and accurate nursing care is important in recognizing GI disorders. Caring for the patient with acute GI issues requires careful assessment, planning, intervention and evaluation. Management plans must be flexible to allow for alterations in the patient's condition, and interventions must be developed using sound evidence-based practice to ensure positive patient outcomes (Cronin & Duffy, 2011).

The chapter will explore the underlying pathophysiology of acute GI conditions, as this knowledge enables nurses to recognise specific disease states and their progress while also guiding assessment and treatment interventions. Nurses identify the holistic needs of the patient through comprehensive assessment, so the key components of GI assessment will be explained. The chapter will then explore appropriate treatment interventions, the purpose of patient education and the processes involved in discharge planning. It will close by discussing how nursing staff can work in a collaboration with other health professionals to ensure patient–centred, holistic care provision for the acutely ill GI patient.

NURSING STANDARDS

The following identifies the national competency standards for the registered nurse from the Nursing and Midwifery Board of Australia (NMBA) and the Nursing Council of New Zealand (NCNZ) that are addressed in this chapter.

Australian Registered Nurse Standards for Practice

Standard 1: Thinks critically and analyses nursing practice

Standard 2: Engages in therapeutic and professional relationships

Standard 3: Maintains the capability for practice

Standard 4: Comprehensively conducts assessments

Standard 5: Develops a plan for nursing practice

Standard 6: Provides safe, appropriate and responsive quality nursing practice

Standard 7: Evaluates outcomes to inform nursing practice.

(NMBA, 2016)

With such a high proportion of acutely unwell patients presenting with, and potentially developing, gastrointestinal complications in the acute care setting, the ability of nursing staff to accurately and critically assess symptoms relating to an acute GI disorder is extremely important. Nurses must have the clinical skills, clinical knowledge and well-developed critical thinking capabilities to recognise acute GI illness, care holistically for patients and make high-quality clinical decisions. Furthermore, looking after the acute GI patient requires nursing care that is evidence based and culturally appropriate, and that adheres to the legal and ethical frameworks that underpin the nursing profession. The provision of safe, effective and timely nursing assessment and care provision aligns with Standard 1.

Pathophysiology, risk factors and prevalence of acute gastrointestinal disorders

Acute gastrointestinal dysfunction in acutely ill patients is common, and carries a high risk of mortality (Martin, 2007). However, there is yet to be a consistent definition of GI illness (Blaser et al., 2012). While some patients may present with a primary GI disease, it is frequently observed that acutely ill patients are at increased risk of developing GI complications during their hospital admission (Martin, 2007). Extensive knowledge of the GI system is fundamental to nursing practice (Cronin & Duffy, 2011), as the GI system is highly complex, due primarily to the large number of organs involved in the processes of ingestion, digestion, absorption and elimination. As there are so many organs involved in the digestive process, it is unsurprising that acute conditions of the GI system are diverse and frequently interrelated. Often acute GI conditions can be life-threatening, thus requiring critical care management or urgent surgical intervention.

GI tract – An organ system of the body that starts with the oral cavity, extends to the pharynx, oesophagus, stomach, intestines and ends with the rectum and anus.

The **GI tract** comprises of the digestive tract, a mucous membrane lined tube that extends from the mouth to the anus (Figure 9.1). This includes the mouth, pharynx, oesophagus, stomach, small and large intestines. The GI tract also includes the accessory organs of the liver, pancreas, and biliary system (Nowicki, Williams & Bradford, 2015). The GI tract includes several different organs and is responsible for multiple bodily functions.

Common acute GI conditions

A range of conditions can affect the GI tract, the clinical manifestations of which are outlined in Table 9.1.

GI bleeding

Upper GI bleeding occurs in the oesophagus, stomach or duodenum (Nurgali & Wildbore, 2015). A high proportion of upper GI bleeding can be attributed to either peptic ulcers or

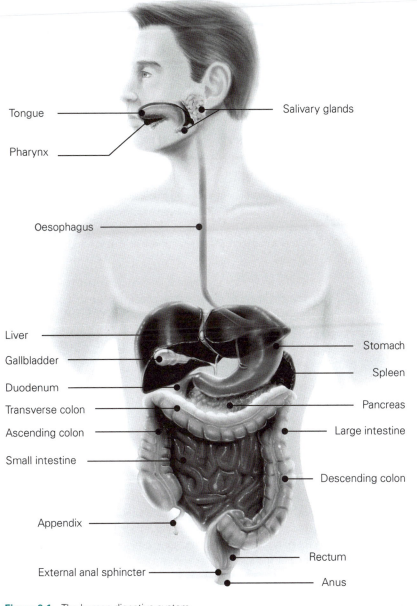

Tongue

Pharynx

Oesophagus

Liver

Gallbladder

Duodenum

Transverse colon

Ascending colon

Small intestine

Appendix

External anal sphincter

Salivary glands

Stomach

Spleen

Pancreas

Large intestine

Descending colon

Rectum

Anus

Figure 9.1 The human digestive system

varices; however, upper GI bleeding can also be caused by damage to the gastric mucosa (Worden & Hanna, 2017). If *Helicobacter pylori* (*H. pylori*) bacteria is present, it damages the gastric epithelium, making the underlying mucosa more susceptible to damage, including atrophy. This bacterium can also cause gastric ulcers. In the presence of peptic ulcer disease, the ulcer erodes large blood vessels, resulting in bleeding (Wilkins et al., 2012). Lower GI bleeding occurs in the jejunum, ileum, colon or rectum. The pathophysiology of lower GI bleeding is dependent on the underlying etiology, which may include inflammatory disease, cancer, diverticular disease or haemorrhoids (Nurgali & Wildbore, 2015). The Agency for Clinical Innovation (2017) states that between 50 and 150 people per 100 000 population develop GI bleeding each year. Upper GI bleeds are four times more likely than lower GI

Table 9.1   Clinical manifestations of acute GI conditions

Acute GI condition	Associated clinical manifestations
GI bleed	Symptoms generally are related to the degree of blood loss and may include: tachycardia, reduced capillary refill, tachypnoea, reduced urine output, confusion, hypotension. Other common symptoms include: melena, hematochezia, and coffee ground vomitus.
Diverticular disease	Abdominal distension, hypo or hyperactive bowel sounds, rebound tenderness, tachycardia, hypotension, shallow respirations, and GI bleeding.
Appendicitis	Symptoms of acute appendicitis will present with right lower quadrant pain which increased on movement, constipation, anorexia, and malaise. If perforation occurs, the patient may experience increased generalised pain, fever and abdominal rigidity.
Pancreatitis	General symptoms may include pain, vomiting, nausea, fever, abdominal distention, hypoactive or absent bowel sounds, ascites and jaundice. As the condition worsens, systemic complications can arise, including hypovolaemic shock, acute respiratory distress syndrome, acute kidney injury, and GI haemorrhage.
Cholecystitis	Regurgitation, flatulence, belching, epigastric discomfort, indigestion, nausea, amber-coloured urine, clay-coloured stools, pruritus, jaundice, steatorrhoea, fever, and pain and the inability to inhale when palpating the gallbladder.
Acute liver failure	Headache, hyperventilation, jaundice, mental status alterations, palmer erythema, spider nevi, increased bruising and oedema.
Intestinal obstruction	Symptoms are dependent on the site and type of obstruction and may include: cramping pain, vomiting, back pain, hiccoughs, belching, constipation, and diminished bowel sounds.
Abdominal compartment syndrome	As a consequence of the underlying pathophysiology, ACS impacts multiple organs and may result in: hypoxia, reduced or no urine output, tachycardia, abdominal distention and hypotension.

Source: Adapted from Fitzgerald Close (2018); Marshall and Gordon (2016); Monahan, Neighbors and Green (2011).

haemorrhages, and risk factors include non-steroidal anti-inflammatory use, *H. pylori* infection, age and male gender (Wilkins et al., 2012).

Diverticular disease

In diverticular disease, diverticula form as the muscles surrounding the large bowel begin to weaken and small bulges of bowel push through the muscle to form pockets

(Ferreira–Aparcio et al., 2012). They are most commonly located in the large intestine and can collect faecal material, which ultimately irritates and inflames the lining of the bowel, resulting in diverticulitis (Nurgali & Wildbore, 2015). The obstructed faecal matter causes bacteria proliferation, and inflammation can ensue, causing oedema that can reduce diverticulum blood flow and cause ischemia. If tissue ischemia is not resolved, perforation of the diverticulum can occur (Monahan, Neighbors & Green, 2011). The prevalence of diverticular disease is increasing, with approximately 50 per cent of Australian adults over 60 years believed to be affected (Weizman & Nguyen, 2011). Risk factors include increasing age, male gender, a low-fibre diet, increased alcohol consumption, smoking, inactivity and obesity (Böhm, 2015).

Appendicitis

Appendicitis is an acute inflammation of the appendix, usually resulting from a blockage in the lumen of the appendix caused by faecal matter, foreign bodies or adhesions. Bacterial infection occurs and the intra-luminal pressure of the organ increases because it cannot drain. Blockage eventuates into hypoxia, ulceration and eventual perforation (Nurgali & Wildbore, 2015). Fitzgerald (2012) states that while appendicitis is the most common cause of acute abdominal pain requiring surgery, there are no known risk factors.

Pancreatitis

Approximately 4.9 to 73.4 people per 100 000 population develop pancreatitis worldwide, with a mortality rate of between 1.2 and 4.2 per cent (Nesvaderani, Eslick & Cox, 2015). When normally inactive pancreatic digestive enzymes become activated early, they cause autodigestion. This can occur through several processes, including obstruction or damage of the pancreatic duct system, alterations to the exocrine cells of the pancreas, infection, ischemia and, in some cases, unknown factors (Fitzgerald Close, 2018). Trypsin is the enzyme that is first activated, and it triggers the release of additional enzymes that can cause increased capillary membrane permeability, leaking of fluid into the interstitium, oedema and hypovolemia. The enzyme elastase is particularly harmful, as it dissolves the elastic fibres of blood vessels and can cause haemorrhage, while lipase can be transported into the systemic circulation and cause necrosis of the pancreas and adjacent tissues (Fitzgerald Close, 2018). Acute pancreatitis can interfere with coagulation and lead to multi-organ failure if left untreated (Nurgali & Wildbore, 2015). Primary risk factors for pancreatitis include gallstones and alcohol consumption (Nesvaderani, Eslick & Cox, 2015).

Cholecystitis

Cholecystitis is the result of obstruction of the common bile duct leading to inflammation of the gallbladder. Often obstruction is due to gallstones; however, stasis, bacterial infection or ischemia of the gallbladder may be responsible (Monahan, Neighbors & Green, 2011). When obstruction occurs, swelling and thickening of the gallbladder walls can occur as oedema develops. Prolonged oedema may scar and fibros the gallbladder tissue, and mucosal irritation will occur due to continual compression of bile. These mechanisms will cause tissue ischemia and necrosis, and possible gangrene or perforation (Monahan, Neighbors & Green, 2011). Risk factors associated with gallstones include ethnicity, age, female gender, family history, obesity, dyslipidemia, diabetes mellitus, metabolic syndrome, drugs, and poor diet, and are estimated to impact between 10 and 15 per cent of the population (Stinton & Shaffer, 2012).

Acute liver failure

Approximately 5.5 million people suffer acute liver failure (ALF) each year (Punzalan & Barry, 2016). A range of aetiologies can result in ALF, with the most common being viral hepatitis and drug reactions (Pyleris, Gianniakopoulos & Dabos, 2010). The condition develops over one to three weeks, and by eight weeks, hepatic encephalopathy is present. Primarily, encephalopathy is resultant from shutdown of the hepatic system and the accumulation of toxins in the bloodstream (Pyleris, Gianniakopoulos & Dabos, 2010). However, multiple pathophysiological mechanisms are involved with ALF, including reduced bilirubin conjugation, reduced production of clotting factors, impaired glucose synthesis and poor lactate clearance (Fitzgerald Close, 2018). Considerable destruction of hepatocytes also occurs as the innate immune system is activated, causing mass production of inflammatory mediators. These then enter the bloodstream, leading to systemic alterations of bodily function (Cardoso et al., 2017).

Intestinal obstruction

When peristalsis of the GI tract ceases, food fails to be digested and absorbed and this is termed an intestinal obstruction. There are three causes of obstruction; simple, whereby there is a blockage of the intestinal contents; strangulation, as the obstruction causes reduced perfusion to the associated tissues; and closed-loop, which occurs when both ends of a section of bowel are occluded and cut off from the balance of the intestine (Springhouse, 2010). Intestinal obstruction increases gastric secretions and the accumulation of fluid, air, and gas, yet fluid absorption reduces causing distention. Distention can stop the flow of venous blood and diminish normal absorptive mechanisms leading to dehydration (Springhouse, 2010). Perforation can also result when the distention reduces organ perfusion, leading to oedema and necrosis (Von Rosenvinge et al., 2013). A small **bowel obstruction** is four times more likely than a large bowel obstruction. Risk factors include abdominal surgery, adhesions, hernias, tumours or inflammatory conditions, and the blockage can be mechanical and block the intestinal lumen, or functional whereby gut motility ceases (paralytic ileus) (Nurgali & Wildbore, 2015).

Bowel obstruction – A blockage of the small or large intestine, which may be mechanical or functional, that prevents products of digestion moving through the intestine.

Abdominal compartment syndrome

Abdominal compartment syndrome (ACS) is a life-threatening GI complication whereby organ function is severely compromised (Bell & Sluys, 2016). ACS can occur secondary to a range of conditions, including sepsis, peritonitis or acute pancreatitis, and refers to a significant increase within the anatomic space of the abdominal cavity. As the pressure within this cavity increases, blood flow to all major organs reduces and tissue ischemia can result. Cardiac output consequently reduces, further impacting on organ perfusion and potentially leading to organ failure (Marshall & Gordon, 2016). Patients who have undergone significant volume resuscitation are most at risk for the development of ACS. Reduced abdominal wall compliance, increased abdominal contents and elevated intraluminal contents are also risk factors for ACS. The incidence of ACS varies, with research indicating that approximately 30 per cent of septic shock patients have the condition (Berry & Fletcher, 2012).

SKILLS IN PRACTICE

Bert's story

Bert is a 78-year-old man, married to Jane, with three adult children. Bert and Jane reside in a small country town. Bert is 180 cm tall, weighs 143 kg and likes to end his day with three or four full-strength beers. Late one evening, after completing his duties on the farm, Bert experiences some mild abdominal discomfort for which he self-administers 400 mg of ibuprofen and goes to bed. Several hours later, the pain becomes so intense that Jane calls for an ambulance. On arrival at the town's multi-purpose health facility, Bert becomes nauseated and starts vomiting. His nurse carries out a comprehensive assessment, which reveals that his abdomen is visibly swollen and firm to touch.

Bert is transferred to a large metropolitan hospital for further investigation and treatment. Following a pancreatic function test, abdominal ultrasound and CT scan, Bert is diagnosed with acute pancreatitis secondary to gallstones. Bert undergoes an endoscopic retrograde cholangio-pancreatography and removal of the gallstones; however, his surgery is complicated and he receives significant fluid resuscitation and blood loss due to haemorrhage. Intra-operatively, he receives 4 L of IV fluid and two blood transfusions. He is admitted to a critical care unit post-operatively, as he is now at high risk for abdominal compartment syndrome.

QUESTIONS

- Bert is obese, with a BMI of 44. What impact will his weight have on his recovery, and what management strategies can the nurse implement to encourage **self-care** behaviours when Bert is discharged home?
- What complications may arise from Bert's fluid resuscitation, and how best would the GI nurse assess fluid status?

Self-care – The process of managing one's own health needs in order to enhance personal wellbeing.

Comprehensive gastrointestinal assessment

The process of assessment aims to gather necessary information about a patient, which is then critically analysed to determine what interventions are required (Patel & Curtis, 2011). Assessment of the gastrointestinal system must be accurate to ensure that the needs of the patient are prioritised appropriately. Failure to do so can place the patient at risk of harm. Nurses must understand that many acute gastrointestinal disorders have a variety of clinical features, and while some may be specific to only a few illnesses, others will be common to a range of conditions.

Health history

Identification of the presenting symptoms is often the first step during a comprehensive assessment of the GI system, and allows the clinician to identify current issues. Common problems include abdominal pain or distention, nausea, vomiting, jaundice, anaemia, indigestion and food intolerances (Crogan, 2013). Past medical history should be obtained, ensuring that any previous GI surgeries are accounted for, and the patient's family history should be established to identify any hereditary GI conditions (Crogan, 2013; Nowicki, Williams & Bradford, 2015).

Medications often have an impact on the GI system, in particular the liver, so any hepatotoxic drugs must be noted. Non-steroidal anti-inflammatory drugs (NSAIDs) are a commonly used drug and can cause upper GI bleeding (Crogan, 2013). Consideration must also be given to any antibiotic use, as this class of drug often affects the bacterial composition of the GI tract and can result in diarrhoea (Nowicki, Williams & Bradford, 2015). An in-depth exploration of nutritional status should be undertaken as adequate nutrition affects patient outcomes. Patients suffering from an acute GI condition may present with metabolic derangement because of acute illness and the inability of the body to meet the increased energy demands (Patel & Curtis, 2011). Elimination patterns should be discussed including the frequency and consistency of stools as alterations in elimination patterns warrant further investigation (Crogan, 2013).

Physical assessment

If possible, the patient's height, weight and body mass index (BMI) should be determined as both malnutrition and malabsorption issues can be indicated via this data. The physical assessment should then progress to inspection of the oral cavity and any distinguishing breath odour should be noted (Crogan, 2013). Abdominal assessment should be systematic, using the techniques of inspection, auscultation, percussion and palpation (Nowicki, Williams & Bradford, 2015). The abdomen is often divided into four quadrants, as this assists in identifying the structures that may be involved in the condition. It is recommended that the patient be examined in the supine position with the knees slightly bent. Inspection of each quadrant may reveal bruising, pulsation, masses or distention (Patel & Curtis, 2011). Auscultation of the abdomen should occur prior to percussion and palpation, as these actions can interfere with bowel sounds (Goolsby & Grubbs, 2011). Bowel sounds should be auscultated and heard approximately every 20 seconds. If no bowel sounds are noted within a five-minute period, then bowel sounds are considered absent (Crogan, 2013). Both hyperactive and hypoactive bowel sounds indicate problems that warrant further investigation (Patel & Curtis, 2011). Normal percussion of the abdomen should sound hollow. The presence of dull sounds can signal possible fluid collection (Patel & Curtis, 2011). Both light and deep palpation enable detection of rebound tenderness, rigidity and guarding, and these symptoms are indicators of abdominal pain. Perform palpation last to minimise discomfort to the patient (Goolsby & Grubbs, 2011), as abdominal pain is a common complaint of the acute GI patient. Clinicians should understand that abdominal pain can be associated with life-threatening issues and therefore must be evaluated carefully (Goolsby & Grubbs, 2011).

Diagnostics

Pathology collected should include a full blood count. GI conditions are often associated with anemia, infection or electrolyte disturbances. Bilirubin testing can determine liver and gallbladder function, while pancreatic enzyme testing can assist in identifying pancreatitis. Occult blood and infection can be detected through stool sampling. (Nowicki, Williams & Bradford, 2015).

Radiological investigations of both the upper and lower GI tract can assist in the diagnosis of strictures, ulcers, tumours, hernias, inflammation, stenosis and obstruction

(Cleary-Holdforth & Leufer, 2013). Abdominal ultrasound uses sound waves technology to produce 2D imagery of the abdominal cavity (Cleary-Holdforth & Leufer, 2013). More invasive diagnosis procedures include endoscopy, laparoscopy and colonoscopy. These procedures allow for the internal lining of the organs involved in the GI to be examined more closely. Tissue and fluid samples can also be obtained to further assist in diagnosis (Nowicki, Williams & Bradford, 2015). Additionally, the patient suffering with an acute GI issue may require computed tomography (CT) of the GI tract, a biopsy or nuclear scanning (Cleary-Holdforth & Leufer, 2013; Nowicki, Williams & Bradford, 2015). The results of diagnostic procedures, coupled with thorough, systematic physical assessment and an extensive patient history, can lead to a definitive diagnosis.

Management of the acute GI patient

Care of the acute GI patient must be systematic to ensure that the comprehensive needs of the patient are addressed. A range of interventions and management strategies will be required to ensure best patient outcomes. Therefore, the acute care nurse is required to understand a range of GI-specific treatment options (Cleary-Holdforth & Leufer, 2013).

Medical intervention

Analgesia

For acute abdominal pain, analgesia should be administered rapidly. In the post-operative period, the main treatment options include both non-opioid and opioid pharmacotherapies. To safety administer analgesics in the event of abdominal pain, the nurse must have an extensive understanding of the potential adverse GI complications that can occur. For example, the use of NSAIDs is considered first-line therapy in acute pancreatitis, but is contraindicated in suspected GI bleeding (Pezzilli, Morselli-Labate & Corinaldesi, 2010). Patient-controlled analgesic devices are often utilised in cases of major surgery, although neuroaxial analgesia via epidural may be preferable as this method also assists in gut motility (Streitberger et al., 2011).

Intravenous fluids

Fluid loss is common in the acute GI patient, particularly in the presence of diarrhoea, vomiting or haemorrhage, placing them at risk of dehydration and electrolyte imbalance (Padhi, Bullock & Stroud, 2013). Clinicians involved in the delivery of intravenous (IV) therapy must understand the physiological changes that can occur and how to appropriately assess an individual's fluid status to ensure safe and effective patient care (Scales, 2014).

Blood transfusions

In the case of significant blood loss, blood transfusion (BT) may be a life-saving treatment. Patients who present with GI bleeding, or those who undergo abdominal surgery, are often recipients of blood products. BTs, however, do carry a level of risk (Higgins & Jones, 2012). Nurses are the primary administrators of blood products, and therefore must be familiar with local and national policy to ensure safe care provision. A knowledge of blood compatibility and the ability to recognise transfusion reactions is also fundamental to the role of the acute care nurse (Higgins & Jones, 2012).

Medications

A range of medications can be used in the treatment of acute GI conditions. These are outlined in Table 9.2.

Table 9.2 Medications used in the treatment of acute GI conditions

Medication class	Purpose	Example
Anti-emetics	Block the neurotransmitters of the vomiting centre. Some anti-emetics also increase gastric emptying and upper GI motility.	Metoclopramide Ondansetron
Gastric acid neutralisers: **Proton-pump inhibitors (PPI)**, H2-receptor antagonists	Neutralise or inhibit the secretion of gastric acid.	Omeprazole (PPI) Ranitidine (H2-RA)
Laxatives	Stimulate the movement of food through the lower GI tract.	Senna Liquid paraffin
Anti-diarrhoeal drugs	Relieve the symptoms of diarrhoea to prevent the loss of fluids and electrolytes.	loperamide
5-aminosalicylates	Anti-inflammatory agent of the lower GI tract.	Sulfasalazine Mesalazine

Source: Bryant and Knights (2015).

Proton-pump inhibitors: (PPI) – a class of medication that inhibits the production of gastric acid.

Nasogastric tube

Nasogastric tube (NGT) – A flexible plastic tube that is placed into the stomach via the nasal passage to allow for abdominal decompression, feeding or medication administration.

The **nasogastric tube (NGT)** can be used for abdominal decompression, delivery of nutritional requirements when the GI tract is dysfunctional and the administration of medications (Curtis, 2013). Prior to the insertion of a NGT, the nurse must understand the anatomy and physiology of the structures of the upper GI system, as potential complications can be severe. Clinicians must remember that radiographic confirmation is the gold standard for correct NGT placement (Walsh & Schub, 2016), as blind insertion carries the risk of misplacement, particularly into the lung (Curtis, 2013). While bedside testing, such as checking the pH level of aspirated gastric contents, may assist in differentiating gastric acid from respiratory fluid, it cannot determine where the tube is located (Curtis, 2013). Insertion of the NGT should only be carried out by healthcare providers who have completed competency training (Walsh & Schub, 2016).

Enteral feeding

Enteral feeding – Refers to the administration of nutrients directly into the gastrointestinal tract.

Hospitalised patients are at risk of developing malnutrition when they suffer acute GI conditions. **Enteral feeding** is a method of avoiding this complication, and is the provision of nutritional requirements via a NGT, or tubes directly into the jejunum or duodenum

(Mula, 2014). Enteral feeding is important for patients who are unable to feed orally, as it maintains gut integrity in addition to promoting gut-associated immunity (Lau & Girard, 2011). Nurses are central to the enteral feeding process, as they are responsible for the administration of feeds (Mula, 2014). Nursing staff must be well versed in the complications and management of enteral feeds.

Stoma care

A patient with a **stoma** may have a colostomy formed from the large bowel (Figure 9.2), or an ileostomy from the small bowel (Figure 9.3). The stoma can be permanent or temporary, and is used for the collection of faecal matter (Burch, 2011).

Stoma – The opening of an organ onto the surface of the abdomen to allow for removal of faecal matter.

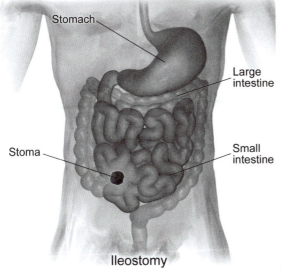

Figure 9.2   Positioning of an ileostomy

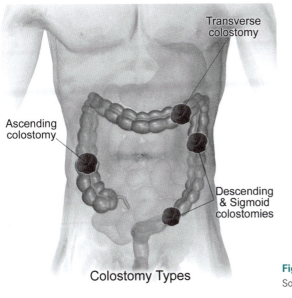

Figure 9.3   Positioning of a colostomy
Source: Blausen (2014).

Ostomy – The surgical creation of an artificial opening in the abdomen to allow for drainage of bodily waste products.

While in the acute care setting, nurses must assess the stomas appearance and surrounding skin for any abnormalities, which should be documented and reported accordingly (Clark et al., 2015). The **ostomy** function should be noted with attention to frequency of flatus, and the appearance and regularity of output (Clark et al., 2015). One of the primary principles of stoma care is to prevent peristomal skin breakdown, but it is the most common complication. Skin breakdown can result from inappropriate sizing of the stoma flange, frequent appliance removal, rough removal of the appliance, a leaking appliance, stomal retraction or prolapse, or diet (Burch, 2010). The formation of a stoma can have a significant impact on the body image and psychological wellbeing of an individual. Therefore, it is important to communicate with the patient about their stoma and address any fears or anxieties that they may have prior to discharge. Additionally, patient education regarding stoma care must commence in the acute setting to ensure that the patient is capable, both physically and psychologically, of managing their stoma at home (Clark et al., 2015).

Wound care

Commonly, the patient who has undergone GI surgery will have a post-operative wound. Appropriate wound care is important to prevent infection. The separation of wound edges, or dehiscence, occurs in roughly 2 per cent of midline abdominal incisions and is associated with increased mortality. Nursing care should focus on wound assessment to identify early signs of infection (Litwack, 2010).

Patient education and discharge planning

Nosbusch, Weiss and Bobay (2010) recognise that the acute care nurse plays an important role is ensuring all patients are successful with at home self-management and care. For this to occur, emphasis must be placed on discharge planning and patient education throughout the hospital admission. Discharge planning should begin at admission and continue until the patient has left the acute care environment (Nosbusch, Weiss & Bobay, 2010). Acute GI patients often require lengthy admissions; consequently, carefully considered discharge planning and quality patient education enable the patient and their family to successfully manage their condition outside the acute care setting.

The importance of self-care in the management of acute GI disorders

Patient education occurs across a range of settings, and nurses must acknowledge that all patient interactions provide a possible teaching opportunity. Education must be relevant, and nurses must confirm that the patient understands their health needs (Massey, Chaboyer & Anderson, 2017; Dillstrom et al., 2017). The specific learning needs of the patient must be identified to guarantee that education focuses on health promotion, risk reduction and post-discharge management. The nurse must also assess the individual's readiness and ability to engage with education (Massey, Chaboyer & Anderson, 2017; Dillstrom et al., 2017).

Patients who can successfully care for themselves following acute hospital admission become empowered in their own healthcare decision-making and treatment regimens (Lawn et al., 2013). It is the responsibility of each member of the multidisciplinary team to provide support and education to the patient to ensure that they are successful in engaging in self-care behaviours once discharged from the acute care setting (Lawn et al., 2013). Providing education to patients around modifiable risk factors, including eating a healthy diet, lowering levels of alcohol consumption, quitting smoking and getting regular exercise (Szoeke et al., 2017) have been discussed widely in both health-education and health-promotion research for many years. To ensure a specific focus on both primary and secondary prevention measures, the gastrointestinal patient should be educated on the modifiable factors shown in Table 9.3.

Table 9.3 Modifiable risk factors for gastrointestinal patient education

Modifiable risk factor	Rationale for education
Non-steroidal anti-inflammatory drugs (NSAIDs)	Chronic use of NSAIDs can elicit significant gastrointestinal irritation, with the potential to cause GI bleeding and ulceration.
Diet	It is widely accepted that eating a balanced diet that is high in fibre can reduce the incidence of acute GI dysfunction.
Inactivity	Increased levels of physical activity directly reduced gastrointestinal symptoms, while higher levels of physical activity can reduce gastrointestinal complaints.
Smoking	Cigarette smoke can cause ulceration and decreased gastric emptying, and alters the blood supply to the gastric mucosa.
Alcohol consumption	Alcohol consumption significantly increases the risk of gastrointestinal bleeding and the risk of developing portal hypertension, liver cirrhosis and liver failure.
Obesity	The risk of developing gastrointestinal disease is greatly increased as a patient's BMI increases. Several gastrointestinal conditions result from obesity, while with others the risk of development or the severity of the condition may be increased significantly due to higher weight.

Source: Adapted from Camilleri, Malhi and Acosta (2017); Rani and Kumar (2016); Somani and Bhanushali (2011); Strate et al. (2016); Vermorken, Andrès and Cui (2016).

REFLECTIVE QUESTION

Consider what resources, both physical and psychological, an 18-year-old male patient would require upon discharge for acute liver failure, secondary to a paracetamol overdose, to ensure successful management of his condition.

Holistic care of the acute gastrointestinal patient

The terms 'patient-centredness' and 'cultural competence' are similar in their purpose, with both seeking to increase healthcare quality. The aim of patient-centred care is to ensure that care provision is individualised and to promote personal relationships between the patient, their family and healthcare providers (Campinha-Bacote, 2011). Conversely, cultural competence is focused on reducing health inequalities that arise from social disadvantage or ethnicity, and the avoidance of stereotypes (Epner & Baile, 2012). However, the primary intention of both concepts is to view the patient as a unique individual (Campinha-Bacote, 2011). When providing appropriate culturally competent patient-centred care to the acute gastrointestinal patient, nurses can determine what aspects of care are the most important to the patient and their individual experience of health (Epner & Baile, 2012).

Collaborative patient-centred care

Holistic care – The treatment of the whole person, not simply their disease process. Holistic care takes into consideration the physical, psychological and social needs of the person.

To ensure that the acute GI patient receives high-quality, safe care, a multidisciplinary team approach should be used. Coordinated collaborative care of a patient ensures a range of disciplines are involved in the **holistic care** of that individual and optimises treatment outcomes (Ben-Ami et al., 2013).

For example, gastrointestinal infections will necessitate consultation and input from a range of highly skilled health professionals as the patient requires complex, coordinated intervention. The treating medical team may include a gastroenterologist and infectious disease specialist. A nephrologist may be required to manage acute kidney failure secondary to acute dehydration, while a cardiologist may be included to combat hypertension or arrhythmias associated with electrolyte imbalances and possible thromboembolic events related to the immobile patient (Elena, 2015).

Additionally, a surgical team may be involved to monitor surgical wounds and possible emergency management of a toxic megacolon. Nurses are in a unique position to partner with the patient and their family to ensure true patient-centred care is provided. Nursing care will be coordinated and collaborative, working in conjunction with the multidisciplinary team to provide holistic care to the patient (Cropley & Duis Sanders, 2013).

Specialist nursing staff may be called upon to care for the gastrointestinal patient. A range of specialist nursing staff from gastrointestinal nurses to stoma therapy nurses, wound care nurses and surgical nursing staff may work alongside the patient to ensure that appropriate holistic care as well as education is provided to the patient and their family (Coyne & Needham, 2012). These nursing specialists would be required to work in conjunction with medical staff, a clinical pharmacist to provide expert pharmacology advice, a dietitian to provide strict nutritional support and the wider nursing team, who would be tasked with providing psychological care, drug administration, appropriate personal hygiene and other aspects of care (Elena, 2015; Lomer, 2014). Irrespective of those involved in the care of the acutely ill GI patient, the key goal of multidisciplinary care is to empower patients through the provision of information from a range of healthcare professionals, thus aligning with the concept of patient-centred care. Nursing staff frequently have excellent assessment and communication skills that can create a link between the multidisciplinary team and the patient to ensure holistic, evidence-based, collaborative care is coordinated for each patient.

As Shah and colleagues (2014) discuss, many gastrointestinal conditions, such as bowel disorders, have correlations with psychological illness. Thus psychological issues can adversely impact the individual's ability to manage their pathophysiological disease, which can lead to a reduction in adherence to medical regimes and medical follow-up. Ultimately, a combination of physical and psychological stress increases the likelihood of poor patient outcomes (Shah et al., 2014). The integration of multidisciplinary teams and collaborative care with such patients is therefore required to ensure that the entire disease spectrum for an individual is assessed, allowing for the whole of the person to be treated rather than simply the disease process (Ghosh, 2013). Collaborative care approaches should be the standard of care for acute gastrointestinal disorders to guarantee that quality care is provided, the disease burden is reduced and improved patient outcomes are achieved (Ghosh, 2013).

Culture

Nurses must understand and acknowledge that culture impacts an individual's perspective of health, disease and illness. Not only can cultural and ethnic factors affect health outcomes, but these personal attributes relating to the patient and their family can impact the patient–health professional relationship, as well as assessment, diagnosis and treatment interventions (Sperber, Drossman & Quigley, 2012). Language and culture can affect the understanding and expression of illness. Issues of communication may be important in the case of IBD, whereby symptoms can be challenging to explain. This can lead to a cross-cultural misinterpretation of information as the patient's way of explaining their symptoms may not accurately correlate with physiological findings; therefore, diagnosis of the actual problem may be difficult, and this potentially can compromise patient safety (Sperber, Drossman & Quigley, 2012). The development of cultural competence will ensure that nurses caring for patients with acute GI conditions can effectively respond to their individual needs (Ignatavicius, 2013).

REFLECTIVE QUESTION

A patient of Indian heritage is admitted with acute diverticulitis. The patient speaks only limited English and the multidisciplinary team cannot understand what the patient is trying to convey to them, which means they often disagree about what the patient's needs are. Consider the impact this communication breakdown will have on the patient's management and health outcomes. How might the multidisciplinary team be able to overcome this issue?

SUMMARY

Learning objective 1: Understand the underlying pathophysiology of a range of gastrointestinal conditions, their prevalence, associated risk factors and clinical manifestations.

The GI system includes a large number or organs. Therefore, a range of conditions can affect this system, including GI bleeding, diverticular disease, appendicitis, pancreatitis, cholecystitis, acute liver failure, intestinal obstruction and abdominal compartment syndrome. These diseases differ in their pathophysiology, prevalence and risk factors; thus, for the acute care nurse to adequately manage the GI patient, an in-depth understanding of this complex system is required to provide safe and effective care.

Learning objective 2: Explain how to undertake a comprehensive gastrointestinal assessment.

Inadequate assessment of the GI system can result in poor patient outcomes. Assessment practices must be thorough and methodical to ensure that all relevant data relating the patient and their presentation are identified. This includes a comprehensive health history, systematic physical assessment and a range of invasive and non-invasive diagnostic techniques. Through assessment, a definitive diagnosis can be determined and individualised interventions implemented.

Learning objective 3: Identify and discuss common evidence-based management strategies for acute gastrointestinal disorders.

Nurses caring for the acutely unwell GI patient must have extensive knowledge about a range of GI-specific clinical skills. Due to the complex nature of GI diseases, interventions and treatment strategies vary. Nurses must have an understanding of common GI medications, blood transfusion administration, IV therapy, pain management, enteral feeding, NGTs, stoma care and wound care.

Learning objective 4: Explore the relevance of quality patient education and outcome-focused discharge planning with acute gastrointestinal conditions.

Patient education for the acute GI patient commences in the hospital setting. Nurses must identify opportunities to engage the patient and provide education as often as possible to ensure that they are prepared for possible health-related challenges once discharged from the acute care setting. Furthermore, patient education provides individuals with the ability to engage in self-care behaviours which leads to patient empowerment, and ultimately, greater patient outcomes. Discharge planning is a multidisciplinary process which requires coordination of a range of services to ensure that the needs of the individual are addressed.

Learning objective 5: Understand the importance of working in collaboration with other healthcare professionals to ensure patient-centred and culturally competent care is provided.

To ensure patient care is holistic, it must be both patient centred and culturally appropriate. Patient-centred care of the GI patient must be a collaborative process between disciplines, and consider the needs and preferences of the patient. To ensure the provision of patient-centred care, both the physical and psychological needs of the patient must be acknowledged. Culture impacts an individual's understanding and experience of health. Therefore, nurses must ensure that they are culturally competent to further address the holistic needs of the patient.

REVIEW QUESTIONS

9.1 Explain how a thorough understanding of the underlying pathophysiology of acute GI conditions assists with care planning.

9.2 Outline the importance of a comprehensive nursing assessment for the acute GI patient, and how an extensive health history and thorough physical exam will assist in the diagnosis of a specific illness.

9.3 Discuss why it is important for nursing staff to have a working understanding of medications that effect the GI system.

9.4 Outline what education strategies you would implement with an elderly patient who has recently suffered a significant lower GI bleed.

9.5 What strategies might you need to employ when caring for a patient who comes from a non-English speaking background and requires an NGT for enteral feeding? Integrate a multidisciplinary approach into your discussion.

RESEARCH TOPIC

Research the impact of a bowel obstruction and long-term colostomy for a 25-year-old male. Explore how this may impact on the patient both physically and psychologically. In your discussion, consider how the patient's self-image and sexual identity may be altered, and whether social media have had any influence on the normalisation of colostomies in contemporary society.

FURTHER READING

Curtis, K. (2013). Caring for adult patients who require nasogastric feeding tubes. *Nursing Standard*, 27(38), 47–56.

Iqbal, F., Kujan, O., Bowley, D.M., Keighley, M.R. & Vaizey, C.J. (2016). Quality of life after ostomy surgery in Muslim patients: A systematic review of the literature and suggestions for clinical practice. *Journal of Wound Ostomy & Continence Nursing*, 43(4), 385–91.

Nurgali, K. & Wildbore. C. (2015). Alterations of digestive function across the lifespan. In J. Craft & C. Gordon (eds), *Understanding Pathophysiology* (2nd ed.). Sydney: Elsevier, pp. 765–819.

Petrov, M. (2013). Nutrition, inflammation, and acute pancreatitis. *ISRN Inflammation*, 341–410. doi:10.1155/2013/341410.

Walsh, K. & Schub, E. (2016). Nasogastric tube: Inserting and verifying placement in the adult patient. Retrieved from https://www.ebscohost.com/assets-sample-content/Nasogastric_Tube_Insertion.pdf.

REFERENCES

Agency for Clinical Innovation (2017). Upper GI bleeding. Retrieved from https://www.aci.health.nsw.gov.au/networks/eci/clinical/clinical-resources/clinical-tools/gastroenterology/upper-gi-bleeding.

Bell, C. & Sluys, P. (2016). Trauma management. In L. Aitken, A. Marshall & W. Chaboyer (eds), *ACCCN's Critical Care Nursing* (3rd ed.). Sydney: Elsevier, pp. 791–828.

Ben-Ami, R., Halaburda, K., Klyasova, G., Metan, G., Torosian, T & Akova, M. (2013). A multidisciplinary team approach to the management of patients with suspected or diagnosed invasive fungal disease. *Journal of Antimicrobial Chemotherapy*, 68(3), 25–33.

Berry, N. & Fletcher, S. (2012). Abdominal compartment syndrome. *Continuing Education in Anesthesia Critical Care and Pain*, 12(3), 110–17.

Blaser, A., Malbrain, M., Starkopf, J., Fruhwald, S., Jakob, S., De Waele, J., … Spies, C. (2012). Gastrointestinal function in intensive care patients: Terminology, definitions and management. Recommendations of the ESICM Working Group on Abdominal Problems. *Intensive Care Medicine*, 38(3), 384–94.

Blausen (2014). Medical Gallery of Blausen Medical. *WikiJournal of Medicine*, 1(2). doi:10.15347/wjm/2014.010. ISSN 2002-4436.

Böhm, S.K. (2015). Risk factors for diverticulosis, diverticulitis, diverticular perforation, and bleeding: A plea for more subtle history taking. *Viszeralmedizin*, 31(2), 84–94.

Bryant, B. & Knights, K. (2015). *Pharmacology for Health Professionals* (4th ed.). Sydney: Mosby Elsevier.

Burch, J. (2010). Management of stoma complications. *Nursing Times*, 107(45), 17–18.

—— (2011). Stoma management: Enhancing patient knowledge. *British Journal of Community Nursing*, 16(4), 162–6.

Camilleri, M., Malhi, H. & Acosta, A. (2017). Gastrointestinal complications of obesity. *Gastroenterology*, 152(7), 1656–70.

Campinha-Bacote, J. (2011). Delivering patient-centred care in the midst of a cultural conflict: The role of cultural competence. *The Online Journal of Issues in Nursing*, 16(2). doi:10.3912/OJIN.Vol16No02Man05.

Cardoso, F., Marcelino, P., Bagulho, L. & Karvellas, C. (2017). Acute liver failure: An up-to-date approach. *Journal of Critical Care*, 39, 25–50.

Clark, L., Gunning, A., Martin, R. & West-Oram, A. (2015). Elimination. In L. Dougherty, S. Lister & A. West-Oram (eds), *The Royal Marsden Manual of Clinical Nursing Procedures* (9th ed.). Chichester: John Wiley & Sons, pp. 127–200.

Cleary-Holdforth, J. & Leufer, T. (2013). Nursing care of conditions related to the digestive system. In A.M. Brady, C. McCabe & M. McCann (eds), *Fundamentals of Medical-Surgical Nursing: A Systems Approach*. Chichester: John Wiley & Sons, pp. 322–49.

Coyne, E. & Needham, J. (2012). Undergraduate nursing students' placement in specialty clinical areas: Understanding the concerns of the student and registered nurse. *Contemporary Nurse*, 42(1), 97–104.

Crogan, A. (2013). Nursing assessment: Gastrointestinal system. In D. Brown & H. Edwards (eds), *Lewis's Medical-Surgical Nursing* (3rd ed.). Sydney: Elsevier Mosby, pp. 4205–83.

Cronin, P. & Duffy, A. (2011). Nursing patients with gastrointestinal, liver and biliary disorders. In C. Brooker & M. Nicol (eds), *Alexander's Nursing Practice* (4th ed.). Sydney: Elsevier, pp. 71–124.

Cropley, S. & Duis Sanders, E. (2013). Care coordination and the essential role of the nurse. *Creative Nursing*, 19(4), 189–94.

Curtis, K. (2013). Caring for adult patients who require nasogastric feeding tubes. *Nursing Standard*, 27(38), 47–56.

Dillstrom, M., Bjersa, K., Engstrom, M. & Sahlgrenska, A. (2017). Patients' experience of acute unplanned surgical reoperation. *Journal of Surgical Research*, 209, 199–205.

Elena, C. (2015). Multidisciplinary approach of the patient with enterocolitis with clostridium difficile – a necessity. *Journal of Colitis & Diverticulitis*, 1(1). doi:10.4172/jcdc.1000e001.

Epner, D. & Baile, W. (2012). Patient-centred care: The key to cultural competence. *Annals of Oncology*, 23(Supplement 3), 33–42.

Ferreira-Aparicio, F.E., Gutiérrez-Vega, R., Gálvez-Molina, Y., Ontiveros-Nevares, P., Athie-Gútierrez, C. & Montalvo-Javé, E.E. (2012). Diverticular disease of the small bowel. *Case Reports in Gastroenterology*, 6(3), 668–76.

Fitzgerald, P. (2010). Gastrointestinal disorders. In T. Buttaro & K. Barba (eds), *Nursing Care of the Hospitalized Older Patient*. Chichester: Wiley-Blackwell.

Fitzgerald Close, J. (2018). Gastrointestinal disorders and therapeutic management. In L. Urden, K. Stacy & M. Lough (eds), *Critical Care Nursing: Diagnosis and Management* (8th ed.). St Louis, MI: Elsevier, pp. 681–704.

Ghosh, S. (2013). Multidisciplinary teams as standard of care in inflammatory bowel disease. *Canadian Journal of Gastroenterology*, 27(4), 199–205.

Goolsby, M. & Grubbs, L. (eds) (2011). *Advanced Assessment: Interpreting Findings and Formulating Differential Diagnoses* (2nd ed.). Philadelphia, PA: F.A. Davis Company.

Higgins, D. & Jones, D. (2012). Ensuring patient safety: Blood transfusion. *Nursing Times*, 109(4), 22–3.

Ignatavicius, D. (2013). Cultural aspects of health and illness. In D. Ignatavicius & L. Workman (eds), *Medical-Surgical Nursing* (7th ed.). St Louis, MI: Elsevier Saunders, pp. 30–8.

Lau, M.T. & Girard, J. (2011). Ensuring safer enteral feeding. *Nursing Management*, 42(12), 39–43.

Lawn, S., Delany, T., Sweet, L., Battersby, M. & Skinner, T. (2013). Control in chronic condition self-care management: How it occurs in the health worker–client relationship and implications for client empowerment. *Journal of Advanced Nursing*, 70(2), 383–94.

Litwack, K. (2010). Care of the surgical patient. In M. Burton & L. Ludwig (eds), *Fundamentals of Nursing Care*. Philadelphia, PA: F. A. Davis Company, pp. 769–804.

Lomer, M. (ed.) (2014). *Advanced Nutrition and Dietetics in Gastroenterology*. Chichester: John Wiley & Sons.

Marshall, A. & Gordon, C. (2016). Gastrointestinal, metabolic and liver alterations. In L. Aitken, A. Marshall & W. Chaboyer (eds), *ACCCN's Critical Care Nursing* (3rd ed.). Sydney: Elsevier, pp. 651–80.

Martin, B, (2007). Prevention of gastrointestinal complications in the critically ill patient. *Advanced Critical Care*, 18(2), 158–66.

Massey, D., Chaboyer, W. & Anderson, V. (2017). What factors influence ward nurses' recognition of and response to patient deterioration? An integrative review of the literature. *Nursing Open*, 4(1), 6–23. doi:10.1002/nop2.53.

Monahan, F., Neighbours, M. & Green, C. (2011). *Swearingen's Manual of Medical-Surgical Nursing: A Care Planning Resource* (7th ed.). St Louis, MO: Elsevier.

Mula, C. (2014). Nurses' competency and challenges in enteral feeding in the intensive care unit (ICU) and high dependency units (HDU) of a referral hospital, Malawi. *Malawi Medical Journal*, 26(3), 55–9.

Nesvaderani, M., Eslick, G. & Cox, M. (2015). Acute pancreatitis: Update on management. *The Medical Journal of Australia*, 202(8), 420–3.

Nosbusch, J., Weiss, M. & Bobay, K. (2010). An integrated review of the literature on challenges confronting the acute care staff nurse in discharge planning. *Journal of Clinical Nursing*, 20(5–6), 754–74.

Nowicki, L., Williams, L. & Bradford, J. (2015). Gastrointestinal, hepatobiliary and pancreatic systems function, assessment, and therapeutic measurement. In L. Williams & P. Hopper (eds), *Understanding Medical Surgical Nursing* (5th ed.). Philadelphia, PA: F.A. Davis Company, pp. 685–716.

Nurgali, K. & Wildbore, C. (2015). Alterations of digestive function across the lifespan. In J. Craft & C. Gordon (eds), *Understanding Pathophysiology* (2nd ed.). Sydney: Elsevier, pp. 765–819.

Nursing Council of New Zealand (NCNZ) ([2007] 2016). *Competencies for Registered Nurses*. Retrieved from http://www.nursingcouncil.org.nz/Nurses.

Nursing and Midwifery Board of Australia (NMBA) (2016). *Registered Nurse Standards for Practice*. Melbourne: Nursing & Midwifery Board of Australia. Retrieved from http://www.nursingmidwiferyboard.gov.au/Codes-Guidelines-Statements/Professional-standards.aspx.

Padhi, S., Bullock, I., Li, L. & Stroud, M. (2013). Intravenous fluid therapy for adults in hospital: Summary of NICE guidance. *British Medical Journal*, 347, f7073.

Patel, L. & Curtis, K. (2011). Patient assessment and essentials of care. In K. Curtis & C. Ramsden (eds), *Emergency and Trauma Care for Nurses and Paramedics*. Sydney: Elsevier, pp. 233–66.

Pezzilli, R., Morselli-Labate, A.M. & Corinaldesi, R. (2010). NSAIDs and acute pancreatitis: A systematic review. *Pharmaceuticals*, 3(3), 558–71.

Punzalan, C. & Barry, C. (2016). Acute liver failure: Diagnosis and management. *Journal of Intensive Care Medicine*, 31(10), 642–53.

Pyleris, E., Giannikopoulos, G. & Dabos, K. (2010). Pathophysiology and management of acute liver failure. *Annals of Gastroenterology*, 23(4), 257–65.

Rani, P. & Kumar, R. (2016). Relation of smoking in the development of mucosal and ulcerative lesions in upper gastrointestinal tract. *Indian Journal of Public Health Research & Development*, 7(4), 130–3.

Scales, K. (2014). NICE CG 174: Intravenous fluid therapy in adults in hospital. *British Journal of Nursing*, 23(8 Supp), S6–7.

Shah, E., Rezaie, A., Riddle, M. & Pimentel, M. (2014). Psychological disorders in gastrointestinal disease: Epiphenomenon, cause or consequence? *Annals of Gastroenterology: Quarterly Publication of the Hellenic Society of Gastroenterology*, 27(3), 224–30.

Soenen, S., Rayner, C., Jones, K. & Horowitz, M. (2016). The ageing gastrointestinal tract. *Current Opinion in Clinical Nutrition and Metabolic Care*, 19(1), 12–18.

Somani, R.R. & Bhanushali, U.V. (2011). Synthesis and evaluation of anti-inflammatory, analgesic and ulcerogenic potential of NSAIDs bearing 1,3,4-oxadiazole scaffold. *Indian Journal of Pharmaceutical Sciences*, 73(6), 634.

Sperber, A., Drossman, D. & Quigley, E. (2012). The global perspective on irritable bowel syndrome: A Rome Foundation–World Gastroenterology Organization symposium. *The American Journal of Gastroenterology*, 107, 1602–9.

Springhouse (2010). *Professional Guide to Pathophysiology* (3rd ed.).Philadelphia, PA: Lippincott Williams & Wilkins.

Stinton, L.M. & Shaffer, E.A. (2012). Epidemiology of gallbladder disease: Cholelithiasis and cancer. *Gut and Liver*, 6(2), 172–87.

Strate, L.L., Singh, P., Boylan, M.R., Piawah, S., Cao, Y. & Chan, A.T. (2016). A prospective study of alcohol consumption and smoking and the risk of major gastrointestinal bleeding in men. *PloS One*, 11(11), e0165278.

Streitberger, K., Stüber, F., Kipfer, B.I. & Stamer, U.M. (2011). Drug therapy of acute and chronic abdominal pain. *Therapeutische Umschau. Revue therapeutique*, 68(8), 435–40.

Szoeke, C., Dang, C., Lehert, P., Hickey, M., Morris, M.E., Dennerstein, L. & Campbell, S. (2017). Unhealthy habits persist: The ongoing presence of modifiable risk factors for disease in women. *PloS One*, 12(4), e0173603.

Vermorken, A.J., Andrès, E. & Cui, Y. (2016). Bowel movement frequency, oxidative stress and disease prevention (Review). *Molecular and Clinical Oncology*, 5(4), 339–42.

Von Rosenvinge, E.C., Song, Y., White, J.R., Maddox, C., Blanchard, T. & Fricke, W.F. (2013). Immune status, antibiotic medication and pH are associated with changes in the stomach fluid microbiota. *ISME Journal*, 7(7), 1354–66.

Walsh, K. & Schub, E. (2016) Nasogastric tube: Insertion and verifying placement in the adult patient. Retrieved from https://www.ebscohost.com/assets-sample-content/Nasogastric_Tube_Insertion.pdf.

Weizman, A.V. & Nguyen, G.C. (2011). Diverticular disease: Epidemiology and management. *Canadian Journal of Gastroenterology*, 25(7), 385–9.

Wilkins, T., Khan, N., Nabh, A. & Schade, R. (2012). Diagnosis and management of upper gastrointestinal bleeding. *American Family Physician*, 85(5), 269–76.

Worden, J. & Hanna, K. (2017). Optimizing proton pump inhibitor therapy for treatment of nonvariceal upper gastrointestinal bleeding. *American Journal of Health System Pharmacists*, 74(3), 109–16.

10 Acute endocrine conditions

Sharon Latimer, Matthew Barton,
Leeane Ford, Julia Gilbert and Nang Sein

LEARNING OBJECTIVES

At the completion of this chapter, you should be able to:

1   define acute endocrine conditions, and identify underlying pathophysiology, risk factors and presentations associated with acute endocrine conditions
2   describe nursing assessment and management strategies for the individual with acute endocrine conditions
3   understand the concepts of patient-centred care and care coordination in relation to acute endocrine conditions
4   identify and discuss the nurse's role in the collaborative management of individuals with acute endocrine conditions
5   understand advanced nursing practice in relation to acute endocrine conditions.

Introduction

Acute endocrine conditions such as diabetes and thyroid disease are potentially life threat-ening, with high mortality rates if they are not detected and treated rapidly. During 2014–15, the prevalence of diabetes among the Australian population was 5.1 per cent, with a mortality rate of 16.3 deaths per 100 000 people (ABS, 2016). Yet for the same period, the mortality rate among Aboriginal and Torres Strait Islander Australians was almost five times higher (76.9 deaths per 100 000 people) (ABS, 2016). The treatment and management of acute endocrine conditions is complex, and requires an individualised approach (Diabetes Australia, 2015a). A multidisciplinary healthcare team is needed to manage these patients, and nurses play a vital role. This chapter discusses the incidence, presentation, clinical mani-festations and treatment of the following acute endocrine conditions: diabetic ketoacidosis, hypoglycaemia, adrenal crisis, hypothyroidism and thyrotoxicosis. In addition, the concepts of patient–centred care and the nurse's role in collaborative care for patients with acute endocrine conditions are discussed.

The nursing care of patients with acute endocrine conditions is complex. Frequent and continuous assessment, monitoring and evaluation of the patient's condition is required. Nurses' decision-making and critical thinking must be underpinned by theoretical knowledge and current evidence-based care. Effective communication and collaboration among the multidisciplinary healthcare team is needed in the delivery of patient-centred care. The following identifies the national practice standards and competencies for registered nurses from the Nursing and Midwifery Board of Australia (NMBA) and the Nursing Council of New Zealand (NCNZ) that are addressed in this chapter.

Australian Registered Nurse Standards for Practice

Standard 1: Thinks critically and analyses nursing practice

Standard 2: Engages in therapeutic and professional relationships

Standard 3: Maintains the capability for practice

Standard 4: Comprehensively conducts assessments

Standard 5: Develops a plan for nursing practice

Standard 6: Provides safe, appropriate and responsive quality nursing practice

Standard 7: Evaluates outcomes to inform nursing practice

(NMBA, 2016)

New Zealand: Competencies for Registered Nurses

Competency 1.1: Accepts responsibility for ensuring that his/her nursing practice and conduct meet the standards of the professional, ethical and relevant legislated requirements

Competency 1.2: Demonstrates the ability to apply the principles of the Treaty of Waitangi/ Te Tiriti o Waitangi to nursing practice

Competency 1.5: Practises nursing in a manner that the health consumer determines as being culturally safe

Competency 4.1: Collaborates and participates with colleagues and members of the health care team to facilitate and coordinate care

Competency 4.2: Recognises and values the roles and skills of all members of the health care team in the delivery of care

(NCNZ, [2007] 2016)

NURSING STANDARDS

Pathophysiology, risk factors and presentations of acute endocrine conditions

The endocrine system is the collection of hormone-producing ductless glands that secrete their respective hormone/s into the circulatory system to act on distant target cells. Affecting almost every human cell, the endocrine hormones are responsible for regulating metabolism, growth and development, tissue function, sexual function, reproduction, sleep and mood. The endocrine system consists of the pituitary gland, thyroid gland, parathyroid glands, adrenal glands, pancreas, ovaries and testes. Diseases of the endocrine system involve these glands, and may be subdivided into three groups:

- endocrine gland hypersecretion (too much hormone)
- endocrine gland hyposecretion (too little hormone)
- tumors of endocrine glands.

The diagnosis of endocrine diseases can be difficult because accurately measuring serum hormone levels is frequently not possible, making the detection and treatment rather challenging. In this chapter, we will only discuss a select number of acute endocrine conditions. However, in reality it is important to remember that the endocrine system works in concert with other body systems (such as the nervous system) to produce key functions such as regulation of blood glucose levels; coordination of the body's responses to stress; and regulation of calcium and phosphate balance. Together, this helps the body to maintain **homeostasis**.

Homeostasis – Balance or equilibrium; an organism's tendency to regulate and stabilise its internal conditions.

Disorders of the pancreas

Diabetes mellitus

The beta-cells, located in the pancreas, secrete the hormone insulin into the circulatory system in response to rises in the body's blood glucose level (American Diabetes, 2013). This hormone has many functions, including facilitating the movement of glucose from the bloodstream into the cells. Without insulin, the glucose would remain in the circulatory system, eventually resulting in catastrophic complications (American Diabetes, 2013). Broadly, **diabetes mellitus (DM)** is a metabolic disorder of carbohydrate, protein and fat metabolism, resulting from defects in insulin secretion, action or both, invariably resulting in **hyperglycaemia** (American Diabetes, 2013). DM is a heterogeneous disorder that is the most common endocrine disease affecting the pancreas. Previously, diabetes was defined according to the patient's age of disease onset: type 1 diabetes – onset in children; and type 2 diabetes – onset in adults; however, this definition is now obsolete. Currently, DM is defined according to its aetiology (cause), and is classified as either type 1 or type 2 DM. The aetiology of type 1 DM is due to the destruction of the beta-cells, leading to absolute insulin deficiency, while type 2 DM is a progressive loss of insulin secretion on a background of insulin receptor resistance (American Diabetes, 2016).

Diabetes mellitus (DM) – A chronic metabolic condition characterised by prolonged elevated blood sugar levels.

Hyperglycaemia – A condition that occurs when an individual's blood glucose levels are elevated above 7 mmol/L (fasting) and 11.0 mmol/L (non-fasting).

In 2015, globally, it was estimated that the DM prevalence rate was 415 million people, with these figures expected to rise to 592 million by 2035 (International Diabetes Federation, 2015). In Australia, approximately 1.7 million people have type 1 and type 2 diabetes (1.2 million known and registered, as well as silent, undiagnosed type 2 diabetes) (Diabetes Australia, 2015a). DM is a chronic disease that, if left unmanaged, can lead to many serious and potentially life-threatening systemic complications. Likewise, disruptions in glucose homeostasis can result in a number of acute complications, which for the patient with DM are equally life-threatening. In the following sections, we discuss three common acute complications of DM: diabetic ketoacidosis; hyperosmolar hyperglycaemic state; and hypoglycaemia.

Diabetic ketoacidosis

Diabetes ketoacidosis (DKA) results from the absence of insulin and/or its functional activity, and increased serum levels of insulin's counter-regulatory hormones (glucagon, cortisol, catecholamines and growth hormone) (Wolfsdorf et al., 2014). This results in a significant increase in serum glucose (hyperglycaemia) due to the body's utilisation of glycogen from the liver and glucose from catabolising proteins. More markedly, fat is also broken down into fatty acids and preferentially converted into ketones, as an alternate energy molecule to glucose, a process known as **ketogenesis**. This biochemical compensatory response will result in the biochemical criteria for DKA diagnosis: hyperglycaemia (>11 mmol/L), metabolic acidosis (venous pH <7.3) and ketonaemia (Wolfsdorf et al., 2014). Typically, those most prone to DKA are people with undiagnosed or poorly managed type 1 DM (due to their complete absence of insulin). However, individuals with type 2 DM can also experience DKA during periods of heightened stress (e.g. surgery, infection), illness or trauma, when their counter-regulatory hormones are increased significantly. DKA is an acute life-threatening complication requiring urgent medical treatment. In addition to hyperglycaemia (>11.0 mmol/L), patients can present with tachycardia, tachypnoea and/or Kussmaul breathing (deep, laboured breathing), thirst, dehydration, nausea/vomiting, serum electrolyte disturbances, abdominal pain, metabolic acidosis and altered levels of consciousness. Without urgent medical intervention, there is a significant risk that the patient may lapse into a coma and eventually die.

Diabetic ketoacidosis (DKA) – An acute, major, life-threatening complication of type 1 diabetes mellitus, characterised by hyperglycaemia, ketoacidosis and ketonuria.

Ketogenesis – The conversion of fats into ketones.

Hyperosmolar hyperglycaemic state

Hyperosmolar hyperglycaemic state (HHS) is a condition characterised by severe hyperglycaemia, serum hyperosmolarity and significant dehydration, without ketogenesis

Hyperosmolar hyperglycaemic state (HHS) – An acute, life-threatening complication of type 2 diabetes mellitus characterised by hyperglycaemia and severe dehydration, resulting in coma and death if left untreated.

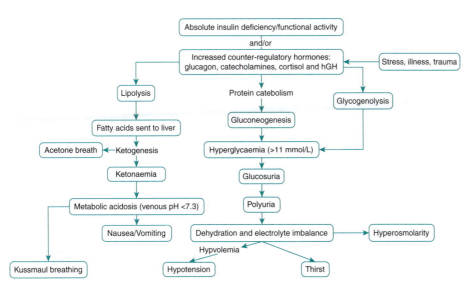

Figure 10.1   Pathogenesis of diabetic ketoacidosis (DKA) and hyperosmolar hyperglycaemic state (HHS)

(the conversion of fats into ketones) (Pasquel & Umpierrez, 2014). Usually, HHS affects patients with type 2 DM, with the elderly particularly vulnerable. HHS is associated with a high mortality rate, which is reported to be up to ten times higher than DKA (Kitabchi et al., 2009). The aetiology of HHS results from an insulin-deficient state on a background of increased levels of counter-regulatory hormones. Hyperglycaemia then develops from the increased conversion of glycogen and proteins into glucose by the liver, but without ketogenesis (Pasquel & Umpierrez, 2014). This is partly due to the higher circulating ratio of insulin/glucagon in HHS when compared with DKA. The diagnosis criteria for HHS include hyperglycaemia (>33.3 mmol/L), serum biocarbonate (>15 mmol/L), effective serum osmolality (>320 mOsm/kg), mild to no ketonaemia, and an altered level of consciousness (Glasgow Coma Scale) (Wolfsdorf et al., 2014). This severe hyperglycaemic state results in glycosuria and subsequent polyuria, due to the osmotic diuresis effect of glucose in the filtrate. This polyuria may go unrecognised for some time until the patient is significantly dehydrated and has profound electrolyte imbalances, which (like DKA) if urgent medical intervention is not instigated, will result in coma and eventually death.

Hypoglycaemia

Hypoglycaemia – A condition that occurs when an individual's blood glucose level falls below 4 mmol/L. Early signs and symptoms may include shaking, trembling, weakness, sweating, hunger, lightheadedness and dizziness.

Hypoglycaemia is an acute complication of insulin treatment in both type 1 and type 2 DM and/or patients receiving glucose-lowering medications that cause serum glucose levels to decreases below a normal range (<4.0 mmol/L) (IABPG, 2017). In a hypoglycaemic event, the insulin serum levels of patients with DM are high relative to the serum glucose levels, due to excessive exogenous insulin loading or from the effects of glucose-lowering medications. In response, the body compensates through the use of its counter-regulatory hormones; however, because the reaction to glucagon is inadequate, the catecholamine hormones predominate (Funk, 2014). Initially, the symptoms and signs of palpitations, tremors, anxiety and sweating are the result of the neurogenic effects of the catecholamines. However, as the serum glucose levels continue to fall, the patient will experience clinical manifestations such as headaches, abnormal behaviour (such as confusion), seizures, an altered level of consciousness, and eventually coma and death.

Nursing assessment and management of diabetes mellitus and hypoglycaemia

The nursing assessment and acute care of patients experiencing hyperglycaemia and hypoglycaemia are outlined below. This is a guide only: in clinical practice, the healthcare organisation's policy and procedure should always be followed.

Health history

Given the individualised nature of DM management and treatment, it is important to complete a comprehensive and detailed patient health history on admission. This patient history should include information about the frequency of blood glucose level (BGL) testing and medications (oral hypoglycaemics and/or insulin), their usual BGL range, the signs and symptoms they experience during a hypoglycaemic or hyperglycaemic episode, the BGL range when they begin the feel these signs and symptoms, and how they manage episodes of hypoglycaemia or hyperglycaemia (IABPG, 2017). The patient's past medical history should also be obtained, including details of recent infections or illnesses. In addition, their current weight and eating patterns should be documented, and a referral to a dietitian is recommended (IABPG, 2017). Finally, obtaining details of their current primary healthcare provider, such as their GP, allows for improved ongoing patient care following discharge (IABPG, 2017).

Any episode of hyperglycaemia or hypoglycaemia is potentially life-threatening. A comprehensive and accurate nursing assessment is vital, so appropriate treatment and/or emergency medical interventions can be prioritised and implemented. In both circumstances, nurses need to assess the patient's blood glucose level (BGL) and carefully monitor their signs and symptoms. Initially, BGL and vital signs should be taken, then repeated every 15 minutes or so, depending on the patient's medical condition (Savage et al., 2011).

Acute patient care for diabetic ketoacidosis

DKA is a medical emergency requiring continuous patient assessment and monitoring. The aim of treatment is to avoid hypovolaemic shock, hypokalaemia and hyperosmolarity, and manage any metabolic acidosis (Goguen & Gilbert, 2013; Savage et al., 2011). Most treatment will be delivered intravenously (IV), and numerous blood samples will be collected for analysis. Following initial assessment, an IV cannula is inserted. Patients experiencing severe dehydration, shock and hypotension require a rapid infusion of IV 0.9% Sodium Chloride (normal saline) of 500 ml to 1000 ml (Goguen & Gilbert, 2013; Savage et al., 2011). Ongoing nursing observation and assessment will include the patient's level of consciousness, fluid input, diuresis and an electrocardiograph (ECG) (Goguen & Gilbert, 2013; Savage et al., 2011). Current guidelines recommend potassium chloride to be added to the IV infusion once the serum potassium level is <5.5 mmol/L (Savage et al., 2011). Metabolic acidosis is treated by administering insulin (short-acting or IV bolus), ceasing the ketone production and allowing the serum glucose to move from the blood into the cells (Goguen & Gilbert, 2013). An IV sodium bicarbonate infusion may be required to maintain the serum pH <7.0 (Goguen & Gilbert, 2013). Hyperosmolarity is treated using an IV saline infusion concentration (Goguen & Gilbert, 2013). During treatment, the target BGL range is 12.0–14.0 mmol/L and, once achieved, an IV glucose infusion is commenced to prevent hypoglycaemia (Goguen & Gilbert, 2013).

Acute patient care for hyperosmolar hyperglycaemic state

HHS is also a medical emergency, with patients requiring continuous assessment and monitoring. These patients receive the same acute patient care outlined for DKA, with metabolic acidosis less likely (Goguen & Gilbert, 2013). The BGL target is 12.0–14.0 mmol/L (Goguen & Gilbert, 2013).

Acute patient care for hypoglycaemia

The aim of treatment is to promptly raise the BGL to 4.0 mmol/L (IABPG, 2017). The treatment and management of hypoglycaemia is determined by two factors: the patient's level of consciousness and their ability to swallow (IABPG, 2017). The following section outlines the acute care of the conscious patient who is able to swallow, the patient who is unconscious, and their post-acute care.

Conscious and able to swallow

The first line of treatment is to administer 15 g of fast-acting carbohydrate, such as three glucose tablets (5 g each), 175 ml regular lemonade or fruit juice, or three teaspoons of sugar or honey (IABPG, 2017). It is important to monitor the patient's BGL every 15 minutes until it reaches >4.0 mmol/L (IABPG, 2017). If, after 15 minutes, the BGL remains <4.0 mmol/L, administer a further 15 g of fast-acting carbohydrate (IABPG, 2017). Retest the BGL in another 15 minutes, and provide a 15 g fast-acting carbohydrate load if the BGL is <4.0 mmol/L (IABPG, 2017). If, after 45 minutes (third BGL retest), the BGL is still <4.0 mmol/L, or if there is a decrease in the patient's level of consciousness, contact the doctor immediately for further advice (IABPG, 2017). Once the BGL reaches ≥4.0 mmol/L, administer a long-acting carbohydrate load such as a small meal or snack (IABPG, 2017).

Unconscious patient

The first priority of care is to contact the medical emergency team (MET), maintain the patient's airway and conduct baseline vital signs (blood pressure, pulse, respirations and oxygen saturations) (IABPG, 2017). A cannula is usually inserted so that IV dextrose can be administered promptly (or intramuscular glucagon may be ordered) (IABPG, 2017). During treatment, the patient's BGL should be retested every 15 minutes until it reaches >4.0 mmol/L (IABPG, 2017). Closely monitor the patient's level of consciousness, and gently reassure them once they become conscious (IABPG, 2017). Be mindful that some patients may become combative during this period, because they may not be aware of the medical emergency that has occurred.

Post-acute episode care

Following the acute care, ongoing monitoring of the patient is required. Accurate documentation of the care provided is a legal requirement, and assists with the continuity of care. Regular BGL testing may be necessary over the next few days, especially if the patient's diabetes management has changed (IABPG, 2017). Exploring the possible causes of the hyperglycaemic or hypoglycaemic episode assists the medical team to make appropriate adjustments to the current management plan (IABPG, 2017). Diabetes management is lifelong, so any sudden change in the patient's condition may result in them experiencing anxiety or depression. Reassurance and education are ways to help patients cope with changes to their current care. For some patients, this medical emergency may trigger an episode of anxiety or depression (Goguen & Gilbert, 2013; Savage et al., 2011), so a referral to a psychologist may be required (Savage et al., 2011).

Discharge planning

Equipment to manage diabetes and hypoglycaemia

Prior to discharge, advise the patient where to source specialised equipment such as BGL monitoring equipment, insulin syringes, insulin pump and so on (Lewis et al., 2016).

Areas of patient education (prior to discharge) include:

- the cause, signs and symptoms, management and prevention of hypoglycaemia (Lewis et al., 2016)
- current medication management (insulin and oral hypoglycaemics), including the correct administration of the insulin (Lewis et al., 2016).

The following procedures should be followed:

- Upon discharge, transport the insulin in the original packaging and in a specially designed refrigerator travel bag (Sofrigam, 2017).
- At home, the insulin should be stored in the middle of the refrigerator (between 2–8°C) as soon as practically possible (Sofrigam, 2017).
- BGL monitoring is vital: check and advise on the frequency and accuracy of the patient's technique (Lewis et al., 2016).
- With regard to insulin storage and equipment, avoid extreme heat and cold, and do not freeze (BD Diabetes Education Center, 2017). Prior to administration, check the insulin by observing it for clumps, stringiness, cloudiness (for clear insulin) and

colour changes (BD Diabetes Education Center, 2017). Discard the insulin if any abnormalities are observed or one month after opening it (BD Diabetes Education Center, 2017).

Multidisciplinary team referrals

The following referrals should be made:

- dietitian: dietary management (Lewis et al., 2016)
- physiotherapist: exercise and activity plan (Lewis et al., 2016)
- podiatrist: foot care and footwear
- diabetic team follow-up and ongoing care (Lewis et al., 2016)
- psychologist: ongoing emotional support (Savage et al., 2011).

Impact on the family

Patients, family, friends and work colleagues should be educated about possible hypoglycaemic episodes, including the signs, symptoms and treatment (Diabetes Queensland, 2017). An emergency care plan to be implemented during a hypoglycaemic episode should be drafted and distributed to family, friends and work colleagues. This plan should include the recommended actions if the patient becomes unconscious, drowsy or unable to swallow. Never feed a drowsy or unconscious patient; rather, lay them on their side, maintain a patent airway and call for an ambulance. Diabetes is a lifelong, chronic medical condition, so counselling support for patients, partners and families may be required.

REFLECTIVE QUESTION

The management of hyperglycaemia and hypoglycaemia is complex, and the care needs to be individualised. Develop an algorithm such as a flow diagram that outlines the differences in the management of these two conditions.

Disorders of the adrenal gland

Adrenal crisis

The adrenal glands produce life-sustaining hormones (glucocorticoids, mineralocorticoids and sex steroids) required during times of stress and critical metabolic functions (Marieb & Hoehn, 2012). **Adrenal crisis (AC)** is a life-threatening pathophysiological event caused by a severe relative insufficiency of adrenal hormones (mineralocorticoids and glucocorticoids) (O'Connell & Siafarikas, 2010). AC occurs in patients with chronic adrenal insufficiency (AI) or adrenal susceptibility, who are experiencing an episode of acute physiological stress (e.g. trauma, surgery, illness) (Allolio, 2015). People with **Addison's disease** (a disorder where the adrenal glands produce insufficient cortisol) are also susceptible to AC during increased stressors such as surgery, emotional stress, infection, burns, myocardial infarction or pregnancy (Salehmohamed, Cuesta & Thompson, 2015).

Illness and infection lead to increases in circulating glucocorticoids levels in healthy subjects, and therefore it has been suggested that glucocorticoids suppress the immune system to prevent the destructive effects of an amplified immune response, most notably

Adrenal crisis (AC) – A potentially life-threatening situation resulting from negligible cortisol levels and requiring immediate emergency treatment.

Addison's disease – A chronic, progressive disorder where the adrenal glands fail to produce sufficient cortisol.

through the pro-inflammatory cytokines (e.g. interleukin 1 (IL6) and tumour necrosis factor alpha (TNFα) (Allolio, 2015). However, in chronic AI or adrenal susceptible patients, their reduced glucocorticoid levels greatly increase the lethal effects of these pro-inflammatory cytokines. Thus, considering TNFα and IL6 have been shown to be key mediators of AC, through their inhibition on glucocorticoid receptor functions they induce a state of relative glucocorticoid resistance (Allolio, 2015). In AC, hypotension occurs because of the inhibition in permissive action of glucocorticoids on adrenergic receptors (e.g. vasoconstriction) and by body fluid depletion caused by a lack of sodium and increased fluid retention due to missing mineralocorticoid activity (Else & Hammer, 2014). Moreover, the hyponatraemia and hyperkalaemia are manifestations of the mineralocorticoid deficiency, while the volume depletion may be worsened by vomiting and diarrhoea (Else & Hammer, 2014).

The onset of AC is often gradual, and may go unnoticed until an acute stressor precipitates it. The most common clinical situations include:

- patients with chronic AI who experience serious infection or other acute stress
- previously undiagnosed patients experiencing a physiological stressor, resulting in AC
- patients with diagnosed AI who are under-replaced therapeutically
- patients experiencing pituitary or adrenal gland destruction (e.g. infarction, haemorrhage)
- patients who are abruptly withdrawn from glucocorticoid therapy (corticosteroids, prednisolone) (Nieman, 2017).

The predominant clinical manifestation of AC is physiological shock, but patients may also present with non-specific symptoms, such as anorexia, nausea/vomiting, abdominal pain, fatigue/lethargy, fever, confusion/coma (Nieman, 2017). Allolio (2015) suggests that for a diagnosis of AC, the patient must present with a profound impairment of general health and at least two of the following conditions: hypotension (systolic blood pressure <100 mmHg), nausea/vomiting, severe fatigue, hyponatraemia, hypoglycaemia or hyperkalaemia. In patients diagnosed with AI, the incidence of AC increases with age and illnesses, especially bacterial infections (gastroenteritis and bronchopulmonary) (Rushworth & Torpy, 2014), whereas, the risk factors for AC in unrecognised AI patients include poor general health, pain states, infection, recent surgery and having received a barbiturate general anaesthetic (Smans et al., 2016).

Nursing assessment and management of adrenal crisis

AC is a medical emergency that requires accurate nursing assessment and immediate treatment (O'Connell & Siafarikas, 2010).

This management guide can vary from individual to individual depending on presentation. The healthcare organisation's policy and procedure should always be consulted and followed. The aim is to support and maintain the vital body functions, closely monitor the vital signs, administer IV medications and fluids, determine the underlying cause and implement treatment.

Monitoring and documentation

Assess the patient's level of consciousness using the Glasgow Coma Scale and maintain their airway, breathing and circulation (Unbound Medicine, 2017). Vital signs, including blood pressure, heart rate, respirations, temperature, oxygen saturations and BGL are monitored regularly (Unbound Medicine, 2017). A baseline ECG will assess for cardiac arrhythmias and myocardial damage due to hyperkalaemia (Emergency Care Institute NSW, 2017). Ongoing telemetry monitoring may be required until the patient's condition stabilises (Emergency Care Institute NSW, 2017). Maintain a strict fluid balance chart (Phipps, 2015).

Insert a cannula and administer IV medications

- A stat dose of IV hydrocortisone 100mg is needed, followed by ongoing IV hydrocortisone 100 mg every six hours until stable. (Emergency Care Institute NSW, 2017). Dexamethasone may also be used if an adrenocorticotrophic hormone (ACTH) stimulation test is being carried out so as not to interfere with the blood result (Klauer, 2017). Fludrocortisone may be administered in patients with hyponatraemia (Klauer, 2017).
- Ninety per cent of patients will present with hypovolaemia, so 2–3 litres of IV fluids (usually 5% dextrose in 0.9% sodium chloride) are administered (Phipps, 2015). A 10% dextrose saline may be ordered depending on the patient's vital signs and BGL (Phipps, 2015).

Assess the underlying cause and implement interventions

- A full blood count and blood cultures will determine whether an infection has precipitated the AC episode. If so, the commencement of an appropriate IV antibiotic is required (Smans et al., 2016).
- Undertake a BGL to assess for hypoglycaemia. IV Glucagon or glucose 10% in 0.9% sodium chloride may be administered (Queensland Health, 2016).
- An ACTH stimulation test will help diagnose whether the patient has AI (Page, 2016). However, in emergency situations, steroidal and fluid treatment is commenced prior to confirmation of results (Klauer, 2017). A blood test prior to administration of a synthetic ACTH is obtained and a blood sample post ACTH injection is obtained to determine whether the adrenal crisis is primary or secondary (NIDDK, 2014).
- Serum potassium levels may indicate hyperkalaemia. This may require the administration of IV calcium gluconate and sodium bicarbonate (Queensland Health, 2016).
- Serum sodium levels may indicate hyponatrameia, requiring the administration of IV fluids (Phipps, 2015). Fludrocortisone causes kidney reabsorption of sodium and excretion of potassium, so it is important to monitor these levels once the patient is stable to ensure over-treatment does not cause congestive heart failure (Unbound Medicine, 2017).
- Blood urea nitrogen (BUN) may be elevated due to hypovolaemia (Unbound Medicine, 2017).
- A CT scan and MRI scan can be performed to diagnose whether the site of damage is at the pituitary gland or the adrenal gland (Campbell-Crofts, 2017). It is also essential to assess for and manage any precipitating factors (Campbell-Crofts, 2017).

Discharge planning

Discharge planning should commence once the patient's medical condition stabilises. The aim of patient education is to minimise the reoccurrence of an AC or promptly implement appropriate treatment. These patients will be discharged on lifelong oral corticosteroid medication (e.g. prednisolone). Patient education about the dangers of abruptly ceasing or missing this medication needs to be reinforced because this may result in an AC (Addison's Clinical Advisory Panel, 2015). Weaning from steroids is vital to allow the hypothalamic-pituitary-adrenal (HPA) axis time to recommence cortisol production (Salehmohamed,

Cuesta & Thompson, 2015). Patients need to aware of the triggers/stressors associated with their condition and to be educated about regulating their oral corticosteroid dose to compensate (Australian Addison's Disease Association, 2017). Wearing a medic alert bracelet is advisable because this may assist in the delivery of prompt medical attention. The immediate administration of IV steroids is paramount to survival, so patients are strongly advised to have immediate access to these medications (NIDDK, 2014). Family members, friends and work colleagues should be aware of the signs and symptoms of a pending AC and know how to administer the required steroids (NIDDK, 2014). Discharge planning requires a multidisciplinary approach, and the patient's GP needs to be informed and involved with care in the community. The patient should know to inform any future surgeons and dentists of their condition (NIDDK, 2014). As the patient has a lifelong diagnosis and dependence on steroids, this can impact heavily on their psychosocial wellbeing, so counselling should be offered. Social workers may also need to be involved if the impact of the disease is such that it interferes with the person's ability to maintain work and financial commitments (Addison's Clinical Advisory Panel, 2015).

SKILLS IN PRACTICE

Michelle's story

For years, Jane's niece Michelle (44) had suffered with migraines, severe fatigue and crippling diarrhoea. Three years ago, she had an appendectomy but took months to recover, experiencing chronic fatigue, abdominal pain and headaches. One day, while at work in a restaurant, Michelle collapsed and was taken to hospital for observation and investigations. Both CT and MRI scans were performed and it was confirmed that Michelle had a prolactinoma on her pituitary gland. Michelle underwent neurosurgery, the tumour was removed and Michelle was told that she would be able to resume her life after a few months. However, she did not improve and experienced symptoms including poor balance, light-headedness, blurred vision and overwhelming fatigue.

Michelle was determined to resume her life as it had been, so she returned to work as a chef. Two days later, she again collapsed at work and was urgently transported to hospital. On arrival, her serum cortisol level was measured and found to be significantly low. Administration of supraphysiologic doses (amounts greater than normally found in the body) is the immediate definitive treatment. Hence she was administered 250 mg IV hydrocortisone immediately, followed by 100 mg hydrocortisone six hourly. In addition to corticosteroid replacement, Michelle was given aggressive fluid replacement, receiving 3 L of IV 5% dextrose saline infusions. Michelle developed coagulopathy, which was reversed by the administration of fresh frozen plasma.

Michelle was diagnosed with secondary adrenal insufficiency hypopituitary disease. She is now corticosteroid dependent, taking four doses of prednisolone every day and additional doses when facing stress or prolonged activity. She has experienced several adrenal crises over the past ten years, requiring emergency hospitalisation and administration of steroids and IV fluids. The nursing staff at the local hospital are familiar with Michelle and administer IV steroids immediately when she presents at the emergency department.

When transported to hospital, the biggest medical challenge Michelle faces is medical and nursing staff who are not familiar with adrenal insufficiency (and subsequent adrenal crisis), and the need for the immediate administration of IV steroids – often within minutes of her admission.

QUESTION
What are the key elements of the clinical management of an individual presenting to an emergency department with AC?

Disorders of the thyroid gland

Subacute thyroiditis, hypothyroidism and thyrotoxicosis

The thyroid gland secretes two main thyroid hormones: T3 (triiodothyronine) and T4 (thyroxine) (Nishihara et al., 2008). These hormones regulate the body's temperature, metabolism and heart rate (Nishihara et al., 2008). Thyroiditis encompasses a diverse group of thyroid disorders characterised by some form of inflammation. **Subacute thyroiditis (SAT)** is one such disorder that is caused by an acute infection that subsequently produces severe thyroid-related pain. A number of alternate names are used to describe SAT, including subacute non-suppurative thyroiditis, De Quervain's thyroiditis and subacute granulomatous thyroiditis. The aetiology of SAT remains unclear; however, it is thought to be a viral-related or post-viral inflammatory process, because most SAT cases are preceded by an upper respiratory infection (Nishihara et al., 2008).

> **Subacute thyroiditis (SAT)** – An acute inflammatory disease of the thyroid, believed to be caused by a virus.

SAT is a self-limiting inflammatory condition, where approximately 90 per cent of patients display a tri-phasic clinical course lasting a few weeks to months. This tri-phasic clinical course is characterised by hyperthyroidism (excessive production of thyroid hormones), hypothyroidism (under-production of thyroid hormones) and then a return to normal thyroid function (Nishihara et al., 2008). The first phase of the condition (hyperthyroidism) typically results in the excessive release of thyroid hormones (T3 and/or T4) into the circulatory system. The elevated thyroid hormone levels can result in the symptoms of thyrotoxicosis (e.g. palpitations, tremors, weight loss and heat intolerance) and suppress the pituitary secretion of thyroid-stimulating hormone (TSH) (Guimaraes, 2006). This hyperthyroid phase continues until the stores of T3 and T4 are depleted from the thyroid gland, resulting in the subsequent hypothyroid phase (phase two). This phase lasts until the thyroid gland regains normal homeostasis and function (phase three). Each phase typically lasts two to eight weeks.

In an analysis of 852 patients with SAT, pain was the presenting symptom in 68 per cent of cases (Nishihara et al., 2008). The onset was typically preceded by an upper respiratory infection, nasal discharge, fever and cough. SAT is not considered a common thyroid disorder when compared with Graves' disease (hyperthyroidism) and Hashimoto's thyroiditis (hypothyroidism); occurring at 20 per cent and 5 per cent of their rates respectively (Guimaraes, 2006). There is little epidemiological data on SAT in Australia; however, a systematic review of SAT's diagnosis in the United States revealed an incidence rate of 4.9 cases per 100 000 (Fatourechi et al., 2003), with similar rates suggested globally. Seasonal variations may influence the incidence rate of SAT, as it has been noted in many countries to be higher in the summer months, correlating strongly with the incidence of some viral infections (Martino et al., 1987; Nishihara et al., 2008). In a study of 160 patients with SAT, 15 per cent of patients eventually developed permanent hypothyroidism (Fatourechi et al., 2003).

Thyrotoxicosis occurs as a result of hyperthyroidism, with common symptoms present in 62 per cent of patients (Nishihara et al., 2008). Although usually mild and transient, it has been associated with serious side-effects such as ventricular tachycardia and **thyroid storm** (Sherman & Ladenson, 2007), a rare and sometimes fatal complication of hyperthyroidism (Australian Thyroid Foundation, 2017).

Thyroid storm – Also known as thyrotoxic crisis; an acute, life-threatening hypermetabolic state resulting from an excessive release of thyroid hormones.

Nursing assessment and management of thyroid conditions

Hypothyroidism

The systemic effect of the thyroid hormone means the nursing assessment must be comprehensive. An accurate health history, physical and psychosocial assessment, including an ECG, will provide the foundation for the appropriate management of this condition (Australian Thyroid Foundation, 2017). Assess the patient's vital signs including blood pressure, pulse rate, temperature, respiratory rate, and oxygen saturation (Australian Thyroid Foundation, 2017). Bradycardia may be associated with hypotension and dizziness, so ensure the patient is safe when moving or mobilising (Australian Thyroid Foundation, 2017). Oral thyroid hormone (e.g. Levothyroxine or Thyroxine) replacement therapy is the mainstay of this lifelong treatment, and is administered in the morning on an empty stomach (Jonklaas et al., 2014; Australian Thyroid Foundation, 2017). Some patients experience iodine deficiency hypothyroidism, so iodine supplements may be prescribed (Walsh, 2016). Psychological support is vital because patients may experience depression and memory problems. Providing reassurance and information about their upcoming care will minimise these issues, and anti-depressant medications may be prescribed for some people (Australian Thyroid Foundation, 2017).

Thyrotoxicosis

The acute nursing care of the patient with thyrotoxicosis is complex. The initial aim is to assess the patient and stabilise their cardiac function (tachycardia, hypertension) (Ross et al., 2016). Beta-adrenergic receptor antagonist (beta-blockers) medications (e.g. Atenolol, Metoprolol) may be administered to treat these cardiovascular symptoms (Ross et al., 2016). Vital signs should be checked every 30 minutes, specifically monitoring heart rate and blood pressure (Ross et al., 2016). In addition, the patient will likely be anxious and frightened, so reassurance is needed or anti-anxiety medications may be prescribed (Australian Thyroid Foundation, 2017). Once the patient is stabilised, the reduction or the elimination of excessive levels of serum thyroid hormones is achieved through a combination of radioactive iodine (RAI) treatment, anti-thyroid drugs (ATD) and/or surgery (Ross et al., 2016).

RAI is a type of radioactive isotope (Iodine-131) administered as a 'once only' medication, targeting and killing the thyroid gland cells, reducing the synthesis of thyroid hormone (Cancer Council NSW, 2015). A reduction of thyroid hormone production is achieved in about 75 per cent of patients, although repeated treatment may be needed (Topliss & Eastman, 2004). ATD (e.g. Carbimazole, Thionamide) block the thyroid gland from synthesising thyroid hormones (Walsh, 2016). This short-term (several months' duration) treatment is recommended for patients with complications of cardiovascular disease (e.g. atrial fibrillation), renal disease or diabetes mellitus (Ross et al., 2016; Walsh, 2016). Surgery – either a partial or full thyroidectomy), whereby part or the entire thyroid gland is removed – reduces or stops the body's production of thyroid hormones (Ross et al., 2016). Total removal of the thyroid gland has a high cure rate for hyperthyroidism, compared with an 8 per cent recurrence of symptoms with a partial thyroidectomy (Ross et al., 2016). In most cases, surgery is performed only after euthyroidism (normal thyroid function) is first achieved with ATD (Ross et al., 2016). Following this treatment, the patient will experience sub-therapeutic serum levels of thyroid hormone, or medically induced hypothyroidism. This requires the lifelong administration of thyroid hormone replacement medication (e.g. Thyroxine) (Ross et al., 2016).

RAI treatment

RAI treatment is administered for the first seven days post treatment. Patients should be advised that RAI treatment means their body secretions are now radioactive for a short period of time. Hence the following precautions must be strictly adhered to:

- Drink fluids to increase urine production and help eliminate the RAI from your body.
- Avoid all contact with pregnant women and children for seven days.
- Maintain a minimum distance of 1 m between you and other people (sit/stand).
- No sexual contact or kissing.
- Minimise contact with people by staying at home in a room on your own.
- Use separate toileting facilities. Triple flush the toilet (seat and lid down) after each use and dispose of all body fluids (saliva, vomit, tissues) down the toilet.
- Shower daily (no baths); no sharing of towels, soap or other hygiene products.
- Do not go to any public places/functions.
- Do not attend work or school.
- Keep your feet covered with socks/slippers at all times.
- Avoid becoming pregnant for a minimum of six months after treatment.

(Society of Nuclear Medicine and Molecular Imaging, 2017)

Anti-thyroid medications

Anti-thyroid medications include Carbimazole and Thionamide. The medication regime is individualised and guided by the disease severity and response to treatment (Ross et al., 2016; Walsh, 2016). Initially, follow-up appointments occur every two to four weeks with the patient's GP or physician to monitor the response to the medication. In the long term, the timing of the follow-up appointments is individualised (Ross et al., 2016; Walsh, 2016). Initial high doses of the medication should gradually be reduced over time until a maintenance dose is achieved (Ross et al., 2016; Walsh, 2016).

Surgery

Surgery could involve either a partial or full thyroidectomy. The patient should follow the individualised discharge plan devised by their surgeon and nurse. General post-surgery advice includes:

- Avoid lifting heavy objects and strenuous activities such as gardening.
- Avoid constipation by eating a nutritious diet and drinking plenty of fluids. Straining

will increase pressure in the throat area and suture line.

- Monitor the suture line for signs of pain, redness and inflammation.
- Monitor for increasing pain, difficulty swallowing or breathing, or shortness of breath, and immediately report this to your doctor.

Discharge planning

Transporting the medication

Upon discharge from hospital, it is vital to protect the thyroxine medication from light, heat and humidity by transporting it in the original foil packaging and in a specially designed refrigerated travel bag (Australian Thyroid Foundation, 2017). Refrigerate the medication as soon as practically possible (Australian Thyroid Foundation, 2017).

Patient education

Patients with hypothyroidism should be reminded that thyroid hormone replacement therapy (e.g. Thyroxine or Levothyroxine) is lifelong (American Thyroid Association, 2013). It may take a number of weeks or months before the serum thyroxine plasma levels are high enough to result in a physiological change felt by the patient (American Thyroid Association, 2013). This also means that achieving the correct medication dosage can take some time. Thyroid hormones should be administered in the morning, with water only, and on an empty stomach. Patients should wait a further 30–60 minutes before eating any food (Australian Thyroid Foundation, 2017). To maintain the potency of the medication, it should be stored in the original foil packaging and in the refrigerator, between 2–8°C (Australian Thyroid Foundation, 2017). Other medications including herbal supplements, vitamins and minerals may interact with the thyroid medications, so patients should consult with their local pharmacist (Australian Thyroid Foundation, 2017). Regular blood tests (usually annually) are required to monitor the patient's thyroid function and serum thyroid hormone levels. Common medication side-effects that the patient may experience include headaches, sleep disturbances, nervousness, irritability and irregular heart rate (Tiziani, 2013). Finally, if the patient experiences feelings of depression, they should consult their GP for treatment and advice (American Thyroid Association, 2013).

Impact on the family

Educating families about hypothyroidism allows them to gain a better awareness of the disease. Until the therapeutic levels of the thyroxine medications are achieved, the patient may continue to experience mood swings and depression (American Thyroid Association, 2013). Advise families that no cure exists for hypothyroidism, and over time there is potential for the condition to worsen (American Thyroid Association, 2013). Counselling support for partners and families may be required (American Thyroid Association, 2013).

REFLECTIVE QUESTION

Patients with thyroid disease face lifelong treatment requirements. Identify some of the barriers to complying with this treatment. What strategies could you implement to encourage patients to engage with their treatment?

Concepts of patient-centred care and care coordination for acute endocrine conditions

Contemporary healthcare practice in Australia embraces patient–centred care (PCC) because it is viewed as an approach that improves the quality and safety of care resulting in fewer adverse events, better health outcomes and an enhanced patient experience (ACSQHC, 2010). The concepts of PCC include information sharing, collaborative decision-making and incorporating patient's care preferences into their care (Luxford, Safran & Delbanco, 2011). These concepts are underpinned by the principles of mutual respect, effective communication, development of partnerships, patient empowerment and self-determination (University of Göteburg, 2014).

The coordination of care is an important aspect of PCC, occurring along the admission-to-discharge continuum. The complex care associated with acute endocrine conditions means a specialist multidisciplinary healthcare team is needed to achieve the best health outcomes for patients. This team consists of specialist doctors, nurses and allied healthcare professionals. The initial acute medical care is provided by doctors and nurses, and continues until discharge. Specialist allied healthcare is also provided by dietitians, pharmacists, physiotherapists, occupational therapists, psychologists and podiatrists (Savage et al., 2011; Lewis et al., 2016). Delivering individualised healthcare is one way to increase the partnership with patients and their engagement in their care (University of Göteburg, 2014).

Throughout the episode of care, involving the patient in all healthcare decisions is an important first step in implementing PCC. Through the delivery of patient education and healthcare information, nurses play a vital role in supporting the patient's ability to make informed decisions about their care (Luxford et al., 2011). Early patient engagement in their self-care should be a priority, given that many endocrine conditions are lifelong. Self-care management is safer for patients, and provides them with a sense of empowerment (University of Göteburg, 2014).

Nurses' role in collaborative management of acute endocrine conditions

Many acute endocrine conditions require either immediate emergency medical intervention and/or complex nursing care. In the management of acute endocrine conditions, nurses work closely with doctors and other healthcare team members in the delivery of this specialised care (Lewis et al., 2016). Nurses have a number of key roles when caring for patients with acute endocrine conditions. Given the large number of acute endocrine disorders and their varied treatment, nurses need to have a good understanding of the pathophysiology, medications and specialist nursing skills associated with each condition (Lewis et al., 2016). Initial and ongoing comprehensive nursing assessment means the nurse can monitor and evaluate the effectiveness of the current management and treatment plan (Lewis et al., 2016). In addition, these assessments permit the nurse to implement timely modifications to the nursing care plan (Lewis et al., 2016).

Of all of the skills and roles nurses have, effective communication (verbal, written and electronic) between the patient, family and healthcare team members is the most important (Lewis et al., 2016). Effective communication reduces adverse events and errors, increases the collaboration between team members and improves the continuity of care (Lewis et al., 2016). Frequently, nurses coordinate the delivery of complex care, requiring problem-solving, clinical decision-making and time-management skills (Lewis et al., 2016). This ensures the healthcare team functions effectively in the management of acute endocrine conditions (Lewis et al., 2016). Delivering patient education that targets the individual needs is another important nursing role, which provides the patient with the knowledge and skills to self-manage their condition (Lewis et al., 2016). Nurses are responsible for early discharge planning and the involvement of community services and primary healthcare providers (GPs) (Lewis et al., 2016). This improves the continuity of care and increases the likelihood of a seamless and successful patient discharge (Lewis et al., 2016).

Advanced nursing practice for acute endocrine conditions

Nurse practitioners and nurse educators are advanced nurse practice specialists involved in the care of patients with acute endocrine conditions. Nurse practitioners are integral members of the healthcare team, and licensed to practise in hospitals, aged care facilities and community settings (Diabetes Australia, 2015b). Nurse practitioners are registered nurses who possess a Master's degree and are endorsed to practise autonomously in an extended clinical practice role (Diabetes Australia, 2015b). As of 2014, in Australia there were 20 nurse practitioners specialising in diabetes management, with many possessing the additional skills of Credentialled Diabetes Educator (Diabetes Australia, 2015b). The role of these nurse practitioners includes patient assessment, diagnostics, referrals and prescribing medications (Diabetes Australia, 2015b). Similarly, many nurse educators across Australia possess Master's degrees and specialise in the delivery of acute endocrine patient care (Endocrine Nurses' Society of Australasia, 2017). Nurse educators practise in hospitals, aged care facilities, schools and community settings, focusing on educating and up-skilling healthcare professionals and patients on the contemporary evidence-based management and treatment of acute endocrine conditions (Endocrine Nurses' Society of Australasia, 2017). Nurse practitioners and nurse educators provide specialised acute care endocrine knowledge and skills to the patient, nursing staff and healthcare team. Through these advanced practice nurses and continued research, clinical costs can be reduced significantly through streamlined clinical coordination, staff up-skilling and improved patient access to specialist services and equipment (Diabetes Australia, 2015b). Finally, the Endocrine Nurses' Society of Australasia (2017) is a professional nursing organisation in Australia and New Zealand that provides a collaborative forum for continued education, development and research across all endocrine disorders.

SUMMARY

Learning objective 1: Define acute endocrine conditions, and identify underlying pathophysiology, risk factors and presentations associated with acute endocrine conditions.

Acute endocrine conditions refer to a group of conditions that involve the endocrine system including diabetes mellitus, thyroid dysfunction, adrenal crisis and endocrine lesions. Nurses need to be able to identify the underlying pathophysiology, risk factors and presentation for each condition.

Learning objective 2: Describe nursing assessment and management strategies for the individual with acute endocrine conditions.

The nurse's role includes assessment and management of the individual with an acute endocrine condition. Nurses provide emergency care, coordinate care, identify early signs of deterioration and support the individual throughout care delivery.

Learning objective 3: Understand the concepts of patient-centred care and care coordination in relation to acute endocrine conditions.

Patient-centred care is central to the management of the individual with an acute endocrine condition and incorporates strategies relating not only to the patient but also their family and the multidisciplinary healthcare team. Through well-developed and seamlessly executed care coordination, the individual needs of the patient will be met.

Learning objective 4: Identify and discuss the nurse's role in the collaborative management of individuals with acute endocrine conditions.

Nurses collaborate with other healthcare team members to form a partnership and negotiate the provision of rapid, holistic, appropriate physical and psychological care to individuals with acute endocrine conditions.

Learning objective 5: Understand advanced nursing practice in relation to acute endocrine conditions.

Advanced nursing practice in this area supports complex therapies, coordinates complex cases and provides education and support to the individual and their support network.

REVIEW QUESTIONS

10.1 What is the pathophysiology of Cushing's syndrome?
10.2 What are the symptoms with which the person with hypothyroidism may present?
10.3 What is hypoglycemia?
10.4 What are the anatomy and physiology of the endocrine system?
10.5 What is diabetes mellitis?

RESEARCH TOPIC

Engage in wider research to identify the impact of ageing on the compromised endocrine system.

FURTHER READING

Funk, J. (2014). Disorders of the endocrine pancreas. In G. Hammer & S. McPhee (eds), *Pathophysiology of Diseases: An Introduction to Clinical Medicine*. New York: McGraw Hill.

Nieman, L.K. (2015). Cushing's syndrome: Update on signs, symptoms and biochemical screening. *European Journal of Endocrinology*, 173(4), M33–M38.

Tucci, V. (2014). The clinical manifestations, diagnosis and treatment of Adrenal Emergencies. *Emergency Medical Clinics of North America*, 32(2), 465–84.

REFERENCES

Addison's Clinical Advisory Panel (2015). Nursing the Addison's patient: Notes for nurses. Retrieved from http://www.addisons.org.uk/forum/index.php?/files/file/75-nursing-the-addison%E2%80%99s-patient-notes-for-nurses.

Allolio, B. (2015). Extensive expertise in endocrinology: Adrenal crisis. *European Journal of Endocrinology*, 172(3), R115–24.

American Diabetes (2013). Diagnosis and classification of diabetes mellitus. *Diabetes Care*, 36(Supplement 1), S67–74.

——(2016). Classification and diagnosis of diabetes. *Diabetes Care*, 39(Supplement 1), S13–22.

American Thyroid Association (2013). *Hypothyroidism: A Booklet for Patients and Their Families*. Retrieved from http://thyroid.org/wp-content/uploads/patients/brochures/Hypothyroidism_web_booklet.pdf.

Australian Addison's Disease Association (2017). What is Addison's Disease? Retrieved from http://addisons.org.au/information/what-is-addisons.

Australian Bureau of Statistics (ABS) (2016). Understanding diabetes mortality on Australia. Retrieved from http://www.abs.gov.au/ausstats/abs@.nsf/Lookup/by%20Subject/3303.0~2015~Main%20Features~Understanding%20diabetes%20mortality%20in%20Australia~5.

Australian Commission on Safety and Quality in Health Care (ACSQHC) (2010). *Patient-centred Care: Improving Quality and Safety by Focusing Care on Patients and Consumers – Discussion paper*. Sydney: ACSQHC. Retrieved from http://www.safetyandquality.gov.au.

Australian Thyroid Foundation (2017). Thyroid treatments. Retrieved from https://www.thyroidfoundation.org.au/page/59/thyroid-treatments.

BD Diabetes Education Center (2017). How to store and handle insulin. Retrieved from http://www.bd.com/us/diabetes/page.aspx?cat=7001&id=7247.

Campbell-Crofts, S. (2017). *Medical-Surgical Nursing: Critical Thinking for Person-Centred Care*. Melbourne: Pearson.

Cancer Council NSW (2015). Radioactive iodine treatment. Retrieved from https://www.cancercouncil.com.au/thyroid-cancer/treatment/radioactive-iodine-treatment.

Diabetes Australia (2015a). Diabetes in Australia. Retrieved from https://www
    .diabetesaustralia.com.au/diabetes-in-australia.

——(2015b). Nurse practitioners. Retrieved from https://www.diabetesaustralia.com.au/
    news/11773?type=articles.

Diabetes Queensland (2017). Managing diabetes. Retrieved from http://www.diabetesqld
    .org.au/managing-diabetes/type-2-diabetes/coping-with-diabetes/hypoglycaemia
    .aspx.

Else, T. & Hammer, G. (2014). Disorders of the adrenal cortex. In G. Hammer &
    S. McPhee (eds), *Pathophysiology of Disease: An Introduction to Clinical Medicine*.
    New York: McGraw Hill, pp. 593–624.

Emergency Care Institute New South Wales (2017). Adrenal crisis treatment. Retrieved
    from https://www.aci.health.nsw.gov.au/networks/eci/clinical/clinical-resources/
    clinical-tools/endocrine/adrenal-crisis-addisonian-crisis/adrenal-crisis–treatment.

Endocrine Nurses' Society of Australasia Inc. (2017). About ENSA. Retrieved from http://
    www.ensa.org.au.

Fatourechi, V., Aniszewski, J.P., Fatourechi, G.Z., Atkinson, E.J. & Jacobsen, S.J. (2003).
    Clinical features and outcome of subacute thyroiditis in an incidence cohort:
    Olmsted County, Minnesota, Study. *Journal Clinical Endocrinology Metabolism*,
    88(5), 2100–5.

Funk, J. (2014). Disorders of the endocrine pancreas. In G. Hammer & S. McPhee (eds),
    Pathophysiology of Diseases: An Introduction to Clinical Medicine. New York:
    McGraw Hill.

Goguen, J. & Gilbert, J. (2013). Hyperglycaemic emergencies in adults. *Canadian Journal of
    Diabetes*, 37(Supplement 1), S72–6.

Guimaraes, V. (2006). Subacute and Riedel's thyroiditis. In L. DeGroot & J. Jameson (eds),
    Endocrinology. Philadelphia, PA: Elsevier, pp. 1595–606.

International Affairs and Best Practice Guidelines (IABPG) (2017). Guidelines for nurses
    on how to manage hypoglycemia. Retrieved from http://pda.rnao.ca/content/
    guidelines-nurses-how-manage-hypoglycemia.

International Diabetes Federation (2015). *IDF Diabetes Atlas*. Brussels: International
    Diabetes Federation.

Jonklaas, J., Bianco, A., Bauer, A., Burman, K., Cappola, A., Celi, F., … Sawka, A. (2014).
    Guidelines for the treatment of hypothyroidism. *Thyroid*, 24(12): 1670–751.

Kitabchi, A.E., Umpierrez, G.E., Miles, J.M. & Fisher, J.N. (2009). Hyperglycemic crises in
    adult patients with diabetes. *Diabetes Care*, 32(7), 1335–43.

Klauer, K. (2017). Adrenal crisis in emergency medicine treatment & management.
    Retrieved from http://www.emedicine.medscape.com/article/765753.medication#2.

Lewis, S.L., Bucher, L., Heitkemper, M.M., Harding, M.M., Kwong, J. & Roberts, D.
    (2016). *Medical-Surgical Nursing e-Book: Assessment and Management of Clinical
    Problems*. Philadelphia, PA: Elsevier.

Luxford, K., Safran, D. & Delbanco, T. (2011). Promoting patient-centered care: A qualitative
    study of facilitators and barriers in healthcare organizations with a reputation for
    improving the patient experience. *International Journal for Quality in Health Care*,
    23(5), 510–15.

Marieb, E. & Hoehn, K. (2012). *Human Anatomy & Physiology* (12th ed.). Boston, MA:
    Pearson.

Martino, E., Buratti, L., Bartalena, L., Mariotti, S., Cupini, C., Aghini-Lombardi, F. & Pinchera,
    A. (1987). High prevalence of subacute thyroiditis during summer season in Italy.
    Journal of Endocrinological Investigation, 10(3), 321–3.

National Institute of Diabetes and Digestive and Kidney Diseases (NIDDK) (2014). Adrenal insufficiency and Addison's disease. Retrieved from https://www.niddk.nih.gov/health-information/endocrine-diseases/adrenal-insufficiency-addisons-disease.

Nieman, L. (2017). *Clinical Manifestations of Adrenal Insufficiency in Adults*. Philadelphia, PA: Wolters Kluwer.

Nishihara, E., Ohye, H., Amino, N., Takata, K., Arishima, T., Kudo, T., … Miyauchi, A. (2008). Clinical characteristics of 852 patients with subacute thyroiditis before treatment. *Internal Medicine Journal*, 47(8), 725–9.

Nursing Council of New Zealand (NCNZ) ([2007] 2016). *Competencies for Registered Nurses*. Retrieved from http://www.nursingcouncil.org.nz/nurses.

Nursing and Midwifery Board of Australia (NMBA) (2016). *Registered Nurse Standards for Practice*. Melbourne: Nursing & Midwifery Board of Australia. Retrieved from http://www.nursingmidwiferyboard.gov.au/Codes-Guidelines-Statements/Professional-standards.aspx.

O'Connell, S. & Siafarikas, A. (2010). Addison's disease: Diagnosis and initial management, *Australian Family Physician,* 39(11), 834–7.

Page, S. (2016). Management guidelines for adrenal crisis in adults. Retrieved from https://www.nuh.nhs.uk/handlers/downloads.ashx?id=63184.

Pasquel, F.J. & Umpierrez, G.E. (2014). Hyperosmolar hyperglycemic state: A historic review of the clinical presentation, diagnosis, and treatment. *Diabetes Care*, 37(11), 3124–31.

Phipps, A. (2015). Adrenal crisis in ED. Retrieved from https://www.emdocs.net/adrenal-crisis-in-the-ed.

Queensland Health (2016). *Clinical Practice Guidelines: Medical/Adrenaline Insufficiency*. Retrieved from https://www.ambulance.qld.gov.au/docs/clinical/cpg/CPG_Adrenal%20insufficiency.pdf.

Ross, D., Burch, H., Cooper, D., Greenlee, M., Laurberg, P., Maia, A., … Walter, M. (2016). American Thyroid Association guidelines for diagnosis and management of hyperthyroidism and other causes of thyrotoxicosis. *Thyroid*, 26(10), 1343–421.

Rushworth, R.L. & Torpy, D.J. (2014). A descriptive study of adrenal crises in adults with adrenal insufficiency: Increased risk with age and in those with bacterial infections. *BMC Endocrine Disorders*, 14, 79.

Salehmohamed, M., Cuesta, M. & Thompson, C. (2015). Adrenal crisis due to steroid withdrawal. Paper presented to 17th European Conference of Endocrinology, Dublin. doi:10.1530/endoabs.37.EP1238.

Savage, M., Dhatariya, K., Kilvert, A., Rayman, G., Rees, J., Courtney, C., Hilton, L., Dyer, P. & Samersley, M. (2011). Joint British Diabetes Societies' guideline for the management of diabetic ketoacidosis in adults. *Diabetic Medicine*, 28(5), 508–15.

Sherman, S.I. & Ladenson, P.W. (2007). Subacute thyroiditis causing thyroid storm. *Thyroid*, 17(3), 283.

Smans, L.C., Van der Valk, E.S., Hermus, A.R. & Zelissen, P.M. (2016). Incidence of adrenal crisis in patients with adrenal insufficiency. *Clinical Endocrinology (Oxf)*, 84(1), 17–22.

Society of Nuclear Medicine and Molecular Imaging (2017). Precautions after out-patient radioactive iodine (I-131) therapy. Retrieved from http://www.snmmi.org/AboutSNMMI/Content.aspx?ItemNumber=5609.

Sofrigam (2017). How to store or transport your insulin safely. Retrieved from http://www.sofrigam.com/store-transport-insulin-safely.

Tiziani, A. (2013). *Harvard's Nursing Guide to Drugs* (9th ed.). Sydney: Elsevier Mosby.

Topliss, D. & Eastman, C. (2004). Diagnosis and management of hyperthyroidism and hypothyroidism. *Medical Journal of Australia*, 180(10), 186–93.

Unbound Medicine (2017). *Adrenal insufficiency (Addison's disease)*. Retrieved from https://nursing.unboundmedicine.com/nursingcentral/view/Diseases-and-Disorders/73511/all/Adrenal_Insufficiency__Addison's_Disease_.

University of Göteburg (2014). *Person-centred care*. Göteburg: University of Göteburg.

Walsh, J. (2016). Managing thyroid disease in general practice. *Medical Journal of Australia*, 205(4), 179–84.

Wolfsdorf, J.I., Allgrove, J., Craig, M.E., Edge, J., Glaser, N., Jain, V., … Hanas, R. (2014). Diabetic ketoacidosis and hyperglycemic hyperosmolar state. *Pediatric Diabetes*, 15(Supplement 20), 154–79.

11 Acute reproductive disorders

Elisabeth Coyne and
Sally-ann de-Vitry Smith

LEARNING OBJECTIVES

At the completion of this chapter, you should be able to:

1 define acute reproductive disorders in males and females
2 discuss the pathophysiology, risk factors and incidence of, and treatment for, acute reproductive disorders
3 explore the nursing considerations involved in the management of testicular disorders, prostate cancer and non-pregnancy and pregnancy-related conditions
4 discuss the role of the nurse in the assessment of reproductive conditions
5 present the nurse's role in interdisciplinary collaboration to achieve patient-centred and culturally competent care.

Introduction

The reproductive system is a body system that shows pronounced changes in structure and function across the lifespan. Reproductive disorders can develop rapidly and may have acute, serious and life-threatening consequences.

Reproductive systems and sexual function are considered 'taboo' in some cultures, and many clients have difficulty talking about them. Therefore, relatively benign conditions are often ignored until they become significant and even life-threatening. The reproductive systems in males and females have both common and unique elements. It is important for the nurse to understand the pathophysiology and care for gender-specific disorders. Cancer of the reproductive organs accounts for the highest percentage of cancer diagnosis in both females and males, with female breast cancer constituting 13 per cent and prostate cancer 23 per cent of all new cancers diagnosed (AIHW, 2017). In Australia in 2015–16, there were 7.5 million emergency department presentations – approximately 20 000 presentations every day – with the most common reasons identified as abdominal and pelvic pain (AIHW, 2017). Genito-urinary system complaints were the reason for 297 368 presentations, and pregnancy, childbirth and the puerperium complaints accounted for 102 451 presentations (AIHW, 2017).

Pelvic pain and vaginal bleeding are common reasons for women to present for emergency care. More than 30 000 males present to emergency departments for reproductive-related issues annually (AIHW, 2017). Reproductive health is also related to capability to reproduce and sexual health, which encompass a broad range of disorders that will not be covered in detail in this chapter.

This chapter discusses the pathophysiology of reproductive conditions, risk factors, incidence and treatment for common acute conditions. The chapter will discuss the role of the nurse and the importance of patient-centred care, cultural competency, client education and discharge planning.

The following national competency standards for the registered nurse from the Nursing and Midwifery Board of Australia (NMBA) and the Nursing Council of New Zealand (NCNZ) are addressed in this chapter.

Australian Registered Nurse Standards for Practice

Standard 1: Thinks critically and analyses nursing practice

Standard 2: Engages in therapeutic and professional relationships

Standard 3: Maintains the capability for practice

Standard 4: Comprehensively conducts assessments

Standard 5: Develops a plan for nursing practice

Standard 6: Provides safe, appropriate and responsive quality nursing practice

Standard 7: Evaluates outcomes to inform nursing practice

(NMBA, 2016)

New Zealand: Competencies for Registered Nurses

Competency 1.1: Accepts responsibility for ensuring that his/her nursing practice and conduct meet the standards of the professional, ethical and relevant legislated requirements

NURSING STANDARDS

Competency 1.2: Demonstrates the ability to apply the principles of the Treaty of Waitangi/ Te Tiriti o Waitangi to nursing practice

Competency 1.5: Practises nursing in a manner that the health consumer determines as being culturally safe

Competency 4.1: Collaborates and participates with colleagues and members of the health care team to facilitate and coordinate care

Competency 4.2: Recognises and values the roles and skills of all members of the health care team in the delivery of care

(NCNZ, [2007] 2016)

Defining common reproductive disorders

Reproductive system – or genital system: a system of internal and external organs that work together for the purpose of sexual reproduction.

When patients present with **reproductive system** disorders, it is important to avoid assumptions related to appearance, behaviours and pre-existing knowledge of reproductive anatomy and physiology. Without awareness of anatomical terminology and basic reproductive physiology, it may be difficult to understand diagnosis, treatment and follow-up. Patients from culturally and linguistically diverse (CALD) populations can find it difficult to discuss reproductive issues, and may require an interpreter if English is their second language. Aboriginal patients may prefer an Aboriginal health worker who understands their culture and can provide support with this sensitive area of health concerns (Waterworth et al., 2014).

Sexual abuse – Undesired sexual behavior inflicted on one person by another, including sexual assault.

Victims of **sexual abuse** may find it distressing to discuss sexual or reproductive health. Patients with a disability may have specific requirements during examination to ensure their comfort. It is therefore very important for the nurse to ensure that confidentiality and privacy are maintained. A patient-centred approach ensures consideration for both gender and trans-gender patients to ensure best practice is maintained (de Silva Joyce et al., 2015).

There are a number of conditions of the male and female reproductive systems which are either primary conditions or disorders occurring as the result of alterations in function of other organs or systems. Men and women presenting with an acute reproductive problem may be concerned about **sexually transmitted infections**, pain, trauma, changes in sexual function and the possibility of infertility. They may also be concerned about their sexuality, fertility and sense of themselves as a man or woman.

Sexually transmitted infections – Infections or diseases passed on during unprotected sex with an infected partner.

Acute reproductive disorders in males

Men are at risk of disorders of the penis, scrotum, testes, prostate gland and breast. Disorders can be inflammatory, structural, benign or malignant, and may pose a risk to fertility, sexual function and urinary function. In some cases, the condition may be serious or life-threatening. Men presenting with symptoms such as swelling (painless or painful), heaviness, lumps, discharge and inflammation in the genital area will require a clinical examination and further testing. The male genitalia are very sensitive, making tests and examination distressing and anxiety provoking. Adolescent males may be particularly apprehensive and embarrassed.

Acute reproductive disorders in females

Females are at risk of disorders of the breasts, uterus, ovaries, adnexa, cervix and vagina, which may involve menstrual disorders, breast disorders that may be inflammatory, structural, benign or malignant bleeding from the reproductive tract, abnormal discharge, lumps and pain, which will require a clinical examination and further testing.

Disorders may pose a risk to fertility, sexual function, urinary function, sexuality, the ability to bear children, sense of self and in some cases may be life-threatening.

Presentation for abnormal uterine bleeding accounts for 30 per cent of outpatient gynaecologist visits (American College of Nurse Midwives, 2016; Sacha & Souter, 2017). In any woman with vaginal bleeding, the acuity and need for resuscitation is the first priority, followed by determining if the bleeding is pregnancy related. Women of reproductive age are at the highest risk of sexually transmitted diseases, **pelvic inflammatory disease**, abnormal uterine bleeding and pregnancy-related disorders (American College of Nurse Midwives, 2016). If bleeding is pregnancy related, the **gestational age**, viability and presenting symptoms determine management. In early pregnancy, ectopic pregnancy and miscarriage (pregnancy loss occurring before 20 weeks' gestation) may occur. After 20 weeks' gestation, uterine bleeding can be related to placental abruption or placenta praevia.

Bleeding may be uterine, or from the vulva, vagina, cervix, ovaries or fallopian tubes. Bleeding from the ovary or fallopian tube may be concealed, intra-peritoneal bleeding. Bleeding from the uterus can be related to menstruation, pregnancy, structural abnormalities such as leiomyoma (fibroids), conditions such as polyps, endometritis, pelvic inflammatory disease and polycystic ovarian syndrome. Cervical bleeding can result from cervicitis, polyps, ectopic pregnancy, pelvic organ prolapse and cervical cancer. Bleeding from the vagina can be from vaginal atrophy, vaginitis, vaginal ulcers, vaginal trauma and vaginal cancer. Vulval bleeding can be related to infection, benign lesions, blistering (genital herpes), vulvar trauma or vulvar cancer. Bleeding may be related to systemic conditions (e.g. hyperprolactinaemia), coagulopathies such as von Willebrand disease or medications such as anti-coagulants (Sacha & Souter, 2017).

Men usually present with acute pain, swelling or disruption to the ability to void. The acuity of the condition and the risks posed to health must be ascertained rapidly.

Pelvic inflammatory disease – An infection of the upper part of the female reproductive system namely the uterus, fallopian tubes and ovaries, and inside of the pelvis.

Gestational age – Used during pregnancy to describe how advanced the pregnancy is in relation to the woman's last menstrual cycle. It is measured in weeks, from the first day of the woman's last menstrual cycle to the current date. A normal pregnancy can range from 38 to 42 weeks. Infants born before 37 weeks are considered premature.

Pathophysiology, risk factors, incidence and treatment of acute reproductive disorders

Acute disorders for the male

Acute reproductive disorders for males frequently involve the penis or scrotum.

Acute penile disorders

The most common disorders occurring in males presenting with acute penile disorders are phimosis, paraphimosis and priapism.

Phimosis

Phimosis is a constriction of the foreskin that makes it too narrow to be retracted enough to expose the glans penis. Severe phimosis can result in painful urination, urine retention, urinary tract infection and infection of the glans penis (Dains, Baumann & Scheibel, 2016). Phimosis can occur in children (congenital phimosis), or be due to injury or infection causing scarring of the foreskin (acquired phimosis). Treatment is urgent if urination is compromised.

Paraphimosis

Paraphimosis is a condition in which the foreskin has been retracted and is stuck behind the glans penis, resulting in pain, swelling and ischaemia. This condition must be corrected promptly or it may result in ischemia and penile necrosis. In infants, the foreskin is adhered to the glans penis and parents should not attempt to retract the foreskin as this can cause injury. The retracted foreskin may not be able to be returned to the normal position covering the glans penis.

Priapism

Priapism is an involuntary, sustained painful erection lasting longer than four hours. Priapism occurs when blood flows into the penis but venous outflow is obstructed causing stasis of blood, resulting in tissue hypoxia (Muneer & Ralph, 2017). Priapism is caused by conditions such as tumours, infections or trauma (primary priapism), blood disorders (leukaemia, sickle cell anaemia), neurological conditions, kidney failure and some medications (secondary priapism). Ischaemic priapism requires urgent treatment to avoid scarring and fibrosis of smooth muscles and subsequent impotence. Treatment is focused on relieving the erection to preserve penile function. Ice packs can assist with the swelling; following local anaesthesia, a needle can be inserted to drain the blood from the penis. Alpha-agonists can be injected into the penis to constrict blood vessels, relieving congestion and swelling.

The acute scrotum

The most common disorders occurring in males presenting with painful scrotal swelling are epididymitis, epididymo-orchitis and testicular torsion (Holden et al., 2010). It is important to ask about the onset of pain, activity at onset, type of pain (aching, sharp, throbbing, etc.), how long it has been present, the severity, location and alleviating or exacerbating factors.

Providing adequate analgesia is important. If surgery is likely, oral analgesia should be avoided. Elevating the scrotum with a rolled towel and using an ice pack may help reduce pain and swelling in patients with epididymitis.

Epididymitis

Epididymitis is an inflammation of the epididymis, a collection of small tubes at the back of each testicle that store sperm. Epididymitis is commonly seen in the outpatient setting. Epididymitis generally begins with slow onset of posterior scrotal pain. Urinary symptoms such as dysuria (painful urination) and frequency are often present. Physical findings include a swollen and tender epididymis with the testis in an anatomically normal position.

Aetiology and treatment are based on patient age and the likely causative organisms. Although the aetiology is largely unknown, reflux of urine into the ejaculatory ducts is considered the most common cause of epididymitis in children younger than fourteen years. Chlamydia trachomatis and Neisseria gonorrhoeae are the most common causes of epididymitis in sexually active males up to 35 years, and a single intramuscular dose of ceftriaxone with ten days of oral doxycycline is the treatment of choice in this age group. In men older than 35 years, epididymitis is usually caused by enteric bacteria transported by reflux of urine into the ejaculatory ducts secondary to bladder outlet obstruction; levofloxacin or ofloxacin alone is sufficient to treat these infections (McConaghy & Panchal, 2016).

Men who practise insertive anal intercourse are also likely to have an enteric organism present, and ceftriaxone with ten days of oral levofloxacin or ofloxacin is the recommended treatment regimen. Because untreated acute epididymitis can lead to infertility and chronic scrotal pain, recognition and therapy are vital to reduce patient morbidity (McConaghy & Panchal, 2016).

Epididymo-orchitis

Epididymitis often occurs with orchitis (inflammation of the testis) and is called epididymo-orchitis. The infection causes pain and scrotal swelling. The cause is usually a urinary tract infection from a sexually transmitted infection (STI). Epididymitis and epididymo-orchitis can impair fertility and cause chronic scrotal pain. Epididymitis requires treatment with antibiotics (McConaghy & Panchal, 2016).

Testicular torsion

Testicular torsion is a twisting of the spermatic cord that stops the blood supply to the testicle, causing unilateral scrotal pain, swelling, vascular engorgement and ischaemia. Testicular torsion is a medical emergency and urgent treatment is required to prevent testicular death from ischaemia (Hazeltine, Panza & Ellsworth, 2017; Huang et al., 2013). It mostly occurs in males under 30, with a spike in incidence in neonates and at puberty. The annual incidence of testicular torsion in males under 18 years is estimated at around one per 4000 people (Hazeltine, Panza & Ellsworth, 2017).

Testicular torsion is generally not present if the cremasteric reflex is intact. This reflex occurs when the cremaster muscle contracts, elevating the testicle when the inner thigh on the same leg is stroked.

Trauma

The testes sit unprotected outside the main body cavity to maintain the cooler temperature required for spermatogenesis. This makes the testes vulnerable to injury from impact or penetrating injuries. A traumatic injury may rupture blood vessels or cause tearing of the testicle.

Prostatitis

Inflammation of the prostate gland is often a chronic condition but may present as an acute bacterial prostatitis. Presentation may include pelvic pain, dysuria, frequency and retention, with systemic signs of infection such as fever, nausea, vomiting and malaise. On examination, the prostate may be boggy, tender and enlarged (Coker & Dierfeldt, 2016). Voiding difficulties may lead to abscesses and sepsis. An abscess requires antibiotics and sometimes surgical drainage (Lee et al., 2016). Urine cultures will provide information on the bacteria and antibiotic sensitivity.

Cancers

Men may develop benign or malignant lesions/tumours of the scrotum, testes, prostate or breast. After skin cancer, prostate cancer is the most common cancer in men, leading to over 300 000 deaths worldwide every year (Zhou et al., 2016). In Australia and New Zealand, prostate cancer accounts for 13 per cent of all cancer deaths and caused the death of 3102 Australian men in 2014 (Australian Cancer Council) (AIHW, 2017; StatsNZ, 2017). Ultrasound, magnetic resonance imaging (MRI), prostate biopsy and new markers are used to diagnose and stage prostate cancer (Harvey & deSouza, 2016). Concerns relating to diagnosis and treatment of prostate cancer have been expressed, as most men diagnosed with prostate cancer will die of other causes, so it is important to determine whether the cancer is aggressive or low risk, and whether prostatectomy, radiotherapy, chemotherapy or systemic therapy is beneficial (Miyahira et al., 2017).

REFLECTIVE QUESTION

Think about how you would ask a male to discuss their fears about prostate surgery. How might you find opportunities to provide post-operative education to the patient and their family? What are the main areas of education required in relation to prostate surgery?

Acute disorders for females

Acute disorders in females range from menstrual cramping to life-threatening disease. There are several disorders that result in women presenting for acute healthcare.

Menstrual disorders

Severe pre-menstrual syndrome (PMS) and dysmenorrhea present with severe physiological and psychological symptoms associated with menstruation. These disorders are more common in teenage girls and young women. Dysfunctional uterine bleeding (DUB) is an excessive amount or prolonged uterine bleeding that may or may not be associated with the menstrual cycle.

Vaginal fistula (abnormal opening or connection)

Vesicovaginal fistula (vagina and urinary bladder) is the formation of an abnormal tract extending between the bladder and vagina. The fistula causes an involuntary discharge of urine from the bladder to the vagina and will require surgical intervention to repair (González León et al., 2017). This condition occurs most frequently in relation to gynaecological surgery but is also uncommon in developed countries.

Cysts

While many cysts are slow to form, large cysts may be infective, cause pain, rupture and bleed.

Bartholin's gland cyst

A Bartholin's gland cyst may be present in one or both sides of the vulva: they can occur due to duct obstruction as a result of non-infectious occlusion or from infection and oedema compressing the duct. Treatment can be surgical excision and drainage or medical treatment (Dankher et al., 2016).

Ovarian cysts

Ovarian cysts are seen commonly in women; they can be functional, benign or malignant. Approximately one in 25 women experiences an ovarian cyst that is symptomatic (Farahani & Datta, 2016). The risk of malignant ovarian cysts increases in post-menopausal women. A thorough history and assessment enable diagnosis and choice of treatment, which could be surgical removal or conservative management (Farahani & Datta, 2016).

Benign and malignant tumours

The following are the most common tumours of the reproductive system in women.

- *Leiomyomas (benign fibroid tumours).* An overgrowth of connective tissue and smooth muscle in the uterus.

- *Cervical cancer.* Most commonly caused by human papilloma virus (HPV). This is the second most common cancer in women worldwide, but the fourteenth most commonly diagnosed in Australia due to screening programs (AIHW, 2001). The incidence is higher among Aboriginal and Torres Strait Islander women due to later diagnostic testing (Saville, 2016).
- *Endometrial cancer.* This is the most common invasive gynaecological cancer, originating in the endometrium. Treatment depends on the degree of spread of the tumour (Morice et al., 2016).
- *Cancer of the vulva.* This is an uncommon tumour, representing just 4 per cent of gynaecologic malignancies. Treatment relates to the stage of the tumour (Hacker, Eifel & van der Velden, 2012).
- *Ovarian cancer.* The eighth most common cancer. Risk increases with age, and limited and vague early signs result in late diagnosis when the disease is more advanced and treatment is less effective (WHO, 2017).
- *Breast cancer.* This is the third most common invasive cancer in Australia and New Zealand (AIHW, 2017; StatsNZ, 2017). Although less prevalent in Aboriginal and Torres Strait Islander, and Māori women compared with Caucasian women, Aboriginal and Torres Strait Islander, and Māori women are more likely to die from the disease because of a reduced participation level in screening programs, resulting in the disease being more advanced at diagnosis.

Dilation and curettage

Dilation and curettage (D&C) is the curettage (or removal) of part of the lining of the uterus to correct dysfunctional uterine bleeding. A D&C may also be completed for removal of products from conception, either early in pregnancy or after the birth, when there may be retained placental fragments. Appropriate support is needed for the client if the D&C is completed for removal of products of conception early in a pregnancy (abortion).

Hysterectomy

Hysterectomy is the removal of the uterus. Hysterectomy is the most common elective surgery for women, particularly between the ages of 40 and 49 years (AIHW, 2017; StatsNZ, 2017). The surgery can be done as a total abdominal hysterectomy (TAH) or by laparoscopically assisted vaginal hysterectomy (LAVH). The vaginal approach leaves no visible scar and is the most common hysterectomy performed. Good communication and rapport with the nurse is needed to ensure the client understands the procedure and expected outcomes (Segaric & Hall, 2015).

Mastectomy

Mastectomy is the surgical removal of the entire breast or part of the breast, depending on size of tumour and reason for surgery. Breast reconstruction may be completed at the time of the mastectomy or as a later surgery, depending on the reason for surgery and the client's decision. Biopsy of the breast or **lumpectomy** is the removal of breast tissue. This can be a simple surgery that is often completed as day surgery.

When considering care for a client who has undergone a mastectomy, it is important to consider the psychosocial impacts of the surgery as well as possible damage to or removal of surrounding tissues. Such tissues will often include axillary lymph nodes.

Removal of lymph nodes has a significant impact on fluid circulation in the associated limb. Nurses should be able to use their knowledge of the function of the lymphatic system to explain possible fluid accumulation in the associated limb, **lymphoedema**. Nurses

Mastectomy – Surgical removal of the whole breast or part of the breast. Can be total, partial, modified or subcutaneous.

Lumpectomy – Removal of abnormal tissue from the breast.

Lymphoedema – The accumulation of excessive amounts of protein-rich fluid, resulting in swelling of one or more regions of the body.

should also be able to list nursing interventions used to reduce the severity of oedema in the affected arm.

SKILLS IN PRACTICE

Breast cancer case scenario: Helena Popovic

Helena is a 42-year-old female patient who has been diagnosed with breast cancer. Helena lives in rural Queensland, 475 km from the treating hospital. Her husband of seventeen years, Stefan, works in the local coal mine driving trucks. His work involves a work roster of ten days' work followed by five days off. Stefan cares for their two children, aged seven and 10, when he is off work, and provides support for the children while Helena is in Brisbane having treatment for the cancer.

Helena had a total mastectomy and removal of axillary nodes nine weeks ago and is now receiving chemotherapy. Her treatment involves six cycles of chemotherapy, which comprise two days of treatment followed by two weeks for recovery. During the treatment weeks, Helena stays at the Cancer Council hostel close to the treating hospital.

After her third cycle, Helena returns home and notices a marked increase in her level of fatigue. She says she is finding it very hard to cope with family demands.

For further information, please see the video, Family Nursing Assessment (oncology patient): Dr Elisabeth Coyne, available on YouTube.

QUESTIONS
- In relation to Helena's mastectomy and your understanding of changes in body image, what assessment and questions would the nurse need to ask Helena in order to understand how she is going after surgery?
- Discuss how the nurse can ensure family-centred care is provided to Helena.
- What education and information can be provided to Helena in relation to her rural location?

The nurse's role in managing acute reproductive disorders

Reproductive disorders in males

In males presenting with an acute scrotum, it is vital to exclude testicular torsion because after four to eight hours permanent damage can occur to the testicle (Sharp & Kieran, 2013). The affected testicle is usually high and the cremasteric reflex is absent; severe unilateral pain accompanied by nausea and vomiting is often present. Surgery should not be delayed to wait for scrotal Doppler ultrasound; manual detorsion is recommended if surgery is not immediately available. Orchiectomy (surgical removal of the testicle) is performed if the testicle is necrotic or non-viable; in boys having surgery for testicular torsion, the orchiectomy rate is 48 per cent (Sharp & Kieran, 2013). With a missed or delayed diagnosis, testicular loss approaches 100 per cent.

With detorsion of testes, surgery needs to occur quickly as after six to eight hours with no blood supply, the testicle will die (Andrology Australia, 2016). During detorsion surgery, both testes are fixed in position to prevent testicular loss and preserve fertility.

If prostate cancer is localised, it may be removed by radical prostatectomy or treated with radiation therapy. A radical prostatectomy is the removal of the entire prostate by open surgery or laparoscopy. Robotic-assisted laparoscopic radical prostatectomy is the most common procedure, with approximately 80 per cent performed this way. Long-term complications can include impotence, urinary incontinence, penile shortening and bladder neck contracture (Agarwal et al., 2015).

Reproductive disorders in females

Non-pregnancy related acute reproductive disorders

Abnormal uterine bleeding

Abnormal uterine bleeding (AUB) refers to a cluster of symptoms, including heavy menstrual bleeding (HMB), inter-menstrual bleeding and prolonged menstrual bleeding (Bradley & Gueye, 2016). Abnormal uterine bleeding affects up to 30 per cent of women, and may be associated with ovulation (e.g. painful periods) or anovulatory, which is more common during menarche, perimenopause and menopause (Farrukh, Towriss, & McKee, 2015).

For women presenting with acute AUB, the focus is on achieving haemodynamic stability with appropriate volume resuscitation (Bradley & Gueye, 2016). If women are severely anaemic, this may need correcting.

The severity of the bleeding will determine treatment. In women who are stable, the first line of treatment is pharmacological, and includes hormonal therapy, non-steroidal anti-inflammatory drugs and anti-fibrinolytics such as Tranexamic acid. Surgical treatment includes endometrial ablation, removal of fibroids by myomectomy or hysterectomy, and uterine artery embolisation.

Dysmenorrhoea

Dysmenorrhoea is pain related to menstruation. Primary dysmenorrhoea occurs in the absence of pelvic pathology. Primary dysmenorrhoea typically occurs in the first six months after menarche, and usually lasts 48–72 hours, with cramping pain radiating to the lower back or thigh. Along with reassurance, treatment includes NSAIDs and oral contraceptives.

Secondary dysmenorrhoea results from identifiable organic conditions. Women with secondary dysmenorrhoea have often had previously painless menstrual cycles, and may have heavy or irregular periods, vaginal discharge and dyspareunia. Investigations may be required to rule out pelvic pathology. Treatment involves correcting the underlying cause and treating pain with NSAIDs such as diclofenac and ibuprofen.

Ovarian cysts

Ovarian cysts often cause no symptoms. Large cysts may cause abdominal and pelvic pain, sometimes radiating to the lower back, abdominal bloating, pressure or fullness, painful bowel movements, dyspareunia, nausea and vomiting, and vaginal bleeding. A ruptured ovarian cyst may cause sudden sharp pain. When a normal follicular cyst ruptures at ovulation, the pain is called mittelschmerz, and will occur in the middle of the menstrual cycle during ovulation. It requires no treatment.

Large ruptured ovarian cysts causing peritoneal bleeding and hypotension require urgent laparoscopic removal (Alammari, Lightfoot & Hur, 2017). Cysts causing persistent pain may also require removal. Ovarian torsion may occur when large cysts are present; this results in acute, severe ischaemic adnexal pain and requires prompt evaluation and possible surgery.

Uterine leiomyomas

Uterine leiomyomas (fibroids) are growths originating from the muscle layer of the uterus. Uterine leiomyomas can cause excessive menstrual bleeding, pelvic pressure, pain, enlarged uterus and problems with fertility. Treatment includes correcting anaemia with iron supplements, pain relief, medical management of heavy bleeding and possibly myomectomy to remove the fibroids. Myomectomy can be performed via small laparoscopic incisions or with a hysteroscope inserted through the cervix.

Endometriosis

Endometriosis effects around 10 per cent of women, and is a chronic inflammatory disease. It occurs when the endometrial tissue that lines the uterus occurs outside the uterus (Endometriosis Australia, 2018). The tissue responds to the menstrual cycle, as does the uterine endometrium; however, the blood and tissue from endometrial growths outside the uterus are unable to leave the body. As a result, endometrial lesions, cysts, fibrosis, adhesions, internal bleeding and inflammation occur outside the uterus in the pelvic region. Women may present for urgent care with pain and non-specific symptoms.

Endometriosis is difficult to diagnosis, and variable symptoms often result in a delayed diagnosis. Common symptoms include pelvic pain, dysmenorrhoea, painful intercourse, pain with bowel movements or urination, diarrhoea, constipation, bloating, nausea, and painful or heavy periods. Gastrointestinal symptoms can lead to endometriosis being misdiagnosed as irritable bowel syndrome, as visceral hypersensitivity is present in both conditions (Moore et al., 2017). Alternatively, the pelvic pain can be similar to pain caused by ovarian cysts or pelvic inflammatory disease. Women may present for urgent care due to their symptoms.

Treatment includes managing pain, medical management with Gonadogtrohin-releasing hormone (GnRH) analogues, ovulation suppression with the levonorgestrel-releasing intrauterine system (LNG-IUD), oral contraceptives, or laparoscopic or excisional surgery to remove endometrioma (Mourad, Brown & Farquhar, 2017).

Pelvic inflammatory disease

Pelvic inflammatory disease (PID) is an acute infection affecting reproductive age women. PID is associated with sexually transmitted lower genital tract infections, most commonly chlamydia trachomatis or Neisseria gonorrhoeae, and affects between 4 and 12 per cent of women (Lee, 2017). The infection spreads upwards through the cervix, causing infection in the uterus (endometritis, parametritis), fallopian tubes (salpingitis), ovaries (oopharitis), fallopian tube/ovarian abscesses and pelvic peritonitis. With chlamydia, the symptoms are often mild and may be ignored. PID may result in complications such as ectopic pregnancy, infertility, tubo-ovarian abscess, chronic pelvic pain, sepsis and Fitz-Hugh-Curtis syndrome (peri-hepatic inflammation). The diagnosis of PID can be difficult, as no single definitive test is available, yet prompt management is important to prevent short- and long-term complications (Vanthuyne & Pittrof, 2016). PID is the main cause of tubal factor infertility and is a risk factor for ectopic pregnancy, particularly with repeated episodes (Price et al., 2017).

Dyspareunia – Painful intercourse

Women with PID may present with lower abdominal pain, **dyspareunia** (pain with intercourse), vaginal discharge, spotting and irregular menses (Simmons, 2015). Severe PID may present with signs of acute infection such as fever, malaise, adnexal tenderness, adnexal mass, nausea and vomiting (Ross, Judlin & Jensen, 2014). Clinical diagnosis can be challenging; however, PID is likely if a combination of the following is present: recent onset of pelvic pain, cervicitis, mucopurulent discharge from cervical os, pain on rocking of cervix, adnexal or fundal tenderness with **bimanual palpation**, adnexal masses, fever greater than 38°C and markers of inflammation, elevated erythrocyte sedimentation rate and C-reactive protein.

Treatment for acute PID is broad-spectrum antibiotics, which cover chlamydia trachomatis, Neisseria gonorrhoeae and anaerobic bacteria (Savaris et al., 2017). Women with severe infections or complications such as an abscess may require hospitalisation and possibly surgery to drain the abscess. Sex partners from the 60 days prior to symptom onset should also be treated with antibiotics.

Sexual assault

Sexual assault is sexual contact occurring without explicit consent or when a person younger than 18 is exposed to sexual activities. In Australia, reports of sexual assault have increased, with 21 380 reports in 2015 or 90 victims per 100 000 persons (AIHW, 2017). Nationally, more than four in five sexual assault victims are female, with women between fifteen and nineteen years seven times more likely to have been a victim (AIHW, 2017). For males, the rate of sexual assault was highest in the ten- to fourteen-year-old age group – 103 per 100 000 persons (AIHW, 2017). Many sexual assaults are not reported, so the numbers are an under-estimate. In the emergency department, adults should be triaged and evaluated for major injury, and referral to the sexual assault service is required for integrated and expert care. If the person is a child or adolescent, mandatory reporting is required. Physical injuries need to be treated, and may include abrasions, lacerations and bruising; females may require screening for STIs and administration of emergency contraception. In women presenting to the Sexual Assault Resource Centre (SARC) in Western Australia, 24.5 per cent with vaginal penetration had genital injuries and 27 per cent with anal penetration had injuries (Zilkens et al., 2017). Male sexual assault has been reported to involve more violence, so injuries may be substantial (RACGP, 2018).

Pregnancy-related reproductive urgent care
Miscarriage

Women experiencing a miscarriage often present to the emergency department with pain and vaginal bleeding. Miscarriage is defined as pregnancy loss prior to 20 weeks' gestation. It is estimated that up to 20 per cent of pregnancies end in miscarriage, with the majority occurring before twelve weeks' gestation (MacWilliams et al., 2016).

Evaluation in the emergency department focuses on determining whether the pregnancy is viable, non-viable or ectopic. The management options for uncomplicated first-trimester miscarriage are expectant (waiting), medical (misoprostol) or surgical dilation and curettage of the uterus (McGee, Diplock & Lucewicz, 2016). Women are often not prepared for the distress, pain, amount of bleeding and lack of emotional support, and are dissatisfied with the care they receive in the emergency department (Edwards et al., 2016; MacWilliams et al., 2016). During this distressing, sensitive and private experience, women often find their privacy is compromised, particularly when only a curtain separates them from other patients (Hartigan et al., 2016). In rural and remote areas, specialist staff and diagnostic imaging may not be available (Edwards et al., 2016). Nurses need to provide emotional support to women experiencing pregnancy loss and to inform them about what to expect at home, such as passing clots and experiencing cramping (MacWilliams et al., 2016).

Bimanual examination – Used to assess the vaginal, uterus and adjoining structures. During the examination, palpation occurs both internally and externally to assess the structures.

Ectopic pregnancy

Ectopic pregnancy occurs when implantation of the fertilised ovum occurs outside of the uterus. The most common site is the fallopian tube, where 90 per cent of ectopic pregnancies occur. Other possible locations include the cervix, ovary, abdomen and a caesarean scar.

The incidence of ectopic pregnancy is approximately eleven per 1000 diagnosed pregnancies. It is the leading cause of maternal morbidity and mortality during the first trimester of pregnancy. The rate of ectopic pregnancy has increased dramatically since the introduction of assisted reproductive technology (ART) and occurs in 1.5 to 2.5 per cent of women undergoing IVF. The signs of ectopic pregnancy are uterine cramping, PV bleeding, pelvic pain, one-sided abdominal pain, dizziness, nausea and vomiting, hypotension, tachycardia, shoulder pain (Szypulski, 2015) and amenorrhoea (Sheele, Bernstein & Counselman, 2016).

Pregnancy should be confirmed with a pregnancy test; however, in early pregnancy or with very dilute urine, a false negative result may occur. If the urine pregnancy test is negative, a serum B-hCG should be taken. An initial trans-vaginal ultrasound (TVUS) will diagnose 70 per cent of ectopic pregnancies, and 90 per cent will be diagnosed on a follow-up scan (Al-Memar, Kirk & Bourne, 2015). An empty uterus can also be present in a very early pregnancy and in non-pregnant women (Richardson et al., 2016).

If, on presentation, a woman is haemodynamically unstable, two large-bore IV cannulas should be inserted, fluid resuscitation commenced, blood taken for group and hold, and preparations made for transfer to theatre. Nurses need to remember to be alert for deteriorating clinical status and to ensure that a woman is cared for with compassion and not treated as merely another emergency. Laparoscopic management is used in preference to laparoscopy (open surgery) if possible (Taheri et al., 2014). Medical management using methotrexate (folic acid antagonist preventing growth of rapidly dividing cells) can be considered If β-hCG <5000 IU/L and ectopic mass <3.5 cm. Accurate diagnosis is vital if methotrexate is used, because it is associated with significant congenital abnormalities.

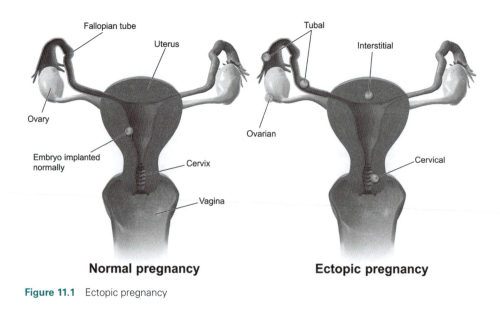

Normal pregnancy   **Ectopic pregnancy**

Figure 11.1 Ectopic pregnancy

Hyperemesis

Women with severe intractable nausea and vomiting during pregnancy require rehydration and anti-emetics such as ondansetron.

Reproductive urgent care after 20 weeks of pregnancy

Antepartum haemorrhage

Placental abruption (premature separation of placenta from the uterine wall) and placental praevia (implantation of the placenta over the cervical os) are common causes of vaginal bleeding and presentation for urgent care in the last half of pregnancy.

Placenta praevia

Placenta praevia occurs when the placenta partially or wholly covers the cervical os. Placenta praevia rates are increasing, and occur in 1.3 per cent of pregnancies (Gibbins, Varner & Silver, 2016) Placenta praevia is characterised by bright-red, painless vaginal bleeding after 20 weeks' gestation. The incidence of haemorrhage is around 20 per cent, and placenta praevia results in increased use of uterotonics, red blood cell transfusion and hysterectomy for haemorrhage (Gibbins, Varner & Silver, 2016).

Placental abruption

Placental abruption is the premature separation of the placenta from the uterine wall. Placental abruption is characterised by vaginal bleeding, abdominal pain, uterine tenderness, hypertonic contractions, increased uterine tone and foetal distress. Blood from a placental abruption may be concealed and a woman's vital signs might indicate hypovolaemia, although the revealed blood loss is minimal. Placental abruption is associated with increased risk of caesarean birth, haemorrhage, red blood cell transfusion and pre-term birth.

Both placenta praevia and placental abruption may require resuscitation for profuse bleeding and an emergency caesarean section may be necessary. Large-bore IV cannulae should be inserted to treat haemodynamic instability and blood collected for cross match, baseline coagulation studies and electrolytes. Rh-negative women will require Rh D immune globulin. The infant is at risk of prematurity, acidosis, encephalopathy, respiratory disorders and needing resuscitation (Downes, Grantz & Shenassa, 2017).

Pre-eclampsia

Women presenting with blood pressures above 160/110 require urgent treatment to control blood pressure and decrease the risk of complications such as seizure, stroke and placental abruption (Lowe et al., 2015). Treatment includes anti-hypertensives and IV magnesium sulphate. Women may present with hypertension, severe headache, visual disturbances, nausea/vomiting, epigastric pain and oliguria. To accurately assess blood pressure, a woman should be seated, the correct size cuff should be used and a manual sphygmomanometer is preferable to an automated machine as it is more accurate when severe hypertension is present (Lowe et al., 2015). If an eclamptic seizure occurs, the airway needs to remain patent, oxygen should be given by mask and IV access should be obtained. Seizures are usually self-limiting; however, if a seizure is prolonged, IV diazepam or clonazepam may be given (Lowe et al., 2015).

Trauma during pregnancy

Trauma is the major cause of indirect maternal mortality and is estimated to complicate 6 to 7 per cent of pregnancies (Downes et al., 2017; Vivian-Taylor et al., 2012). Research on maternal trauma during pregnancy found an incidence of ten admissions per 1000 births (van der Knoop et al., 2017). As many as 11 per cent of women do not survive, foetal mortality is up to 65 per cent and is highest when maternal death occurs, with the best foetal survival rates occurring when mothers also survive (Mowry, 2017). Most foetal morbidity and mortality are related to placental abruption and pre-term birth. Trauma may be unintentional (motor vehicle accident or falling) (Vivian-Taylor et al., 2012) or intentional (assault, intimate partner violence) (Gartland et al., 2016). Due to changes in gait and joint laxity, falling is more common during pregnancy, and women hospitalised after a fall have an increased risk of pre-term labour and placental abruption (Foroutan & Ashmead, 2014).

The physiological changes of pregnancy can make detection of maternal compromise more difficult. The pregnancy-related increase in blood volume means women may not show signs of shock until they have lost 1500 to 2000 ml, or around 30 per cent of their blood volume; when blood loss exceeds 2500 ml, the maternal condition deteriorates rapidly (Mowry, 2017). The bladder is displaced upwards, making it vulnerable to abdominal trauma; the enlarged uterus alters the respiratory system, decreasing chest compliance and making CPR more difficult.

The nurse must also be alert to women who present for urgent care as a result of intimate partner violence. An Australian longitudinal study found 19.5 per cent of women experienced intimate partner violence in the year following the birth of a child and 28.2 per cent in the four years following the birth of their first child (Gartland et al., 2016).

Care of pregnant women with trauma requires the same principles of primary and secondary survey, with oxygen and fluid resuscitation as necessary. Auscultation of the foetal heart with a Doppler should be included in the vital signs. The mother should be placed in a left lateral tilt to avoid supine hypotension syndrome from aorto-caval compression. During emergency care for maternal trauma, the risks of anaesthesia, antibiotics, anti-coagulants and radiation from x-rays must be considered (Tejwani et al., 2017). Surgery may be required to treat fractures or other acute injuries. Collaboration from the healthcare team is essential for the best outcome for both mother and foetus. Any woman with bleeding who has an Rh-negative blood group will require anti-D (RhoGAM) and a Kleihauer–Betke to assess the degree of maternal–foetal haemorrhage if bleeding occurs. The foetus should be assessed with continuous electronic foetal monitoring (EFM) for at least four hours.

REFLECTIVE QUESTION

You are working in emergency and a young female presents with vaginal bleeding after a fall. She explains that she is sixteen weeks pregnant. When starting the assessment, how can you establish a rapport with the patient? What is your priority for the assessment? Should you ask about domestic violence as part of your assessment and how would you include this?

The nurse's role in the assessment of reproductive conditions

For many clients, it may be embarrassing and difficult to talk about issues related to their reproductive system and genitalia, and this may interfere with their willingness to seek medical advice or disclose important information. It is important to provide explanations, ensure privacy and protect the client's modesty throughout all assessments.

The assessments required depend on the client's presenting condition, underlying conditions and current status. Nursing assessments include the primary survey to identify life-threatening risks and vital signs including pain. The secondary survey is then conducted and a focused assessment carried out that relates to the specific area of complaint. A systematic head-to-toe assessment is performed and extended as needed – for example, physical examination of palpable lumps, or swollen or inflamed genitalia. Assessment includes a history of the current or presenting situation, the impact on activities of daily life as well as an overall health and medication history.

As with any condition, ongoing assessment and documentation are required, including intravenous devices, drains and wounds.

Health history

First obtain a general health history, including past illnesses, pre-existing conditions, prior surgery and medications. Data should be collected on menstrual history (for women), sexual history, contraception, abnormal discharge, environmental exposures, discharge, odour, itching, urinary function (frequency, urgency, incontinence, haematuria), fertility treatments, history of physical or sexual abuse and mental health issues. The results of prior screening tests, including PSA or pap smear, should be noted in the health history.

Physical assessment

Physical examination involves visual inspection of the external genitalia, and may involve palpation of structures and organs. An examination of the reproductive system can be uncomfortable and emotionally distressing. It is important to provide information, explain the procedure and gain consent for the examination. Always be sure to respect privacy and ensure that drapes are used to minimise exposure and decrease possible embarrassment.

Breast assessment is similar for the male and female. Both the breast and axilla should be inspected for dimpled or irregular skin and systematically palpated for the existence of lumps or cysts. The nipple and areola are also inspected for swelling and/or discharge. In males, gyaecomastia refers to enlarged glandular tissue around the areola. Obese men may have enlarged breasts due to increased fatty tissue.

Assessment of the male reproductive system

Commence with an inspection for visible abnormalities. The scrotum is palpated for masses, nodules and inflammation. During testicular examination, the technique of testicular self-examination can be demonstrated. The penis is inspected and palpated for lesions, inflammation and discharge. A digital rectal examination examines the size, shape and consistency of the prostate gland and notes any tenderness.

Urine samples and swabs may need to be collected. These can include a first-void urine sample for chlamydia and gonorrhoea, a blood sample to check the prostate specific antigen and throat, urethral, rectal or ulcer swabs.

Assessment of the female reproductive system

Ensure women have an empty bladder, as this can make palpation difficult and uncomfortable. The supine lithotomy position is most commonly used but a Sim's position (left side with right leg bent to a 90 degree angle) may be used for women unable to lie supine. Begin by inspecting the external genitalia for structural changes, lesions, colour changes, swelling or discharge. A speculum is inserted to inspect the vaginal and cervix; swabs may be taken at this time. A bimanual examination may be performed to assess the size, position and any pain or tenderness of the uterus and adnexae.

The nurse's role in the delivery of patient-centred and culturally competent care

Nursing care responsibilities when caring for patients with reproductive disorders include coordination of safe, holistic, evidence-based patient-centred care. The nurse must understand the disorder and assessment process to enable priorities of care to be delivered. Priorities of care are similar to those for other medical and surgical disorders, with specific attention paid to the comfort and understanding of the patient and their family.

The nurse is the key point of contact for the interdisciplinary team and the patient's family, provides current information and acts as the liaison between the patient, family and health professional team (Coyne et al., 2017).

The nurse assesses and monitors the client's condition. Assessment and ongoing monitoring informs the plan of care, which is evaluated to ensure patient and family needs are met during the hospital stay and after discharge. To ensure the delivery of evidence-based care that meets registration standards, nurses are expected to have knowledge of medications, including expected effects, potential side-effects and complications. Accurate documentation and prompt reporting of deterioration are also essential. Although it is the medical officer's responsibility to provide medical information and gain client consent for specific procedures, it the role of the nurse to ensure that the client is provided with education about all aspects of the treatment and care (the nurse as educator). Detailed information for each test and procedure is usually accessible within the clinical area, and it is the nurse's responsibility to review information in order to remain well informed. The nurse needs to ensure that privacy and respect for the client's culture, values and preferences are maintained during any procedures and during hospital admission.

The nurse is also responsible for preparation for discharge, including medications (in liaison with the pharmacist) and follow-up care, and education about any relevant physical or lifestyle changes and alterations in physical functioning. Disorders of the reproductive system may have implications for a client's ongoing fertility, sexuality, sense of self and ability to engage in sexual relationships; therefore, it is important to allow time for open discussion with the patient and family (Dieperink, Mark & Mikkelsen, 2016). Psychosocial support, education and resources should be made available to the patient and their family. Links to specific websites can also be helpful after cancer diagnosis (Cancer Council, 2017).

Interdisciplinary care

Although some disorders are more common in certain age groups, disorders of the reproductive system, including cancers, may happen at any age. The patient will often have a range of health professionals involved with their care, from surgeon, physician and obstetrician to allied health professional – particularly physiotherapists and occupational therapists. After surgery – particularly after mastectomy, hysterectomy and prostate surgery, where post-surgical complications and fatigue can be reduced with planned exercise routines – the physiotherapist will guide the patient with exercises (Du et al., 2015). Leadership and communication are key aspects of providing tailored interdisciplinary care for the patient. Reproductive conditions occur across the lifespan, and patients will often have complex needs. The approach to care should be focused on the patient outcomes and, with clear patient decision-making, an interdisciplinary team enables comprehensive care to be delivered to the patient (Nancarrow et al., 2013).

SUMMARY

Learning objective 1: Define acute reproductive disorders in males and females.

Acute reproductive disorders are related to the reproductive system's anatomy and physiology. In males, this includes the breasts, penis, scrotum, testes and prostate gland. In females, it includes the breasts, uterus, ovaries, adnexae, cervix and vagina.

Learning objective 2: Discuss the pathophysiology, risk factors and incidence of, and treatment for, acute reproductive disorders.

Nurses need to understand the pathophysiology, risk factors and incidence of, and treatment for, acute reproductive disorders. Acute reproductive disorders in males and females can be primary conditions, or secondary disorders from a disturbance in other organs or body systems. The disorders may be related to inflammatory, structural, benign or malignant processes. Risk factors can be related to early life events or to lifestyle factors such as sexual practice, and may have a genetic component as in breast cancer. Risk varies depending on age, gender and history, with reproductive issues being a common cause of presentation for urgent treatment. Urgent treatment is required for significant bleeding in females (e.g. ectopic pregnancy) and for the threat of loss of function in males (e.g. testicular torsion). Antibiotics are used to treat infections, and chemotherapy and radiotherapy are used for malignant conditions.

Learning objective 3: Explore the nursing considerations involved in the management of testicular disorders, prostate cancer and non-pregnancy and pregnancy-related conditions.

Nursing considerations are an important part of the management of testicular disorders, prostate cancer and non-pregnancy and pregnancy-related conditions. Reproductive disorders are intimately related to sexuality and the ability to reproduce. When patients present for care, they are often in pain and emotionally distressed. Therefore, the nurse needs to be sensitive to their situation, recognise the possible implications quickly and provide competent, evidence-based care.

Learning objective 4: Discuss the role of the nurse in the assessment of reproductive conditions.

Nurses have an important role to play in the assessment of reproductive conditions. This includes taking vital signs, patient history, physical examination, collection of samples for pathology and documentation.

Learning objective 5: Present the nurse's role in interdisciplinary collaboration to achieve patient-centred and culturally competent care.

Interdisciplinary collaboration and cultural competence are a vital part of patient-centred care. The nurse liaises with the patient, their family and members of the interdisciplinary team to ensure holistic care is provided. This includes ensuring that patients are well informed and understand their condition and treatment options. Nurses must be aware of the cultural needs of Aboriginal and Torres Strait Islander people and patients from culturally diverse backgrounds or marginalised groups.

REVIEW QUESTIONS

11.1 List the most common causes of scrotal pain and swelling.

11.2 Prostate cancer is a common cancer in males; discuss the age of males most likely to be affected and what symptoms they may present with.

11.3 Vulval cysts are a common infective disorder of the female reproductive system. Outline the treatment for this type of cyst.

11.4 Abnormal uterine bleeding occurs in up to 30 per cent of women; list the common reasons for abnormal uterine bleeding.

11.5 Dyspareunia is often associated with what acute female disorder?

RESEARCH TOPIC

Menstrual bleeding is a normal part of life for most women; however, for some this becomes a concern and influences their quality of life. Abnormal uterine bleeding can have serious effects on a woman's life. Review the articles and discuss how nurses can be more aware of menstrual concerns when working with acute reproductive disorders in females.

FURTHER READING

Coyne, E., & Borbasi, S. (2006). Hold it all together: Breast cancer and its impact on life for younger women. *Contemporary Nurse*, 23(2), 157–69.

Dieperink, K.B., Coyne, E., Creedy, D. & Ostergaard, B. (2016). Family functioning and perceived support from nurses during cancer treatment among Danish and Australian patients and their families. *Journal of Clinical Nursing*, 27(1–2), e154–61.

Dieperink, K.B., Mark, K. & Mikkelsen, T.B. (2016). Marital rehabilitation after prostate cancer: A matter of intimacy. *International Journal of Urological Nursing*, 10(1), 21–9.

Dieperink, K.B., Wagner, L., Hansen, S. & Hansen, O. (2013). Embracing life after prostate cancer: A male perspective on treatment and rehabilitation. *European Journal of Cancer Care*, 22(4), 549–58.

Fraser, I.S., Mansour, D., Breymann, C., Hoffman, C., Mezzacasa, A. & Petraglia, F. (2015). Prevalence of heavy menstrual bleeding and experiences of affected women in a European patient survey. *International Journal of Gynecology & Obstetrics*, 128(3), 196–200.

Karlsson, T.S., Marions, L.B. & Edlund, M.G. (2014). Heavy menstrual bleeding significantly affects quality of life. *Acta Obstetricia et Gynecologica Scandinavica*, 93(1), 52–7.

REFERENCES

Agarwal, G., Valderrama, O., Luchey, A.M. & Pow-Sang, J.M. (2015). Robotic-assisted laparoscopic radical prostatectomy. *Cancer Control*, 22(3), 283–90.

Al-Memar, M., Kirk, E. & Bourne, T. (2015). The role of ultrasonography in the diagnosis and management of early pregnancy complications. *Obstetrician & Gynaecologist*, 17(3), 173–81.

Alammari, R., Lightfoot, M. & Hur, H.C. (2017). Impact of cystectomy on ovarian reserve: Review of the literature. *Journal of Minimally Invasive Gynecology*, 24(2), 247–57.

American College of Nurse Midwives (2016). Abnormal uterine bleeding. *Journal of Midwifery & Women's Health*, 61(4), 522–7.

Andrology Australia (2016). Testes problems. Retrieved from https://www.andrologyaustralia .org/testes-problems.

Australian Institute of Health and Welfare (AIHW) (2001). *Cancer in Australia 2001*. Retrieved from http://www.aihw.gov.au/publications/can/ca01/ca01.pdf.

——(2017). *Australia's Welfare 2017*. Retrieved from https://www.aihw.gov.au/reports/ australias-welfare/australias-welfare-2017/contents/table-of-contents.

Bradley, L.D. & Gueye, N.A. (2016). The medical management of abnormal uterine bleeding in reproductive-aged women. *American Journal of Obstetrics & Gynecology*, 214(1), 31–44.

Cancer Council (2017). Cancer Council Queensland. Retrieved from http://www.cancerqld .org.au.

Coker, T.J. & Dierfeldt, D.M. (2016). Acute bacterial prostatitis: Diagnosis and management. *American Family Physician*, 93(2), 114–20.

Coyne, E., Grafton, E., Reid, A. & Marshall, A. (2017). Understanding family assessment in the Australian context: What are adult oncology nursing practices? *Collegian*, 24(2), 175–82.

Dains, J.E., Baumann, L.C. & Scheibel, P. (2016). *Advanced Health Assessment and Clinical Diagnosis in Primary Care* (5th ed.). St Louis, MO: Elsevier.

Dankher, S., Zutshi, V., Bachani, S. & Arora, R. (2016). Bartholin's gland cyst presenting as anterior vaginal wall cyst: An unusual presentation. *International Journal of Reproduction*, 5(9), 3216–17.

de Silva Joyce, H., Slade, D., Bateson, D., Scheeres, H., McGregor, J. & Weisberg, E. (2015). Patient-centred discourse in sexual and reproductive health consultations. *Discourse & Communication*, 9(3), 275–92.

Dieperink, K.B., Mark, K. & Mikkelsen, T.B. (2016). Marital rehabilitation after prostate cancer: A matter of intimacy. *International Journal of Urological Nursing*, 10(1), 21–9.

Downes, K.L., Grantz, K.L. & Shenassa, E.D. (2017). Maternal, labor, delivery, and perinatal outcomes associated with placental abruption: A systematic review. *American Journal of Perinatology*, 34(10), 935–57.

Du, S., Hu, L., Dong, J., Xu, G., Jin, S., Zhang, H. & Yin, H. (2015). Patient education programs for cancer-related fatigue: A systematic review. *Patient Education and Counseling*, 98(11), 1308–19.

Edwards, S., Birks, M., Chapman, Y. & Yates, K. (2016). Miscarriage in Australia: The geographical inequity of healthcare services. *Australasian Emergency Nursing Journal*, 19(2), 106–11.

Endometriosis Australia (2018). About endometriosis. Retrieved from https://www .endometriosisaustralia.org/about-endometriosis.

Farahani, L. & Datta, S. (2016). Benign ovarian cysts. *Obstetrics, Gynaecology and Reproductive Medicine*, 26(9), 271–5.

Farrukh, J.B., Towriss, K. & McKee, N. (2015). Abnormal uterine bleeding: Taking the stress out of controlling the flow. *Canadian Family Physician*, 61(8), 693–7.

Foroutan, J. & Ashmead, G. (2014). Trauma in pregnancy. *Postgraduate Obstetrics & Gynecology*, 34(14), 1–6.

Gartland, D., Woolhouse, H., Giallo, R., McDonald, E., Hegarty, K., Mensah, F., … Brown, S.J. (2016). Vulnerability to intimate partner violence and poor mental health in the first 4-year postpartum among mothers reporting childhood abuse: An Australian pregnancy cohort study. *Archives of Women's Mental Health*, 19(6), 1091–100.

Gibbins, K.J., Varner, M.W. & Silver, R.M. (2016). Quantifying maternal morbidity associated with placenta previa. *American Journal of Obstetrics & Gynecology*, 214, S18–19.

González León, T., Rodríguez Romero, M., Barreras González, J.E., Amelibia Alvaro, Z. & Darías Martin, J.L. (2017). Laparoscopic transperitoneal vesicovaginal fistula repair. *Journal of Gynecologic Surgery*, 33(5), 175–9.

Hacker, N.F., Eifel, P.J. & van der Velden, J. (2012). Cancer of the vulva. *International Journal of Gynecology & Obstetrics*, 119(2), S90–6.

Hartigan, L., Cussen, L., Meaney, S. & O'Donoghue, K. (2016). Pregnancy loss in the emergency room: Why a walled room is better than a curtained cubicle. *Journal of Pain & Symptom Management*, 52(6), e138.

Harvey, H. & deSouza, N.M. (2016). The role of imaging in the diagnosis of primary prostate cancer. *Journal of Clinical Urology*, 9(2 Supp), 11–17.

Hazeltine, M., Panza, A. & Ellsworth, P. (2017). Testicular torsion: Current evaluation and management. *Urologic Nursing*, 37(2), 61–71.

Holden, C.A., McLachlan, R.I., Pitts, M., Cumming, R., Wittert, G., Ehsani, J.P., … Handelsman, D.J. (2010). Determinants of male reproductive health disorders: The men in Australia telephone survey (MATeS). *BMC Public Health*, 10(1), 96.

Huang, W.Y., Chen, Y.F., Chang, H.C., Yang, T.K., Hsieh, J.T. & Huang, K.H. (2013). The incidence rate and characteristics in patients with testicular torsion: A nationwide, population-based study. *Acta Paediatrica*, 102(8), e363–7.

Lee, D.S., Choe, H.S., Kim, H.Y., Kim, S.W., Bae, S.R., Yoon, B.I. & Lee, S.J. (2016). Acute bacterial prostatitis and abscess formation. *BMC Urology*, 16(1), 38.

Lee, L. (2017). Pelvic inflammatory disease. *JAAPA: Journal of the American Academy of Physician Assistants*, 30(2), 47–8.

Lowe, S.A., Bowyer, L., Lust, K., McMahon, L.P., Morton, M., North, R.A., … Said, J.M. (2015). SOMANZ guidelines for the management of hypertensive disorders of pregnancy. *Australian & New Zealand Journal of Obstetrics & Gynaecology*, 55(5), e1–29.

MacWilliams, K., Hughes, J., Aston, M., Field, S. & Moffatt, F.W. (2016). Understanding the experience of miscarriage in the emergency department. *Journal of Emergency Nursing*, 42(6), 504–12.

McConaghy, J. & Panchal, B. (2016). Epididymitis: An overview. *American Family Physician*, 94(9), 723–6.

McGee, T.M., Diplock, H. & Lucewicz, A. (2016). Sublingual misoprostol for management of empty sac or missed miscarriage: The first two years' experience at a metropolitan Australian hospital. *Australian & New Zealand Journal of Obstetrics & Gynaecology*, 56(4), 414–19.

Miyahira, A.K., Roychowdhury, S., Goswami, S., Ippolito, J.E., Priceman, S.J., Pritchard, C. C., … Soule, H.R. (2017). Beyond seed and soil: Understanding and targeting metastatic prostate cancer: Report from the 2016 Coffey-Holden Prostate Cancer Academy Meeting. *The Prostate*, 77(2), 123–44.

Moore, J.S., Gibson, P.R., Perry, R.E. & Burgell, R.E. (2017). Endometriosis in patients with irritable bowel syndrome: Specific symptomatic and demographic profile, and response to the low FODMAP diet. *Australian & New Zealand Journal of Obstetrics & Gynaecology*, 57(2), 201–5.

Morice, P., Leary, A., Creutzberg, C., Abu-Rustum, N. & Darai, E. (2016). Endometrial cancer. *The Lancet*, 387(10023), 1094–108.

Mourad, S., Brown, J. & Farquhar, C. (2017). Interventions for the prevention of OHSS in ART cycles: An overview of Cochrane reviews. *Cochrane Database of Systemic Reviews*, 1, CD012103.

Mowry, M. (2017). Obstetrical trauma with maternal death and fetal survival. *Critical Care Nursing Quarterly*, 40(1), 36–40.

Muneer, A. & Ralph, D. (2017). Guideline of guidelines: Priapism. *BJU International*, 119(2), 204–8.

Nancarrow, S.A., Booth, A., Ariss, S., Smith, T., Enderby, P. & Roots, A. (2013). Ten principles of good interdisciplinary team work. *Human Resources for Health*, 11(1), 19.

Nursing Council of New Zealand (NCNZ) ([2007] 2016). *Competencies for Registered Nurses*. Retrieved from http://www.nursingcouncil.org.nz/Nurses.

Nursing and Midwifery Board of Australia (NMBA) (2016). *Registered Nurse Standards for Practice*. Melbourne: Nursing & Midwifery Board of Australia. Retrieved from http://www.nursingmidwiferyboard.gov.au/Codes-Guidelines-Statements/Professional-standards.aspx.

Price, M.J., Ades, A.E., Welton, N.J., Simms, I. & Horner, P.J. (2017). Pelvic inflammatory disease and salpingitis: Incidence of primary and repeat episodes in England. *Epidemiology & Infection*, 145(1), 208–15.

RACGP (2018). Sexual assault. In *Clinical Guidelines*. Retrieved from https://www.racgp.org.au/your-practice/guidelines/whitebook/chapter-9-sexual-assault.

Richardson, A., Gallos, I., Dobson, S., Campbell, B.K., Coomarasamy, A. & Raine-Fenning, N. (2016). Accuracy of first-trimester ultrasound in diagnosis of tubal ectopic pregnancy in the absence of an obvious extrauterine embryo: Systematic review and meta-analysis. *Ultrasound in Obstetrics & Gynecology*, 47(1), 28–37.

Ross, J., Judlin, P. & Jensen, J. (2014). 2012 European guideline for the management of pelvic inflammatory disease. *International Journal of STDs and AIDS*, 25(1), 1–7.

Sacha, C.R. & Souter, I. (2017). Abnormal uterine bleeding in women with infertility. *Current Obstetrics and Gynecology Reports*, 6(1), 42–50.

Savaris, R.F., Fuhrich, D.G., Duarte, R.V., Franik, S. & Ross, J. (2017). Antibiotic therapy for pelvic inflammatory disease. *Cochrane Database of Systemic Reviews*, 4, CD010285.

Saville, A.M. (2016). Cervical cancer prevention in Australia: Planning for the future. *Cancer Cytopathology*, 124(4), 235–40.

Segaric, C.A. & Hall, W.A. (2015). Progressively engaging: Constructing nurse, patient, and family relationships in acute care settings. *Journal of Family Nursing*, 21(1), 35–56.

Sharp, V.J. & Kieran, K. (2013). Testicular torsion: Diagnosis, evaluation, and management. *American Family Physician*, 88(12), 835–40.

Sheele, J.M., Bernstein, R. & Counselman, F.L. (2016). A ruptured ectopic pregnancy presenting with a negative urine pregnancy test. *Case Reports in Emergency Medicine*, 7154713.

Simmons, S. (2015). Understanding pelvic inflammatory disease. *Nursing*, 45(2), 65–6.

StatsNZ (2017). Website. Retrieved from http://www.stats.govt.nz.

Szypulski, H. (2015). Practice guideline to prevent ectopic pregnancy rupture. *International Journal of Childbirth Education*, 30(1), 59–62.

Taheri, M., Bharathan, R., Subramaniam, A. & Kelly, T. (2014). A United Kingdom national survey of trends in ectopic pregnancy management. *Journal of Obstetrics & Gynaecology*, 34(6), 508–11.

Tejwani, N., Klifto, K., Looze, C. & Klifto, C.S. (2017). Treatment of pregnant patients with orthopaedic trauma. *Journal of the American Academy of Orthopaedic Surgeons*, 25(5), e90–e101.

van der Knoop, B.J., Zonnenberg, I.A., Otten, V.M., van Weissenbruch, M.M. & de Vries, J.I. (2017). Trauma in pregnancy, obstetrical outcome in a tertiary centre in the Netherlands. *Journal of Maternal Fetal Neonatal Medicine*. doi:10.1080/14767058.2 017.1285891.

Vanthuyne, A. & Pittrof, R. (2016). Diagnosis and treatment of pelvic inflammatory disease. *Prescriber*, 27(10), 47–50.

Vivian-Taylor, J., Roberts, C.L., Chen, J.S. & Ford, J.B. (2012). Motor vehicle accidents during pregnancy: A population-based study. *BJOG: An International Journal of Obstetrics & Gynaecology*, 119(4), 499–503.

Waterworth, P., Rosenberg, M., Braham, R., Pescud, M. & Dimmock, J. (2014). The effect of social support on the health of Indigenous Australians in a metropolitan community. *Social Science & Medicine*, 119, 139–46.

World Health Organization (WHO) (2017). Cancer. Retrieved from http://www.who.int/ mediacentre/factsheets/fs297/en.

Zhou, C.K., Check, D.P., Lortet-Tieulent, J., Laversanne, M., Jemal, A., Ferlay, J., … Devesa, S.S. (2016). Prostate cancer incidence in 43 populations worldwide: An analysis of time trends overall and by age group. *International Journal of Cancer*, 138(6), 1388–400.

Zilkens, R.R., Smith, D.A., Phillips, M.A., Mukhtar, S.A., Semmens, J.B. & Kelly, M.C. (2017). Genital and anal injuries: A cross-sectional Australian study of 1266 women alleging recent sexual assault. *Forensic Science International*, 275, 195–202.

12 Health emergencies

Elicia Kunst, Jasmine Wadham,
Monica Peddle, Susanne Thompson, Elizabeth Elder,
Ann-Marie Brown and Amy Johnston

LEARNING OBJECTIVES

At the completion of this chapter, you should be able to:

1 identify and discuss the role of the nurse in recognising and reporting a deteriorating patient
2 define and discuss common health emergencies, including pathophysiology
3 demonstrate the provision of patient-centred care with respect to preparation for treatment of health emergencies
4 outline the role of the nurse as a collaborative member of an inter-professional team in dealing with health emergencies.

Introduction

This chapter focuses on the nursing care of patients who experience a health emergency. It addresses the role of nurses in the assessment, recognition and reporting of patient deterioration, with a focus on triage and the implementation of primary and secondary surveys. Strategies used to escalate care in the acute clinical setting are identified, along with the common categories of health emergencies experienced by patients in the clinical setting. Legal, ethical and cultural concerns are addressed. The chapter also explores concepts of inter-professional teamwork and the team focus on patient safety during health emergencies. The importance of effective teamwork and the impact of teamwork on patient outcomes in the clinical setting is outlined. It summarises the role of medical emergency teams in health emergencies and examines the importance of role clarification in high-functioning acute clinical teams. The chapter is not a definitive 'how to' guide, but rather is intended to highlight and explain some key components of health emergencies and provide key ideas, concepts and components that each nurse or nursing student should follow up using policy and procedure documents in every institution in which they practise clinically.

When caring for a patient experiencing a health emergency, the nurse uses a variety of critical thinking strategies along with current evidence to make decisions. The nurse engages in effective therapeutic and professional relationships and is an important member of the healthcare team. Nurses are required to conduct comprehensive systematic, evidence-based and informed assessments and to analyse the significance of findings to determine an appropriate plan of care. Care is implemented efficiently and effectively in accordance with evidence and guidelines, with timely responses addressing the rapidly changing patient needs. Patient progress and outcomes, as well as professional practice are evaluated, with reference to scope, evidence and practice guidelines.

Competency 1.5: Practises nursing in a manner that the health consumer determines as being culturally safe

Competency 4.1: Collaborates and participates with colleagues and members of the health care team to facilitate and coordinate care

Competency 4.2: Recognises and values the roles and skills of all members of the health care team in the delivery of care

(NCNZ, [2007] 2016)

The nurse's role in recognising health emergencies

In the acute healthcare environment, a nurse is likely to have more direct contact with the patient than any other healthcare professional. This places the nurse crucially at the centre of care, with responsibility for identifying patients whose physiological health is deteriorating. Recognising and responding appropriately to a health emergency is a critical role.

Patient assessment in health emergencies

Patient assessment is a continuous process that begins from the first moment of patient contact, beginning with visual observation, physical observation or a verbal history (see Chapter 2). This history-taking informs the nurse's clinical decision-making. In the early learning stages of nursing practice, patient assessment can be daunting because of the complexity of a patient's clinical picture. The nurse will be looking out for key indicators in the assessment or history to help understand the physiological compromise in each individual patient (Curtis & Ramsden, 2016).

Regular documentation can help a nurse to recognise physiological changes in patients and to 'trend' or 'track' those changes. This, in turn, will enable clear and systematic handover to other health professionals, including medical, rapid response or emergency care teams to ensure seamless transition of care. An updated nursing assessment is required during admission, during and soon after shift or change of care, and whenever a particular concern is identified.

Triage

At its most simple, triage is a process of sorting or ordering patients for care delivery. Triage in emergency settings is typically a process of assigning urgency of illness or injury to individuals who require medical attention using a predefined scale or sorting system.

The Australasian Triage Scale (ATS) is a five-tier numerical clinical tool that incorporates the patient's own description of their complaint along with an objective assessment of signs and symptoms (Department of Health, 2009; FitzGerald et al., 2010). Triage is typically a role allocated to an experienced nurse, as it can test the nurse's capacity to direct assessment requirements (Curtis & Ramsden, 2016). Like a detective, the nurse is continually seeking clues and data to provide evidence about the patient. A patient's triage category can change, depending on patient deterioration or improvement. This system is designed to optimise time-appropriate care allocation to ensure that emergency resources are used appropriately to improve patient outcomes (Evans, Hughes & Ferguson, 2017; FitzGerald et al., 2010). Key communication points include remaining calm, listening, interpreting, explaining with care and checking back to ensure under-standing (Department of Health, 2009).

There are five categories of acuity:

1 immediately life-/limb-threatening (immediate attention)
2 imminently life-/limb-threatening (<10 minutes to medical intervention)
3 potentially life-threatening, important, time critical or severe pain (<30 minutes to medical intervention)
4 Potentially life-serious or situational urgency (<60 minutes to medical intervention)
5 Non-urgent (<2 hours to medical intervention) (Department of Health, 2009).

To address the need for continual reassessment, many emergency departments have imple-mented a clinical initiative nurse role (CIN), who typically works in the patient waiting areas undertaking ongoing assessment, including assessing physiological vital signs, under-taking physical examinations and initiating treatments such as wound care or analgesia when required.

Primary survey

Primary survey is the term used to describe the initial patient assessment for all critically unwell or **deteriorating patients**. At its simplest level, it can include looking at a patient and thinking logically about what can be seen. It is a short, rapid and systematic assessment of a patient, to help determine the urgency of treatment required and help the team iden-tify the appropriate diagnostic tools and resources that might be needed. This assessment involves the following key points:

Danger: Consideration of the risk to self or patient.

Response: Assessment of the patient's level of alertness.

Situation: Assessment of the situation to determine what is required for urgent care of the patient. This includes requesting further support (sending for help).

Airway: Assessment of patency of airway and providing supportive care when the airway has been compromised.

Breathing: Observation of the rate, regularity, depth, symmetry of chest wall movement and work of breathing.

Circulation: Assessment of circulation and perfusion to vital organs and provision of nursing care to support circulation.

Disability: Assessment of other factors that could be causing reduced consciousness or reduced function.

Exposure: Looking beyond the immediate life-threatening concerns for additional information, including signs of further injury or disease pathology not seen during the initial phases.

Secondary survey

The secondary survey occurs when the primary survey is complete, the immediate or criti-cal clinical issues arising from the primary survey (ABCDE) have been addressed and the patient is considered stable enough to proceed with a further examination. The secondary survey in an emergency context is also a rapid assessment, involving direct inspection of a patient's entire body from head to toe. The secondary assessment aims to identify injuries, issues and other concerns requiring intervention for which immediate treatment is neces-sary. This includes examination for areas of deformity, swelling, bruising, tenderness, wounds and loss of sensation or function. In an emergency situation, secondary interventions may include taking a full set of vital signs, plain film radiography, computerised tomography

Deteriorating patient – Changes that may be detrimental to the individual. It is a crucial clinical skill for nurses to recognise physical signs that show a patient may be deteriorating.

(CT) scans, additional pathology tests including blood electrolyte, renal and liver function, cell count and arterial blood gas tests, and initiation of supportive intravenous therapy. Many of these secondary survey components must be undertaken with a facility-specific nurse-initiation protocol or a medical order. Attention to the patient's airway, breathing and circulation continues to be a priority throughout the secondary survey and if deterioration is detected, the focus of nursing care must return to the primary survey (ABCDE) until the patient is stabilised. Consideration should be given to the expected 'normal' measures or values from each assessment, based on the age and comorbidities of the patient.

Recognising and reporting patient deterioration

Recent advances to optimise patient safety within healthcare systems have highlighted patient assessment as a key indicator for preventing, recognising and implementing early treatment interventions in critically unwell and deteriorating patients. These studies have identified that deterioration is not often a sudden event and early warning signs can be found through the process of competent assessment (Massey, Chaboyer & Anderson, 2017).

Information obtained during a thorough, systematic and high-quality assessment can be passed forward (handed over) to a more senior or experienced nurse or medical doctor. Early warning recognition and response tools have been widely implemented to identify changes in a patient's clinical condition, while providing clear prompts for timely action and care plan escalation as an integral part of the patient's ongoing assessment. This can assist all nurses in the provision of safe and competent patient care. It supports nurses' integration of clinical information with a critical thinking approach to ensure that the appropriate actions for high-quality, safe patient care are delivered. A single set of **vital signs** only provides information about a single moment in time. Frequency of vital sign observation must be adjusted to the individual patient situation; increasing the frequency of monitoring is not only an essential component of critical clinical thinking skills, but also establishes documented trends (Osborne et al., 2015; Preece et al., 2010). It is critical that a nurse uses assessment and recording of vital signs as part of building a holistic picture of their patient, rather than just as tasks that should be completed (Massey, Osborne & Johnston, 2017).

Vital signs – A person's blood pressure, pulse rate, body temperature and rate of respiration; checked to obtain a rapid assessment of someone's physical state.

Escalation of care

Emergency care processes are guided by policies, directing when and how to best escalate care to a provider of higher acuity care or to another facility. It is the responsibility of all care providers to be aware of these policies and processes, and to respond appropriately when a patient deteriorates. (Boots et al., 2016; Zegers et al., 2016). Patients' needs and wishes must be respected when planning care and responding to clinical deterioration. Some patients will have indicated their wishes clearly in the event that their health deteriorates, but others have not. In this situation, it is important to be aware of and follow the relevant health facility policy for health professionals, including policies set out for responsible nurses, senior nurses and medical staff to communicate with the patient and family to co-determine the most appropriate healthcare plan. In this situation, health professionals are governed by legal and ethical decision-making processes and can be guided by the facility protocols.

Patients, families and carers can escalate care in Australian healthcare facilities, including by obtaining an independent second opinion. The role of family/carer contribution in recognising patient deterioration has increased on the background of paediatric cases in which it was deemed by the courts that the parental concerns about their child's wellbeing were not addressed by healthcare professionals (Gill, Leslie & Marshall, 2016). An example of this policy in action is 'Ryan's Rule' (Queensland Health, 2017). This ensures that family members and caregivers can act where they feel that a patient known to them is physiologically or psychologically deteriorating and is not receiving the healthcare that they feel is necessary.

Categories of health emergencies

The initial focus of health emergencies managed by health professionals is on maintaining cardiac and cerebral perfusion, respiratory function and, as much as possible, tissue integrity to maintain, cardiac, circulatory (vascular) and central nervous system function. There is very limited regenerative and even compensatory capacity in many adult tissues, particularly cardiac and central nervous system tissue. Just three minutes of lack of oxygen supply to brain tissue can be sufficient to cause long-term loss of function; these are typically the primary foci of emergency interventions. Part of the nursing role in acute emergency situations is consideration of the broader wellbeing of a patient.

Hypoxia/hypoxaemia

Hypoxaemia describes a physiological condition where the relative concentration of oxygen in arterial blood, described as partial pressure or PaO_2, falls below the normal level (between 80 and 100 mmHg). Hypoxia describes cyanosis, both peripherally and centrally, which is observed in a blue/grey tinge in the skin and in mucous membranes that typically accompanies hypoxaemia. Hypoxia can be clinically observed but not objectively assessed.

Factors that contribute to hypoxaemia include reduced capacity to inspire, being in a low-oxygen environment, airway obstruction, disruption of gas exchange in the alveoli in lungs, anaemia (inadequate blood haemoglobin), disruption of oxygen transportation by blood (for example, in carbon monoxide poisoning where the haemoglobin selectively takes up carbon monoxide molecules so there is no space left to carry oxygen molecules) and some very unusual conditions where extremes of blood temperature and pH (acidity) limit oxygen transport. Falling levels of oxygen and/or elevated levels of carbon dioxide can lead to respiratory failure and death (Craft et al., 2017).

Principles of nursing management

Nursing management of hypoxaemia aims to help address, correct or compensate for whatever factor is impeding blood oxygen content. This may include providing supplemental oxygen – usually with a medical order (Cousins, Wark & McDonald, 2016). It may also include enhancing airway patency pharmacologically, with bronchodilatory, anti-inflammatory or surfactant drugs, or physically, using high flow oxygen delivery or positive pressure ventilatory support, or by altering the patient's positioning; and clearing obstructions with suctioning, deep breathing and coughing exercises or forms of inspiratory spirometry. In the case of low haemoglobin, a whole-blood or packed red blood cell transfusion may be administered. The aim is always to increase blood oxygen concentration or functional perfusion.

Arterial or venous blood gas samples are taken to test blood acidity, known as pH, and the partial pressure of both oxygen and carbon dioxide (PaO_2 and $PaCO_2$), along with bicarbonate (HCO_3). This provides an indication of the severity of illness, the likely mechanism – metabolic or respiratory – and the level of compensation that the body's processes are undertaking to maintain homeostasis. When the compensation is great, the patient is at significant risk of severe deterioration and mortality.

Airway support can be provided through the use of adjuncts. These can include invasive adjuncts, like endotracheal intubation, and non-invasive adjuncts, like an oropharyngeal airway or non-invasive ventilation through CPAP. These should always be applied in keeping with the policy and procedure requirements of the health facility and in accordance with the clinical scope of the healthcare practitioner, and should include establishing that there are minimal contraindications for the respiratory support selected (Patel, Gillon & Jones, 2017).

Hypotension

Hypotension describes the clinical scenario where blood pressure falls below the usual range for systolic and diastolic blood pressure for a patient, based on age and gender. This can result in inadequate perfusion of tissues (insufficient oxygen and other nutrient supply, inadequate removal of waste products) so that their integrity and viability can become compromised.

The pressure of blood against the walls of arteries is generated by a number of factors, including the vessel elasticity and level of arteriolar smooth muscle contraction of the artery walls, the ease of flow through the arteries, the 'push' generated by active contraction of the heart, the volume of blood in the blood vessels and the viscosity of blood. When change occurs with inadequate compensation, hypotension will result. This can occur as a result of compensation for other conditions, including over-heating or changing position from supine to standing rapidly (postural hypotension) (Wieling et al., 2007). Hypotension may also result from the onset of shock – anaphylactic or circulatory.

Principles of nursing management

The primary aim of nursing management for a patient with hypotension is to prevent further harm, and to attempt to restore physiological homeostasis or return the patient to the range of blood pressure that is normal for them (Jevon, 2010). This is particularly critical in hypotension as syncope – a sudden loss of consciousness due to inadequate cerebral oxygen supply – increases the risk of falls, and a lack of respiratory and circulatory control. One of the more common management strategies for hypotension is to increase circulatory pressure by increasing circulatory volume through increased fluid intake, or by pharmacologically increasing the contraction of smooth muscle around arterial vessel walls (vasopressors). This is typically accompanied by positional support of the patient (supine/prone) and undertaking a secondary survey to reveal other possible sinister findings that might require more specific medical intervention.

Hypertension

Hypertension describes the clinical scenario where blood pressure is elevated above normal range. Acute and chronic forms of management of hypertension are critical to maintain ongoing circulatory function. Without hypertensive control, a person is at elevated risk of vessel wall damage (aneurism), vessel wall scar tissue formation (stenosis), vessel plaque formation, vessel wall rupture, central nervous system damage (haemorrhagic stroke), clot formation and consequential ischaemic stroke, pulmonary or renal embolus, myocardial infarction and myocardial damage, including cardiomyopathy.

Principles of nursing management

Many factors can lead to acute hypertension, and often the management will include removal of the extrinsic causative factors and a cautious 'wait and see' approach. However, in the case of hypertensive emergency, the aim is to reduce blood pressure rapidly. This can include a range of measures including pharmacologically regulating (reducing) the volume of circulating fluid (blood) by reducing fluid intake (fluid restrictions) and increasing fluid loss from the body using diuretics, increasing the space inside blood vessels to hold fluid using vasodilatory agents and protecting the heart from overwork by reducing the work of the cardiac muscle (calcium channel blockers and beta-blockers). All these measures are undertaken as part of a multidisciplinary clinical team effort, and under medical direction.

Alteration in conscious state

A decreased level of consciousness can range from mild confusion or irritability through to advanced neurological impairment with unresponsiveness to stimuli, known as a coma. The severity of the change in level of consciousness experienced by an individual will depend on the underlying cause or mechanism of injury. Causes of impaired consciousness include structural issues, like lack of blood flow leading to hypoxia, or non-structural issues, like metabolic disturbance such as hypoglycaemia or drug toxicity. Consciousness stems from the cerebral cortex, the grey matter on the outer surface of the brain, and the reticular activating system, found in the mid-brain and brain stem.

Diagnosis of underlying cause will involve a thorough neurological assessment, and may include a general physical assessment, blood electrolytes, glucose and gases to exclude metabolic cause, imaging including CT and MRI scans of the brain to exclude structural disorders like lesions or haemorrhage, lumbar puncture and examination of cerebrospinal fluid (CSF) for pathogens. If results are inconclusive, an electroencephalogram (EEG) can be undertaken to assess electrical activity.

Principles of nursing management

Regular ongoing assessment for changes in level of consciousness is vital to ensure that any further deterioration in brain function can trigger an immediate response. The **Glasgow Coma Scale (GCS)** measures should be performed frequently (usually every 30 minutes) until GCS equal to 15 is sustained (Teasdale, 2014). Nursing management of people with reduced GCS has one clear goal: to maintain wellbeing by managing and supporting the usual daily functions. This may include, but is not limited to, maintenance of airway to ensure adequate ventilation; regular hygiene and skin care, including mouth and eye care, and pressure area care; managing elimination of urine and faeces; provision of adequate hydration and nutrition; and passive exercise of joints and limbs to maintain function. In addition, support for family and significant others of the unconscious patient is a very important part of the nursing role.

Glasgow Coma Scale (GCS) – A neurological assessment that measures a person's level of consciousness or alertness.

Patient experiencing chest pain

Chest pain is frequently encountered in acute care settings. Chest pain is used to describe any form of pain or discomfort arising within the thoracic region, often – but not exclusively – left-sided or sub-sternal. Cardiac pain is often caused by myocardial hypoxia, as a result of angina, spasm or occlusion of the coronary arteries. Myocardial infarction describes the partial or full occlusion of the coronary artery, resulting in tissue hypoxia and death. Chest pain can also originate from the respiratory system (pulmonary embolism, pneumothorax or lung infections), and can often be differentiated by the description of pain – for example, if the pain is worse on inspiration. Other causes can be related to trauma such as pulmonary contusions or bony fractures or from the musculoskeletal system, such as muscle strains or costochondritis (inflammation of the rib cartilage). Some patients also describe pain arising from the epigastric region as chest pain.

Principles of nursing management

Excluding acute myocardial infarction is a priority in managing chest pain. This is done through a thorough chest pain assessment, blood tests for troponin level, vital sign monitoring and review of a 12-lead ECG. Troponin enzymes are released into the blood stream when myocardial damage occurs. Pain management is a priority, but the method used will depend on the cause of the pain. The scope of the nurse will vary and actions will be guided by experience, area of practice and governing organisational policies and procedures.

For all new-onset chest pain, rapid assessment is required to eliminate the possibility of potentially life-threatening causes. The use of the 'PQRST' mnemonic (Table 12.1) provides clinicians with a framework for comprehensively assessing pain. Initiating the **medical emergency team (MET)** protocol will usually occur in acute care environments.

Medical emergency team (MET) – A contingency team that has evolved in acute care hospitals to review and treat at-risk patients in the early stages of deterioration.

Table 12.1 Pain assessment PQRST mnemonic

P	Palliative factors	What factors make the pain better? What helps the pain to subside?
	Provocative factors	What factors make the pain worse? What precipitates the pain?
Q	Quality	Describe the pain. What does the pain feel like? What are its characteristics?
R	Region/radiation	Where is the pain? What area of the body is affected? Does it radiate? Where else do you feel the pain?
S	Severity	Can you rate the severity of the pain on a scale from 1 to 10? How does this pain compare with other pain you have experienced? Is the pain staying at the same level or getting better or worse?
T	Timing	When did the pain begin? How long have you had the pain? How often do you experience pain? Did the pain come on suddenly or develop gradually?

Source: Adapted from Stayner et al. (2016).

Cardiac-related pain may require the use of medication such as nitro-glycerine to vasodilate the coronary vessels. Opioid drugs are also commonly used during the acute phase, acting on pain-modulating receptors in the nervous system as well as reducing cardiac preload through vasodilation. This can lead to hypotension, so close and careful monitoring of blood pressure is required. Simple analgesia may be considered for non-cardiac causes of chest pain. Non-pharmacological interventions include having the patient brace a pillow to the chest wall when encouraging them to deep breathe or cough (Winzenberg, Jones & Callisaya, 2015). Patient education is also a key component of managing any form of pain and, where possible, should commence from the first interaction with the patient.

Alteration in fluid balance

Maintaining adequate fluid balance is essential for homeostasis. Hypovolaemia occurs when there is reduced intravascular volume, and can result in hypotension and poor perfusion of the tissues with oxygenated blood. Hypervolaemia, inversely, is excessive fluid volume, which may result in fluid shifting to the interstitial or transcellular spaces, like peripheral oedema, ascites or pleural effusion. The kidneys are primarily responsible for fluid balance, influenced by the adrenal glands and the brain. Normal fluid balance can be affected by many factors, including loss through blood or elimination, abnormal electrolyte balance, excessive blood glucose, reduced fluid intake or organ dysfunction.

Principles of nursing management

Maintaining a record of fluid intake and output, particularly for patients at high risk of compromise, is important. This includes educating patients about maintaining fluid intake restriction and careful documentation of urine, vomit, surgical drain, nasogastric and bowel output (especially in the case of high-functioning ileostomy with large liquid output). Concerns about excessive fluid loss or gain should be escalated to the medical team, to reduce the risk of patient deterioration.

Mental health emergency

According to the Department of Health (2013), psychotic illness, depressive illness, attempted suicide, suicidal thoughts, anxiety, acute situational crisis, substance-induced disorders and physical symptoms in the absence of illness are the most common mental health presentations in the emergency department. These account for a significant proportion of Australian and New Zealand health emergencies. The same primary-survey approach should be used in assessing all patients presenting to the emergency department, prior to commencing mental health assessment. Mental health triage categories are based on assessment of an individual's appearance, behaviour and conversation. Assessment may include the patient's and/or family members' or others' accounts of the presenting complaint and presenting history. The triage code is based on the mental health triage tool, which describes acute behavioural disturbances along with risk of harm to self or others.

   While acute mental health assessment should be undertaken by healthcare professionals with specialised skills, all health carers should be able to recognise signs of risk and establish a safe response. Many nurses lack the confidence and skill to provide mental healthcare at a basic level (Moxham et al., 2011). A brief assessment (Table 12.2) can identify risk of harm to self or others. In addition, it is important to recognise that not all aggressive behaviour is associated with mental illness. Physical illnesses such as hypoglycaemia, delirium, acquired brain injury or intoxication can cause changes to mood and behaviour.

Table 12.2   The ABCs of a mental health assessment

Appearance
What does the patient look like?   • Are they dishevelled, unkempt or well presented?   • Are they wearing clothing appropriate for the weather?   • Do they look malnourished or dehydrated?   • Are they showing any visible injuries?   • Do they appear intoxicated, flushed, with dilated or pinpoint pupils?   • Are they tense, slumped over, displaying bizarre postures or facial grimaces?   This information provides cues when assessing the person's mood, thoughts and ability to self-care.

(cont.)

Table 12.2 (cont.)

Affect
What is your observation of the patient's current emotional state?

- Are they flat, downcast, tearful, distressed or anxious?
- Is their expression of emotion changing rapidly?
- Is their emotion inconsistent with what they are talking about?
- Are they excessively happy?

This information provides cues when assessing the person's mood.

Behaviour

How is the patient behaving?

- Are they restless, agitated, hyperventilating or tremulous?
- Are they displaying bizarre, odd or unpredictable actions?
- Are they orientated?

How is the patient reacting?

- Are they angry, hostile, uncooperative, over-familiar, suspicious, guarded, withdrawn, inappropriate or fearful?
- Are they responding to unheard voices or sounds, or unseen people or objects?
- Are they attentive or refusing to talk?

Conversation and mood

- What language is being spoken?
- Is an interpreter needed?

Conversation

How is the patient talking?

Does their conversation make sense?

- Is it rapid, repetitive, slow or uninterruptible, or are they mute?
- Are they speaking loudly, quietly or whispering?
- Are they speaking clearly or slurring?
- Are they speaking with anger?
- Are they using obscene language?
- Do they stop in the middle of a sentence?
- Do you think the patient's speech is being interrupted because they are hearing voices?
- Do they know what day and time it is and how they got to the emergency department?

Mood

How does the patient describe their mood? Do they say they feel:

- Down, worthless, depressed or sad?
- Angry or irritable?
- Anxious, fearful or scared?
- Sad, really happy or high?
- Like they cannot stop crying all the time?

What do you think is the risk of suicide/homicide?

For example, does the patient tell you that they are thinking about suicide, wanting to hurt others, worrying about what people think about them, worrying that their thoughts don't make sense, afraid that they are losing control, feeling that something dreadful is going to happen to them, and/or feeling unable to cope with everything that has happened to them lately in relation to recent stressors?

Source: Department of Health (2009, pp. 39–40).

Principles of nursing management

A key nursing role in mental healthcare can be stabilisation of the frightened or psychologically stimulated patient. Maintaining a calm, therapeutic relationship with the patient and their family or friend is essential for effective care. Comprehensive assessment is important, using good communication skills with open questioning techniques and de-escalation strategies where necessary. This should include consideration of physiological causes of psychological disturbance. Anticipating patient needs for information, treating pain and simple things like food and drink can build rapport and trust (NSW Health, 2015). Privacy, reducing environmental stimuli like noise, lights and activity, and timeliness of care are all key issues in mental healthcare in acute settings (Morphet et al, 2012).

Patient experiencing trauma

A critical factor in trauma management is time. Early intervention, effective teamwork and a comprehensive assessment within the first hour after injury have been demonstrated to provide the best opportunity to reverse life-threatening conditions. Providing quality definitive management within the 'Golden Hour' reduces morbidity and secondary injury.

Principles of nursing management

The trauma team should have clear and effective leadership, with each member assigned to a specific role; however, while there should be an awareness of their own role, each member should also have an understanding of other team members' roles. The team should be resilient, and have the flexibility to manage a rapidly changing patient condition. The team should have very effective communication, using closed-loop communication (Figure 12.1) to reduce ambiguity.

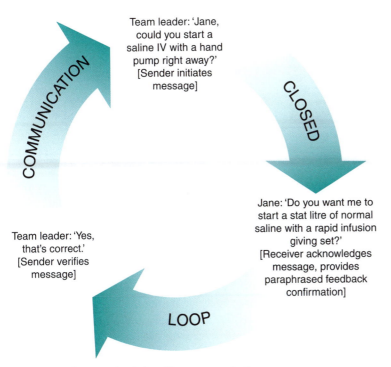

Figure 12.1 An example of closed-loop communication

Resuscitation

Basic life support (BLS) is the maintenance of life by the initial establishment and maintenance of airway, breathing and circulation. This also includes the use of an automated external defibrillator (AED) (Australian Resuscitation Council and New Zealand Resuscitation Council, 2016a).

Principles of nursing management

Basic life support training is widely available to members of the public; however, there is an expectation that nurses will have expert-level skill in the recommended techniques for airway management and chest compression. Nurses are expected to maintain their skills with regular practice and annual assessment of competence. The focus of resuscitation has evolved over the years away from complex interventions to maintenance of perfusion to brain and myocardium through early, uninterrupted and effective chest compressions. This aims to restore oxygen delivery to the myocardium to allow restoration of normal rhythm. In addition, defibrillation has moved up in priority to become a first-line response. AEDs are now widely available and designed to be used even by the untrained bystander. Figure 12.2 shows a basic life-support flowchart.

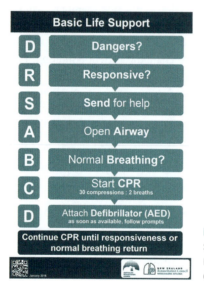

Figure 12.2 ARC basic life-support flowchart
Source: Reproduced with the permission of the Australian Resuscitation Council and New Zealand Resuscitation Council (2016b).

Debriefing after a critical incident is important, as it can lead to practice improvement. There are two key methods of debriefing the team following a critical incident: immediate or delayed. Immediate debriefing occurs immediately after the event. Feedback is based on team members' immediate recall of events, and this means that the effectiveness of the debriefing can be limited while emotions are still high. In contrast, debriefing with feedback within hours or days after the event has been shown to improve the process of managing a critical event and, in turn, patient outcomes. Recall of team performance can be supported by objective data that have been collected during the event, such as defibrillator records or other documented processes, like the resuscitation record form. Both verbal debriefing in groups and individual written feedback have been associated with an improvement in performance.

REFLECTIVE QUESTION

REFLECTIVE QUESTION

You are called to an emergency on your ward. The patient is day 1 post-operative, with two surgical drains in situ, and has collapsed in the bathroom after a shower. What are the risks to the safety of the patient, yourself and other members of the healthcare team?

Patient-centred care in health emergencies

Cultural competency

Effective care during a health emergency relies on both accurate, evidence-based clinical practice and cultural competence. 'Cultural competence' is a broad term that refers to acknowledging, respecting, being responsive to and being inclusive of the patient's cultural perspective (Flowers, 2004). Both the Nursing and Midwifery Board of Australia (2016) and the Nursing Council of New Zealand (2007) set guidelines and standards requiring all registered nurses to practise cultural competence as part of their nursing care. Examples of this include not stereotyping or making assumptions about a particular patient based on their gender or their ethnic, cultural or religious background. Clarifying the needs and desires of the patient is important, but in a health emergency this may not always be possible. In this situation, the practitioner may need to rely on the patient's family or other nominated person to provide this information. In some instances, religious clergy are also available to help the healthcare team to address some of the religious aspects of cultural competence.

Legal and ethical concerns

Health emergencies can present the practitioner with many ethical and legal challenges. Advancing technologies, changes to treatment protocols and the shift to patient-centred care have all contributed to the increase in ethical and legal challenges faced by health practitioners.

Autonomy refers to the patient's right control their care and the decision-making process around their care (Lee & Lin, 2010). Beneficence refers to preventing harm or promoting good, whereas non-maleficence refers to doing no harm (Kinsinger, 2009). During the delivery and provision of healthcare, practitioners can be morally and ethically challenged in the course of their work. It is important to ensure at all times that you refer to and practise under organisational policy and governing legislation while respecting the wishes of the patient during health emergencies.

Advance care planning/advanced health directives

One way to ensure that the patient's voice remains heard during a health emergency is through advance care planning. This can be undertaken as part of a patient's admission into the healthcare facility (for example a 'not for resuscitation order') or as something the individual undertakes of their own accord prior to becoming unwell, after consultation with a medical officer. An advance care directive is a legal document stating the patient's wishes relating to their health and healthcare treatment in the event that they become incapacitated and are unable to make an informed decision or provide consent (Queensland Government, 2016). The advance care directive might only state goals of care or provide very specific instructions – for example, goals of care may consider concepts such as 'comfort measures' or 'privacy measures', whereas very specific instructions might state that the patient is happy to receive intravenous fluids, CPR and be defibrillated, but does not wish to be intubated in the event that their condition deteriorates. Some religious and cultural groups may have an advance care directive, as they do not wish to receive blood or blood products as part of their care (West, 2014). This may present some challenges for the treating healthcare team, particularly if the patient becomes incapacitated before clearly communicating their wishes or if the patient involved is either a minor or unable to provide consent from the beginning of care. Health practitioners who are aware that a patient for whom they are caring has an advance care directive need to include this as key information in their handover. It is important to follow the organisational policy and state legislation under which you are practising to ensure that you comply with the legal aspects of your practice while supporting the patient's wishes in the event that they become incapacitated.

Nursing management of unexpected death

The purpose of the state coroner is to investigate reportable deaths (Queensland Courts, 2017; NSW Department of Justice, 2017). It is the responsibility of the healthcare practitioner to forward information about all reportable deaths to the authorities unless they believe this has already been undertaken by another person (Queensland Courts, 2017; NSW Department of Justice, 2017. The role of the coroner is not to lay blame or establish guilt, but rather to determine potential causes and contributing factors (Curtis & Ramsden, 2016). Further to this, the coroner also makes recommendations to change practice or processes to prevent future deaths of this nature (Queensland Courts, 2017; NSW Department of Justice, 2017). Legislation and guidelines relating to the care of the deceased vary depending on the state or territory. It is recommended that any devices connected to the patient (for example, intravenous cannula, in-dwelling catheters) be left in-situ (Curtis & Ramsden, 2016; Queensland Courts, 2017), but consideration must be given to family wellbeing, as viewing the attached medical devices may cause psychological harm (Office of the State Coroner Queensland, 2017). If devices are either removed or disconnected for whatever reason, then it is imperative that the action is documented in the deceased patient's medical notes (Queensland Courts, 2017). The preservation of evidence is an important aspect of any forensic investigation; however, the Coroner's Court also acknowledges that healthcare facilities have the competing priority of maintaining patient flow and continuing the perseveration of care for other patients as well as minimising the distress of the family. In most cases, unless deemed a crime scene, the patient can be transferred to the mortuary and witness statements, evidence collected from the deceased and their medical file will help to inform the investigation (Queensland Courts, 2017). It is important to remember, however, that policy and legislation are under constant review and each health practitioner should consistently refer to the latest governing policies and legislation to ensure that they are working within the legal parameters and expectations of their role.

SKILLS IN PRACTICE

Managing an acute respiratory emergency

Bill Jones is a 71-year-old man who lives at home with his wife of 48 years, Marion. Bill has presented to the emergency department with shortness of breath, which came on suddenly at home. He was driven in to the hospital by his wife, and has managed to walk inside from the car, but is leaning on the triage counter and appears to be distressed. He is able to talk in short sentences, but is flustered when you ask for further details of his medical conditions. Marion discloses that he takes medications for his heart, blood pressure, cholesterol and diabetes, including insulin twice a day.

The triage nurse will commence the primary survey, assessing for danger to self or to patient, and note that he is responding appropriately. However, he is slightly agitated, which might indicate early confusion associated with cerebral hypoxia. Airway assessment will note that he has air entry, but does have a slight wheeze on inspiration and appears to be 'sucking in' a deeper breath intermittently, which might indicate airflow restriction. His respiratory rate is 22 per minute, and he is rounding his shoulders and positioning himself to maximise air entry into the posterior lung, known as tripod positioning. His radial pulse is palpated and is found to be irregular, with a rate of 89 per minute. His skin is cool and dry. His peripheral oxygen saturation level is 94 per cent. His blood pressure is slightly elevated (130/90 mmHg). BSL is 6.8 mmol/L.

Bill is triaged as a category 3, which means treatment should be commenced within 30 minutes to reduce the risk of further deterioration. When a bed becomes available, the nurse helps him to undress and change into a hospital gown, where it is noted that he has bilateral ankle oedema. When questioned about his urinary habits, Bill states that he is supposed to take 'tablets to make him pee', but he hasn't taken them for the past few days as he has been out of the house every day and he has to rush to get to the toilet when he takes those tablets.

QUESTIONS

- What are the key features of this case?
- What could be the underlying pathophysiology causing Bill's symptoms?
- What further assessments may be needed for this patient?
- What treatment will most likely be initiated?
- What might be appropriate education for Bill and Marion?

Inter-professional teams in health emergencies

Teamwork is a central tenet of most high-risk industries, including aviation, oil and gas, and healthcare (Crichton, O'Connor & Flin, 2013). In healthcare settings, patients can receive care from teams comprising members of multiple professions (Weller, Boyd & Cumin, 2014), so it is important that these teams function efficiently and effectively to maximise patient outcomes. Poor team performance, lack of leadership and clear and well-understood roles, and inadequate communication can negatively affect the quality and safety of patient care (Manser, 2008; Paige, 2010), and can directly increase the risk of complications or death (Mazzocco et al., 2009).

What is a team?

The definition of a team, according to Salas et al. (1992, p. 4), is:

> a distinguishable set of two or more people who interact, dynamically, interdependently, and adaptively toward a common and valued goal/objective/mission, who have each been assigned specific roles or functions to perform, and who have a limited life-span of membership.
>
> (Cited in Crichton et al., 2013, p. 94)

Characteristics of teams in healthcare

Healthcare teams can be inter-professional, comprising individuals from varied professions, or intra-professional, consisting of individuals from a single profession collaborating to meet agreed patient goals. Team membership is often ad hoc, with members changing frequently, often working together for short periods of time in dynamic and constantly changing environments (Manser, 2009).

Strategies for effective teamwork in health emergencies

To achieve team tasks, teams must function effectively from the moment they are formed (Crichton et al., 2013). Five key factors have been proposed for effective teams: team leadership, mutual performance monitoring, back-up behaviour, adaptability and team orientation (Weller, Boyd & Cumin, 2014). These factors are supported by the underpinning concepts of mutual trust, closed-loop communication and shared mental models (Weller, Boyd & Cumin, 2014) (Table 12.3).

Table 12.3 Key factors for effective teams

Key factors		Underpinning concepts
Team leadership	Task coordination and planning Development of team motivation	• Mutual trust – members of the team must respect and trust each other in order to give and receive feedback on their performance (Weller, Boyd & Cumin, 2014).
Mutual performance monitoring	Monitoring of other team members to identify lapses or task overload	• Closed-loop communication – a three-step sequence whereby a message is sent by a team member, another team member provides feedback regarding the received message and the originating team member then verifies that the intended message was received (Crichton et al., 2013).
Back-up behaviour	Have sufficient understanding of others' tasks	
	Behaviour among team members that indicates both the competence and willingness to help, and be helped by, other team members (Crichton et al., 2013)	• Shared metal models – individually held knowledge structures that help team members function collaboratively in their environments (McComb & Simpson, 2014).

Key factors		Underpinning concepts
Adaptability	Change patient management plan in response to the environment	
Team orientation	Beliefs that the team goals are more important than those of individuals	
	Willingness to take others' perspectives into account	

Source: Adapted from Weller, Boyd and Cumin (2014).

The exchange of information during patient handovers in health emergencies across professional boundaries can be incomplete and inadequate, leading to preventable adverse patient events (Roberts et al., 2014). It is suggested that a multifactorial approach is required to address team communication in order to maintain patient safety (Weller, Boyd & Cumin, 2014) (Table 12.4).

Table 12.4   Strategies to improve communication

Tool	Brief description
Step-back (call-out)	Stepping back from, and taking an overview of, the situation, the health professional who is leading the team calls the attention of the team and provides an update of the situation and the plan, and invites suggestions.
Closed-loop communication	This three-step strategy involves the sender directing the instruction to the intended receiver, using their name where possible; the receiver confirming what was communicated as a check on hearing and understanding the instruction, seeking clarification if required; and the sender verifying that the message has been received and interpreted correctly.
Structured information transmission (SBAR/ ISBAR)[1]	This is a widely used acronym to help structure verbal information at handover or patient referral. The original version (SBAR) has been expanded in some reports to **ISBAR**, starting with Identify yourself: Identify →Situation→Background→Assessment→Recommendation
Structured handover	Simple templates for summarising important patient information at handover
Graded assertion (PACE)	Escalating concern (Probe, Alert, Challenge, Emergency)

ISBAR – A standardised format for communicating patient information in the clinical setting. The aim of this mnemonic is to ensure that communication is clear and details aren't missed or overlooked.

[1] Please note that these terms – SBAR/ISBAR/ISOBAR – vary slightly across health systems; however the basic principle of effective communication remains unchanged.

Source: Reproduced from Weller, Boyd and Cumin (2014, p. 151).

Conflict in teams

Conflict in teams has been identified as a significant contributor to poor patient outcomes (Almost et al., 2016). Conflict in teams can lead to disagreement and can create barriers that hinder the attainment of team goals (Almost et al., 2016). Specific communication strategies enable communication that is clear, concise and timely, to maximise patient outcomes (Sexton & Orchard, 2016) (Table 12.5).

Table 12.5 Strategies to express concern in healthcare teams

CUS	A three-step process for assisting people to stop a problematic activity	I am **C**oncerned. I am **U**ncomfortable. This is a **S**afety issue.
DESC script	A constructive process for resolving conflicts	**D**escribe the specific situation or behaviour and provide concrete evidence or data. **E**xpress how the situation makes you feel and what your concerns are. **S**uggest other alternatives and seek agreement. **C**onsequences should be stated in terms of their effect on established team goals or patient safety.

Source: AHRQ (2018).

Leadership and teamwork in medical emergency teams

Medical emergency teams (MET), also known as rapid response teams, have evolved in acute care hospitals to review and treat at-risk patients in the early stages of deterioration. This contingency team consists of professionals with different backgrounds, skills and roles coming together to manage health emergencies; they must immediately be able to coordinate actions in changeable situations (Schmutz et al., 2015).

A MET situation is typically highly stressful, characterised by uncertainty, a high information load, risk and complex tasks that are time sensitive (Schmutz et al., 2015). Clear leadership improves adherence to frameworks and guidelines, and rapid formulation of patient management plans (Wallin et al., 2007). Leadership and role clarity can support coordination of the tasks and distribution of sub-tasks within the team according to team members' knowledge and skill (Schmutz et al., 2015).

REFLECTIVE QUESTION

Reflect on your most recent clinical experience. Identify a healthcare team that was present. Did you observe team leadership? Did the team members demonstrate mutual performance monitoring and back-up behaviours? What effective communication strategies were utilised?

SUMMARY

Learning objective 1: Identify and discuss the role of the nurse in recognising and reporting a deteriorating patient.

The nurse is responsible for recognising and responding appropriately to patient deterioration. Part of this responsibility is regular patient assessment and documentation of findings. Nurses should have skills in assessing and managing a range of health issues that may occur in the acute care setting, including both physical and psychological distress. Advanced assessment skills are needed to undertake triage or complex trauma management in the emergency care setting.

Learning objective 2: Define and discuss common health emergencies, including pathophysiology.

Nurses need to have a good understanding of the causes of health deterioration and how these can be managed. This will lead to better outcomes and reduce the risk of morbidity and mortality arising from complex conditions.

Learning objective 3: Demonstrate the provision of patient-centred care with respect to preparation for the treatment of health emergencies.

Nurses need to consider the wider social and cultural context when caring for patients in acute emergencies. Respect for the patient and their significant others, including provision of culturally sensitive care, should be paramount. This includes reviewing legal considerations like advance care directives for instructions regarding resuscitation and other interventions. In addition, when an adverse event – like the death of a patient – occurs, nurses need to consider their legal responsibilities around reporting the death to the coroner.

Learning objective 4: Outline the role of the nurse as a collaborative member of an inter-professional team in dealing with health emergencies.

In healthcare settings, patients receive care from teams comprising members of multiple professions, so it is important that these teams function efficiently and effectively to maximise patient outcomes. It is important that team members are aware of team factors, including team leadership, mutual performance monitoring, back-up behaviour, adaptability, and team orientation and team communication strategies such as step-back (call-out), closed-loop communication, structured information transmission and graded assertion approaches.

REVIEW QUESTIONS

12.1 Describe the process of a primary survey assessment from the nurse's perspective.
12.2 What are the key issues in the nursing management of hypoxaemia?
12.3 List three considerations in managing the care of a deceased patient in the emergency department.
12.4 Discuss the role of inter-professional teamwork in maintaining safe patient outcomes.

12.5 Name the key nursing considerations when preparing a patient for discharge from the emergency department to home.

RESEARCH TOPIC

Family presence in resuscitation is gradually becoming accepted practice in emergency department settings. Reviewing the literature, there are a number of arguments presented for and against family presence during resuscitation. Provide a summary of the evidence for both sides of the argument. In your response, you should consider broader issues like age of the patient, cultural considerations, and the ethical and legal factors that may influence this issue.

FURTHER READING

Australian Commission on Safety and Quality in Health Care (ACSQHC) (2018). *ISBAR Revisited: Identifying and Solving BARriers to Effective Handover in Inter-hospital Transfer – Hunter New England Area Health Service*. Retrieved from https://www .safetyandquality.gov.au/implementation-toolkit-resource-portal/interface/additional-clinical-handover-resources/national-clinical-handover-initiative-pilot-program/isbar-revisited-hunter-new-england-ahs.html.

Department of Health (2009). *Emergency Triage Education Kit*. Canberra: Australian Government. Retrieved from http://www.health.gov.au/internet/main/publishing.nsf/Content/casemix-ED-Triage+Review+Fact+Sheet+Documents.

Preece, M.H.W., Horswill, M.S., Hill, A. & Watson, M.O. (2010). *The Development of the Adult Deterioration Detection System (ADDS) Chart*. Retrieved from https://www .safetyandquality.gov.au/wp-content/uploads/2012/01/35981-ChartDevelopment.pdf.

REFERENCES

Agency for Healthcare Research and Quality (AHCRQ) (2018). *Pocket Guide TeamSTEPPS 2.0*. Retrieved from https://www.ahrq.gov/teamstepps/instructor/essentials/pocketguide.html.

Almost, J., Wolff, A.C., Stewart-Pyne, A., McCormick, L.G., Strachan, D. & D'Souza, C. (2016). Managing and mitigating conflict in healthcare teams: An integrative review. *Journal of Advanced Nursing*, 72(7), 1490–505.

Australian Resuscitation Council and New Zealand Resuscitation Council (2016a). *ANZCOR Guideline 7: Automated External Defibrillation in Basic Life Support*. Retrieved from https://resus.org.au/guidelines.

——(2016b). Flowcharts. Retrieved from https://resus.org.au/guidelines/flowcharts-3.

Boots, R., Carter, A., Erickson, S., Hawker, F., Jones, D., Nicholls, M., … & Barrett, J. (2016). Joint Position Statement on Rapid Response Systems in Australia and New Zealand and the Roles of Intensive Care. Retrieved from https://www.cicm.org.au.

Cousins, J.L., Wark, P.A. & McDonald, V.M. (2016). Acute oxygen therapy: A review of prescribing and delivery practices. *International Journal of Chronic Obstructive Pulmonary Disease*, 11, 1067–75.

Craft, J., Gordon, C., Huether, S.E., McCance, K.L. & Brashers, V.L. (2017). *Understanding Pathophysiology: ANZ Adaptation* (2nd ed.). Sydney: Elsevier.

Crichton, M., O'Connor, P. & Flin, R. (2013). *Safety at the Sharp End: A Guide to Non-Technical Skills*. Aldershot: Ashgate.

Curtis, K. & Ramsden, C. (2016). *Emergency and Trauma Care for Nurses and Paramedics (Australia and New Zealand edition)* (2nd ed.). Sydney: Elsevier.

Department of Health (2009). *Emergency Triage Education Kit*. Canberra: Australian Government. Retrieved from http://www.health.gov.au/internet/main/publishing.nsf/Content/casemix-ED-Triage+Review+Fact+Sheet+Documents.

Evans, C., Hughes, C. & Ferguson, J. (2017). Improving patient safety through the introduction of a formal triage process. *Emergency Nurse*, 24(9), 19–25.

FitzGerald, G., Jelinek, G., Scott, D. & Gerdtz, M. (2010). Emergency department triage revisited. *Emergency Medicine Journal*, 27, 86–92.

Flowers, D.L. (2004). Culturally competent nursing care: A challenge for the 21st century. *Critical Care Nurse*, 24(4), 48–52.

Gill, F.J., Leslie, G.D. & Marshall, A.P. (2016). The impact of implementation of family-initiated escalation of care for the deteriorating patient in hospital: A systematic review. *Worldviews on Evidence-Based Nursing*, 13(4), 303–13.

Jevon, A. (2010). How to ensure observations lead to prompt identification and management of hypotension. *Nursing Times*, 106(5), 9–13.

Kinsinger, F.S. (2009). Beneficence and the professional's moral imperative. *Journal of Chiropractic Humanities*, 16(1),44–6.

Lee, Y.-Y. & Lin, J.L. (2010). Do patient autonomy preferences matter? Linking patient-centered care to patient–physician relationships and health outcomes. *Social Science & Medicine*, 71(10), 1811–18.

Manser, T.P. (2008). Team performance assessment in healthcare: Facing the challenge. *Simulation in Healthcare: The Journal of the Society for Simulation in Healthcare Spring*, 3(1), 1–3.

——(2009). Teamwork and patient safety in dynamic domains of healthcare: A review of the literature. *Acta Anaesthesiologica Scandinavica*, 53(2), 143–51.

Massey, D., Chaboyer, W. & Anderson, V. (2017). What factors influence ward nurses' recognition of and response to patient deterioration? An integrative review of the literature. *Nursing Open*, 4(1), 6–23.

Massey, D., Osborne, D. & Johnston, A.N.B. (2017). *Chuck Out the Obs*. London: Hive.

Mazzocco, K., Petitti, D.B., Fong, K.T., Bonacum, D., Brookey, J., Graham, S., … Thomas, E.J. (2009). Surgical team behaviors and patient outcomes. *The American Journal of Surgery*, 197(5), 678–85.

McComb, S. & Simpson, V. (2014). The concept of shared mental models in healthcare collaboration. *Journal of Advanced Nursing*, 70(7), 1479–88.

Morphet, J., Innes, K., Munro, I., O'Brien, A., Gaskin, C.J., Reed, F. & Kudinoff, T. (2012). Managing people with mental health presentations in emergency departments: A service exploration of the issues surrounding responsiveness from a mental health care consumer and carer perspective. *Australasian Emergency Nursing Journal*, 15(3), 148–55.

Moxham, L., McCann, T., Usher, K., Farrell, G. & Crookes, P. (2011). Mental health nursing education in preregistration nursing curricula: A national report. *International Journal of Mental Health Nursing*, 20(4), 232–6.

NSW Health (2015). *Mental Health for Emergency Departments: A Reference Guide*. Sydney: NSW Health. Retrieved from http://www.health.nsw.gov.au/mentalhealth/publications/Publications/mental-health-ed-guide.pdf.

Nursing Council of New Zealand (NCNZ) ([2007] 2016). *Competencies for Registered Nurses*. Retrieved from http://www.nursingcouncil.org.nz/Nurses.

Nursing and Midwifery Board of Australia (NMBA) (2016). *National Competency Standards for the Registered Nurse*. Melbourne: Nursing & Midwifery Board of Australia. Retrieved from http://www.nursingmidwiferyboard.gov.au.

NSW Department of Justice (2017). State Coroner's Court of New South Wales. Retrieved from http://www.coroners.justice.nsw.gov.au.

Office of the State Coroner Queensland (2017). *Information for Health Professionals*. Brisbane: OSCQ. Retrieved from http://www.courts.qld.gov.au/__data/assets/pdf_file/0006/92868/m-osc-fs-information-for-health-professionals.pdf.

Osborne, S., Douglas, C., Reid, C., Jones, L. & Gardner, G. (2015). The primacy of vital signs: Acute care nurses' and midwives' use of physical assessment skills: A cross-sectional study. *International Journal of Nursing Studies*, 52(5), 951–62.

Paige, J.T. (2010). Surgical team training: Promoting high reliability with nontechnical skills. *Surgical Clinics of North America*, 90(3), 569–81.

Patel, S., Gillon, S.A. & Jones, D.A. (2017). Rapid response systems: Recognition and rescue of the deteriorating hospital patient. *British Journal of Hospital Medicine*, 78(3), 143–8.

Preece, M.H., Horswill, M.S., Hill, A. & Watson, M.O. (2010). *The Development of the Adult Deterioration Detection System (ADDS) Chart*. Brisbane: School of Psychology, University of Queensland.

Queensland Courts (2017). *Reportable Deaths*. Brisbane: Office of the State Coroner. Retrieved from http://www.courts.qld.gov.au/courts/coroners-court/coroners-process/reportable-deaths.

Queensland Government (2016). Advanced health directive. Retrieved from https://www.qld.gov.au/law/legal-mediation-and-justice-of-the-peace/power-of-attorney-and-making-decisions-for-others/advance-health-directive.

Queensland Health (2017). *Ryan's Rule – patient, family and carer escalation process*. Brisbane: Queensland Government. Retrieved from https://www.health.qld.gov.au/psu/ryans-rule-patient,-family-and-carer-escalation-process.

Roberts, N.K., Williams, R.G., Schwind, C.J., Sutyak, J.A., McDowell, C., Griffen, D., … Meier, A.H. (2014). The impact of brief team communication, leadership and team behavior training on ad hoc team performance in trauma care settings. *The American Journal of Surgery*, 207(2), 170–8.

Salas, E., Dickinson, T., Converse, S.A. & Tannenbaum, S.I. (1992). Toward an understanding of team performance and training. In R.W. Swezey & E. Salas (eds), *Teams: Their Training and Performance*. Norwood, NJ: Ablex, pp. 3–29.

Schmutz, J., Hoffmann, F., Heimberg, E. & Manser, T. (2015). Effective coordination in medical emergency teams: The moderating role of task type. *European Journal of Work and Organizational Psychology*, 24(5), 761–76.

Sexton, M. & Orchard, C. (2016). Understanding healthcare professionals' self-efficacy to resolve interprofessional conflict. *Journal of Interprofessional Care*, 30(3), 316–23.

Stayner, R.S., Ramezani, A., Prasad, R. & Mahajan, G. (2016). Chronic pain and psychiatric illness: Managing comorbid conditions – pay close attention to risk and benefit when planning pain management. *Current Psychiatry*, 15(2), 26–33.

Teasdale, G. (2014). Forty years on: Updating the Glasgow Coma Scale. *Nursing Times*, 110(42), 12–16.

Wallin, C.J., Meurling, L., Hedman, L., Hedegård, J. & Felländer-Tsai, L. (2007). Target-focused medical emergency team training using a human patient simulator: Effects on behaviour and attitude. *Medical Education*, 41(2), 173–80.

Weller, J., Boyd, M. & Cumin, D. (2014). Teams, tribes and patient safety: Overcoming barriers to effective teamwork in healthcare. *Postgraduate Medical Journal*, 90(1061), 149–54.

West, J.M. (2014). Ethical issues in the care of Jehovah's Witnesses. *Current Opinion in Anaesthesiology*, 27(2), 170–6.

Wieling, W., Krediet, C.P., Van Dijk, N., Linzer, M. & Tschakovsky, M.E. (2007). Initial orthostatic hypotension: Review of a forgotten condition. *Clinical Science*, 112(3), 157–65.

Winzenberg, T., Jones, G. & Callisaya, M. (2015). Musculoskeletal chest wall pain. *Australian Family Physician*, 44(8), 540–4.

Zegers, M., Hesselink, G., Geense, W., Vincent, C. & Wollersheim, H. (2016). Evidence-based interventions to reduce adverse events in hospitals: A systematic review of systematic reviews. *BMJ Open*, 6(9), e012555.

Index

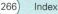